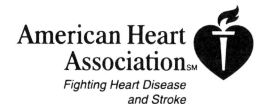

American Heart Associationsm

Fighting Heart Disease and Stroke

Monograph Series

SUDDEN CARDIAC DEATH

PAST, PRESENT, AND FUTURE

Previously published:

Cardiovascular Applications of Magnetic Resonance
Edited by Gerald M. Pohost, MD

Cardiovascular Response to Exercise
Edited by Gerald F. Fletcher, MD

Congestive Heart Failure: Current Clinical Issues
Edited by Gemma T. Kennedy, RN, PhD,
and Michael H. Crawford, MD

Atrial Arrhythmias: State of the Art
Edited by John P. DiMarco, MD, PhD
and Eric N. Prystowsky, MD

Invasive Cardiology: Current Diagnostic
and Therapeutic Issues
Edited by George W. Vetrovec, MD
and Blase Carabello, MD

Syndromes of Atherosclerosis:
Correlations of Clinical Imaging and Pathology
Edited by Valentin Fuster, MD, PhD

Exercise and Heart Failure
Edited by Gary J. Balady, MD
and Ileana L. Piña, MD

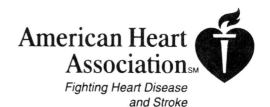

American Heart Association℠

Fighting Heart Disease and Stroke

Monograph Series

SUDDEN CARDIAC DEATH

PAST, PRESENT, AND FUTURE

Edited by

Sandra B. Dunbar, RN, DSN

*Nell Hodgson Woodruff School of Nursing
Emory University
Atlanta, Georgia*

Kenneth A. Ellenbogen, MD

*Medical College of Virginia
McGuire Veterans Affairs Medical Center
Richmond, Virginia*

Andrew E. Epstein, MD

*University of Alabama at Birmingham
Birmingham, Alabama*

**Futura Publishing
Company, Inc.**
Armonk, NY

Library of Congress Cataloging-in-Publication Data
Sudden cardiac death : past, present, and future / edited by
  Sandra B. Dunbar, Kenneth A. Ellenbogen, Andrew E. Epstein.
      p.   cm. — (American Heart Association monograph series)
  Includes bibliographical references and index.
  ISBN 0-87993-666-5
  1. Cardiac arrest.   I. Dunbar, Sandra Byars.   II. Ellenbogen,
  Kenneth A.   III. Epstein, Andrew E.   IV. Series.
  [DNLM: 1. Death, Sudden. Cardiac—prevention & control.
  2. Death, Sudden, Cardiac—etiology.   3. Heart Arrest—therapy.
  WG 205 S9417 1997]
  RC685.C173S8125   1997
  616.1'23025—DC21
  DNLM/DLC
  for Library of Congress   96-47804
                                                                        CIP

Copyright © 1997
Futura Publishing Company, Inc.

Published by
Futura Publishing Company, Inc.
135 Bedford Road
Armonk, New York 10504

LC #: 96-47804
ISBN #: 0-87993-666-5

Every effort has been made to ensure that the information in this book is as up to date and accurate as possible at the time of publication. However, due to the constant developments in medicine, neither the author, nor the editor, nor the publisher can accept any legal or any other responsibility for any errors or omissions that may occur.

Printed in the United States of America on acid-free paper.

Preface

Sudden cardiac death continues to be a major healthcare problem in the United States, claiming the lives of 350 000 patients each year. Numerous physicians, nurses, and scientists continue to work to better understand the syndrome of sudden cardiac death, improve the clinical management of survivors of cardiac arrest, and develop primary prevention strategies. Our understanding of this problem has evolved, largely as a result of the commitment of physicians, nurses, and scientists; however, much remains to be learned.

This book makes a unique contribution to this field. The Committee on Sudden Cardiac Death of the American Heart Association and the Councils on Clinical Cardiology, Nursing, and Basic Science have joined together to produce this state-of-the-art summary of basic and clinical investigation in this area. The physicians, nurses, and scientists who contributed to this volume have all worked hard to advance our understanding of sudden cardiac death.

The editors wish to thank and acknowledge the scholarly contributions of the participants in this symposium. We also thank the staff of the American Heart Association and Futura Publishing Company who helped make this volume on sudden cardiac death possible. The support and encouragement of our families have further helped to provide the time to make this volume a reality. We believe this book will allow the reader an opportunity to review many exciting new developments in this field.

Sandra B. Dunbar, RN, DSN
Nell Hodgson Woodruff School of Nursing,
Emory University, Atlanta, Ga

Kenneth A. Ellenbogen, MD
Medical College of Virginia and McGuire
Veterans Affairs Medical Center, Richmond, Va

Andrew E. Epstein, MD
University of Alabama at Birmingham, Birmingham, Ala

Guest Preface

Sudden, unexpected, premature, arrhythmic cardiac death is always a triple tragedy when it occurs—a tragedy for the individual, for the family, and for the medical profession for having failed to prevent the sudden death. During the past few years, the knowledge base for understanding the mechanisms of lethal cardiac arrhythmias, the factors that precipitate ventricular fibrillation including many routine prescription drugs, and the improved modalities for preventing and emergently treating (aborting) life-threatening arrhythmias has increased enormously. Major progress has been made on many fronts, from identification of the genes that code for myocellular ionic sodium and potassium channels to third-generation implantable defibrillator devices that can effectively diagnose and terminate ventricular tachycardia and fibrillation within seconds of the onset of a life-threatening arrhythmia. In addition, public access defibrillation and the current availability of the "smart" automatic external defibrillator are increasingly saving lives in communities throughout the country.

As we approach the 21st century, we have a responsibility to translate the new information about sudden death and its prevention into concrete action. This book provides a wealth of up-to-date information on the clinical, epidemiologic, basic science, genetic, psychologic, preventive, and postarrest aspects of sudden death. The editors have chosen the leaders in the field to author 23 concise, well-focused chapters on relevant aspects of the problem, and they have accomplished their tasks admirably.

The American Heart Association is committed to significantly reducing sudden cardiac death during the closing part of the 20th century. The valuable scientific information contained in this book will contribute to the success of the American Heart Association's goal. It has been said that he (she) who saves one life saves the world. I congratulate the authors, the editors, and the publisher for putting together this superb book that provides direction for preventing sudden cardiac death in the future.

Arthur J. Moss, MD
Professor of Medicine
University of Rochester School of Medicine & Dentistry
Rochester, New York

vii

Contributors

Masood Akhtar, MD   Professor of Medicine, University of Wisconsin-Milwaukee, Milwaukee, Wisconsin

Steffen Behrens, MD   Research Fellow, VA Medical Center, Washington, DC

Alfred E. Buxton, MD   Professor of Medicine and Cardiology, Temple University School of Medicine, Philadelphia, Pennsylvania

David J. Callans, MD   Associate Professor of Medicine, Allegheny University of the Health Sciences, Philadelphia, Pennsylvania

Agustin Castellanos, MD   Professor of Medicine, University of Miami School of Medicine, Miami, Florida

Marie J. Cowan, PhD, RN   Professor and Dean, School of Nursing, University of California at Los Angeles, Los Angeles, California

Susan M. Daunch, RN, BSN   Clinical Nurse Specialist, Cleveland Clinic Foundation, Cleveland, Ohio

Sanjay Deshpande, MD   Assistant Professor of Medicine, University of Wisconsin-Milwaukee, Milwaukee, Wisconsin

Kathleen Dracup, RN, DNSc   LW Hassenplug Professor of Nursing, University of California, Los Angeles, Los Angeles, California

Barbara J. Drew, RN, PhD   Associate Professor and Vice Chair of Academic Programs, University of California, San Francisco, San Francisco, California

Milou-Daniel Drici, MD, PhD   Fellow in Clinical Pharmacology Georgetown University Medical Center, Washington, DC

William N. Dudley, PhD   Biostatistician, Emory University Nell Hodgson Woodruff School of Nursing, Atlanta, Georgia

Sandra B. Dunbar, RN, DSN   Professor, Emory University, Ne Hodgson Woodruff School of Nursing, Atlanta, Georgia

Debra S. Echt, MD   Cardiac Pathways Corporation, Sunnyvale, California

Kenneth A. Ellenbogen, MD   Professor of Medicine, Medical College of Virginia, Richmond, Virginia

Andrew Epstein, MD   Professor of Medicine, Department of Medicine, University of Alabama at Birmingham, Birmingham, Alabama

Gerald F. Fletcher, MD   Professor of Medicine, Mayo Clinic Medical School, Jacksonville, Florida

David A. Flockhart, MD   Assistant Professor of Medicine and Pharmacology, Georgetown University Medical Center, Washington, DC

Michael R. Franz, MD, PhD   Associate Professor of Medicine and Pharmacology, Georgetown University Medical School, VA Medical Center, Washington, DC

Charles D. Gottlieb, MD   Professor of Medicine, Allegheny University of the Health Science, Philadelphia, Pennsylvania

John Collins Harvey, MD, PhD   Professor of Medicine, Emeritus, Senior Research Scholar, Kennedy Institute of Ethics, Center for Clinical Bioethics, Georgetown University, Washington, DC

Mary Hawthorne, RN, PhD   Assistant Professor, Duke University School of Nursing, Durham, North Carolina

Raymond E. Ideker, MD, PhD   Professor of Medicine, Pathology, and Biomedical Engineering, University of Alabama at Birmingham, Birmingham, Alabama

Louise Sherman Jenkins, RN, PhD   Professor, University of Maryland School of Nursing, Baltimore, Maryland

Bruce H. KenKnight, PhD   Cardiac Pacemakers, Inc., St. Paul, Minnesota

Kenneth M. Kessler, MD   Professor of Medicine, University of Miami School of Medicine, Miami, Florida

Larry S. Liebovitch, PhD   Associate Professor, Florida Atlantic University, Boca Raton, Florida

David C. Man, MD   Clinical Fellow in Electrophysiology, Allegheny University of the Health Sciences, Philadelphia, Pennsylvania

Francis E. Marchlinski, MD   Professor of Medicine, Allegheny University of the Health Sciences, Philadelphia, Pennsylvania

Robert J. Myerburg, MD   Professor of Medicine, University of Miami School of Medicine, Miami, Florida

Laura Porter, RN, PhD   Assistant Professor, Nell Hodgson Woodruff School of Nursing, Emory University, Atlanta, Georgia

Barbara Reigel, DNSc, RN, CS   Associate Professor of Nursing, San Diego State University, San Diego, California

Mary Jane Sauvé, DNSc, RN   University of California, Davis Health Systems, Center of Nursing Research, Sacramento, California

David Schwartzman, MD   Associate Professor of Medicine, Allegheny University of the Health Sciences, Philadelphia, Pennsylvania

Pippa M. Simpson, PhD   Associate Professor of Pediatrics, Biostatistician, Wayne State University, Detroit, Michigan

Brian H. Sarter, MD   Clinical Fellow in Electrophysiology, Allegheny University of the Health Sciences, Philadelphia, Pennsylvania

Angelo T. Todorov, PhD   Postdoctoral Fellow, Florida Atlantic University, Boca Raton, Florida

G. Michael Vincent, MD   Professor of Medicine, University of Utah School of Medicine, Salt Lake City, Utah

Gregory P. Walcott, MD   Assistant Professor of Medicine, University of Alabama at Birmingham, Birmingham, Alabama

John A. Walker, PhD   Associate Clinical Professor, University of California, San Francisco, California

Gayle R. Whitman, RN, MSN   Clinical Nurse Specialist, Cleveland Clinic Foundation, Cleveland, Ohio

Mary A. Woo, DNSc, RN   Assistant Professor, UCLA School of Nursing, Los Angeles, California

Mark A. Wood, MD   Associate Professor of Medicine, Medical College of Virginia, Richmond, Virginia

Raymond L. Woosley, MD, PhD   Professor of Medicine and Pharmacology, Georgetown University Medical Center, Washington, DC

D. George Wyse, MD, PhD   Associate Dean for Clinical Affairs and Professor of Medicine, The University of Calgary/Foothills Hospital, Calgary, Alberta, Canada

Dina R. Yazmajian, MD   Clinical Fellow in Electrophysiology, Allegheny University of the Health Sciences, Philadelphia, Pennsylvania

Erica S. Zado, PA-C   Physician's Assistant, Allegheny University of the Health Sciences, Philadelphia, Pennsylvania

Xiaohong Zhou, MD   Assistant Professor of Medicine, University of Alabama at Birmingham, Birmingham, Alabama

Contents

Chapter 1

Sudden Cardiac Death:
Magnitude of the Problem

Sanjay Deshpande, MD, and Masood Akhtar, MD

Sudden cardiac death remains one of the continuing challenges to the modern clinician. Currently, it accounts for the death of the majority of people with cardiovascular disease, affecting more than 350 000 individuals in the United States,[1,2] and has enormous socioeconomic implications. The usual mechanism of sudden cardiac death is ventricular tachyarrhythmias, and bradycardia or nonarrhythmic causes are responsible for a minority of deaths.[3,4] In the adult population, coronary artery disease represents the most common cardiac substrate.[5,6] Unfortunately, a high proportion of sudden cardiac deaths occur as a first expression of undetected heart disease or a previous silent myocardial infarction,[7] and a substantial proportion occur outside the hospital.[2] Up to 50% of deaths in patients with congestive heart failure are reported to be sudden.[8,9] Although on the basis of the temporal course of death, sudden cardiac death is assumed to be arrhythmic, definitions of sudden cardiac death[10–12] that are time-based (death within 1 to 24 hours of symptom onset) do not require documentation of the rhythm present at the onset of the terminal event, which renders this definition somewhat frail.[13,14] Because of the variability in the definition of sudden cardiac death used by investigators in the past, a succinct definition is lacking, and this affects the collection and interpretation of epidemiological data.

Although epidemiological studies show a strong correlation between major risk factors such as hypertension, hypercholesterolemia, and smoking and the incidence of coronary artery disease,[15] a specific risk factor has not been identified for sudden

From: Dunbar SB, Ellenbogen KA, Epstein AE, (eds). *Sudden Cardiac Death: Past, Present, and Future.* Armonk, NY: Futura Publishing Company, Inc.; © 1997.

cardiac death, which limits the efficiency of preventive interventions. This highlights the fact that sudden cardiac death is not a distinct clinical entity but rather a unique outcome of a spectrum of cardiac diseases. In this chapter, after an overview of sudden cardiac death as an entity, issues specific to disease states associated with it will be addressed.

Overview of the Problem

Ventricular fibrillation is the rhythm initially documented by rescue personnel in 65% to 85% of out-of-hospital cardiac arrests.[2,16] Bradyarrhythmias or asystole are encountered in about 20% to 30%, and these victims have the worst outcome.[5] A minority of victims have ventricular tachycardia at the time of initial contact; they have the best outcome in terms of survival.[5] Despite the availability of cardiopulmonary resuscitation in some communities, by bystanders and out-of-hospital defibrillation, at least 80% of these cardiac arrest victims will not survive to hospital discharge.[17] Of those who do survive, 50% will be dead within 3 years.[17,18] Although women are at decreased risk at all ages, they are more likely to suffer a cardiac arrest as the first manifestation of heart disease.[19,20] Targeting this most visible segment of the cardiac arrest population alone and not the relatively invisible larger population who are at risk, therefore, will not significantly affect sudden cardiac death mortality.[21–23] Instead, a multifaceted approach encompassing primary prevention of heart disease, recognition of the patient at high risk, and early intervention aimed at reducing this risk as well as community awareness and education in cardiopulmonary resuscitation should be the ideal goal.[23]

Since the majority of sudden cardiac deaths occur in individuals with heart disease, substrate-oriented interventions would logically have the greatest impact. Epidemiological data regarding primary prevention of coronary artery disease are encouraging in this regard, as reflected by a steady decline in the prevalence of coronary artery disease and consequent reduction in sudden cardiac death over the past decade.[24,25] This trend has been primarily a result of coronary risk factor modification.[26] A significant reduction in cardiac events has been achieved with the use of cholesterol-lowering agents not only in those with established coronary artery disease[27] but also in those without prior documented disease.[28] Long-term follow-up is as yet lacking to confirm the anticipated consequential reduction in sudden cardiac death mortality.

The risk of sudden cardiac death after myocardial infarction is highest in the first year,[29,30] and hence, medical therapy directed toward this evolving substrate might conceptually be most important during this time. The use of β-adrenergic receptor–blocking agents after myocardial infarction, especially in the population with reduced left ventricular function and complex ventricular ectopy, can lead to a significant reduction in sudden cardiac death.[31,32] In contrast, the use of antiarrhythmic drugs before and during the Cardiac Arrhythmia Suppression Trial (CAST) have shown no benefit in survival.[33] This demonstrates the futility of drug suppression in an evolving substrate characterized by myocardial remodeling, neurohormonal influences, and progression of coronary disease. Few data support the role of amiodarone in the post–myocardial infarction phase for sudden death risk reduction,[34] although the long-term benefit is curiously limited to those patients with ejection fractions >40%.[35] Amiodarone was not helpful in reducing sudden death mortality in patients with heart failure in a large randomized controlled study in the United States, although it was successful in the subset of patients with nonischemic cardiomyopathy.[36] In contrast, in the Grupo de Estudio de Sobrevida en Insuficiencia Cardiaca en Argentina (GESICA), trial, amiodarone did extend survival, but patients with and without ischemic heart disease were not analyzed separately.[37] The role of amiodarone in hypertrophic cardiomyopathy is unclear because of conflicting data.[38-40] There is, however, compelling evidence that mortality reduction is possible with the use of hydralazine, nitrates, or angiotensin-converting enzyme inhibitors[41-45] in patients with reduced left ventricular function. Differences in the magnitude of sudden cardiac death mortality reduction in these trials are most likely due to differences in the patient populations and the definitions of sudden cardiac death.

Long-term data from the Coronary Artery Surgery Study (CASS)[46] demonstrate a favorable sudden death risk reduction with surgical myocardial revascularization compared with medical management in patients with triple-vessel disease and reduced left ventricular function (9% incidence of sudden death versus 31% over a 5-year period). In addition, reperfusion and revascularization with thrombolytics and catheter interventions aimed at infarct size reduction and opening the infarct-related artery even well beyond the phase of myocardial salvage have contributed to the decline in sudden cardiac death mortality.[47-50] This benefit is presumably extended by limiting infarct size, preserving ischemic myocardium, altering ventricular remodeling, and stabilizing the electrophysiological matrix.

Secondary prevention of recurrent cardiac arrest has a high profile but less impact on the overall magnitude of reduction of sudden cardiac death. Smaller trials and large ongoing and completed trials have demonstrated important limitations to antiarrhythmic drug therapy, including amiodarone, when prescribed empirically and guided by electrophysiological testing.[51–53] The results of the Cardiac Arrest Study Hamburg (CASH),[52] which compared metoprolol, amiodarone, propafenone, and the implantable cardioverter-defibrillator, showed device therapy to be superior to propafenone in prevention of sudden death or recurrent cardiac arrest. In the Cardiac Arrest in Seattle: Conventional Versus Amiodarone Drug Evaluation (CASCADE)[53] trial, amiodarone was shown to be superior to other drugs selected by electrophysiologically guided therapy in reducing sudden death. However, with longer follow-up, the apparently comparable impact on total mortality leads to a reluctance to accept the role of the implantable cardioverter-defibrillator as unquestionable in this population.[13,54] The role of empirical amiodarone compared with the use of the implantable cardioverter-defibrillator will be clarified in the Canadian Implantable Defibrillator Study (CIDS)[54] and the Antiarrhythmics Versus Implantable Defibrillator (AVID) trials.[13]

Although the Electrophysiologic Study Versus Electrocardiographic Monitoring (ESVEM) Study[55] found the two methods of evaluation of drug efficacy comparable and found sotalol to be more effective than other drugs,[56] long-term follow-up indicates that a more accurate conclusion would be that neither method was accurate in prediction of drug efficacy, since 58% experienced a recurrence of arrhythmia at 2 years of follow-up. More importantly, sudden death rates were significantly higher than those achieved with the use of the implantable cardioverter-defibrillator in comparable populations.[57–59]

Sudden cardiac death rates at 5-year follow-up with the implantable cardioverter-defibrillator have been reported to be impressively low ($\approx 4.5\%$),[57–59] yet total mortality reduction has not been as significant. The AVID[13] and CIDS[54] trials are anticipated to determine the relative efficacy and impact of the implantable cardioverter-defibrillator versus drug therapy with regard to total mortality.

Sudden Cardiac Death in Coronary Artery Disease

Coronary artery disease accounts for more than half of all cardiovascular deaths, and about half of these deaths are sudden.[60] Although women are at decreased risk at all ages, they are more likely to suffer a cardiac arrest as the first manifestation of heart disease; yet interestingly, they are less likely to have underlying coronary artery disease and more likely to have other forms of heart disease or apparently normal hearts.[20] Sudden cardiac death may occur in coronary artery disease during the period of acute ischemia or at some future point after the index myocardial infarction.

The pathophysiology of acute myocardial infarction in the majority of cases involves coronary thrombosis overlying a disrupted atherosclerotic plaque.[60,61] Serial angiographic studies have shown that this usually occurs in a mildly to moderately narrowed artery on the initial angiogram.[62,63] An old myocardial infarction is evident in about 40% to 80% of patients who suffer sudden cardiac death,[64–66] although a coexisting active coronary lesion with occlusive or nonocclusive coronary thrombosis[67,68] may be responsible for the arrhythmic death. The typical arrhythmic sequence leading to sudden cardiac death is the development of ventricular tachycardia that degenerates to ventricular fibrillation, or else ventricular fibrillation is the initial rhythm. The arrhythmic mechanism underlying this sequence is primarily intramyocardial reentry in the ischemic or infarcted area or within its perimeter. Modulating factors such as fluctuating autonomic tone, electrolyte abnormalities, antiarrhythmic drug therapy, ventricular filling pressures, and variations in cycle length with ectopy can exert a triggering influence on a previously stable substrate.

The issue of sudden cardiac death in coronary artery disease may be addressed in two populations: first, in individuals who have experienced a myocardial infarction, and second, in those who have coronary artery disease but have not yet suffered a myocardial infarction. This latter population is a large and relatively "silent" segment of the individuals at risk. Identification of the individual with coronary artery disease and a prior myocardial infarction who may be at high risk for sudden cardiac death is based on assessment and delineation of risk factors.[69–72] Although no single factor is predictive alone, combination of these data usually provides a better clinical perspective.

Left ventricular systolic function is the most powerful predictor of overall survival[3,69–72] and of arrhythmic outcome in this population, although it cannot predict the mode of cardiac death. Patients with depressed left ventricular function who do not have an inducible ventricular tachycardia or other demonstrable cause for the initial cardiac arrest have a risk of recurrence >30% over a 1- to 3-year period.[73,74] If ventricular tachycardia is inducible and is implicated as the mechanism, the risk of recurrent arrest remains between 15% and 50% over the next 2 to 3 years even if arrhythmia suppression is achieved by electrophysiologically guided therapy.[73,75] Even if cardiac arrest in this population was attributed to a reversible cause, such as hypoxia or proarrhythmia, the risk of recurrence is reportedly 39% over the next year despite efforts to control the triggers.[76] For unclear reasons, left ventricular ejection fraction is not as accurately predictive for mortality in women after myocardial infarction or cardiac arrest.[20] The use of signal-averaged electrocardiography to detect evidence of the underlying substrate of ventricular arrhythmias in the post–myocardial infarction population has been validated in several studies.[77-79] The presence of late potential has been shown to correlate with an increased incidence of sudden death, and the combined influence of an ejection fraction <40% confers a 34% risk of arrhythmic events at a median follow-up of 14 months.[77] Conversely, absence of late potentials and a normal ejection fraction imply a favorable prognosis.[77] Unfortunately, limitations persist with regard to its application in patients with baseline intraventricular conduction abnormalities and anterior infarction.

Autonomic nervous dysfunction is believed to facilitate sudden cardiac death.[80-85] Although there is compelling evidence for this association, the mechanism by which it occurs is as yet unclear. This sympathovagal imbalance is reflected clinically as an attenuation of overall heart rate variability and reflects a reduced vagal output and enhanced adrenergic tone. Abnormal heart rate variability has been suggested to be an independent risk factor for sudden death in the post–myocardial infarction population.[83] Baroreceptor sensitivity and measurement of electrical alternans have recently been suggested as alternative noninvasive tests for risk stratification; however, they are yet to be validated in large-scale trials.[84,85]

The detection of ventricular ectopy by long-term ambulatory monitoring after myocardial infarction also has been associated with an increased risk of sudden cardiac death.[86,87] The sensitivity and positive predictive value of this test are relatively poor. The naive assumption that suppression of this ectopy would translate into reduction of sudden death was dispelled by the CAST data.[33] Ambulatory monitoring has been used to channel high-risk patients for risk stratification by programmed electrical stimulation on the basis of inducibility.[88] Routine electrophysiologically guided risk stratification of infarct survivors has a low positive predictive value, especially in the low-risk group, but appears to have a high negative predictive value.[89,90] Instead, the focus has been shifted to further risk stratification of the population with reduced left ventricular function into those with and those without inducible ventricular tachycardia. Two ongoing multicenter trials are examining the role of electrophysiologically guided drug therapy (Multicenter Unsustained Tachycardia Trial)[91] or a prophylactic implantable defibrillator (Multicenter Automatic Defibrillator Trial)[92] on survival. A third ongoing multicenter study (CABG Patch)[93] is evaluating the impact on total mortality of prophylactic use of the implantable cardioverter-defibrillator in patients undergoing coronary artery bypass surgery who have reduced left ventricular function. Historically, this population has a mortality rate of 30% at 3 years, and a significant proportion of these deaths are sudden.[94]

Risk factors for sudden cardiac death have been well established for those individuals who have already experienced a myocardial infarction, as addressed above. The larger population of patients with coronary artery disease who have not yet experienced a myocardial infarction is more difficult to identify. Although symptoms of myocardial ischemia or provocative stress testing and coronary angiography may identify and quantify the disease, clinicians are limited in their ability to predict, on the basis of angiographic findings, which specific plaque is likely to transform into an unstable plaque or manifest endothelial dysfunction and potentially cause sudden cardiac death.[95-97] It is believed that silent ischemia detected by ambulatory monitoring may identify a subset of individuals who have biologically unstable disease and a higher risk for adverse outcome during short-term follow-up.[97]

Sudden Cardiac Death in Idiopathic Dilated Cardiomyopathy

Nonischemic cardiomyopathy is increasingly being recognized as an important entity in the underlying spectrum of cardiac diseases associated with sudden cardiac death. The disease has a grim prognosis, with reported annual mortality between 25% and 45%,[98,99] and ≈30% of deaths are sudden.[98-100] Implementation of vasodilator therapy has made a significant impact in reduction of total mortality, although its influence on risk of sudden death is less clear.[41,45] This population of patients constitutes a significant fraction of individuals who are referred for cardiac transplantation.[101,102]

Although there is a high prevalence of ventricular arrhythmias[103] and a high risk of sudden[98-100] cardiac death with this disease, the relationship remains controversial. The mechanism of death is usually a ventricular tachyarrhythmia, although bradyarrhythmias and electromechanical dissociation are also observed in patients with advanced left ventricular dysfunction.[3,4] Patchy ventricular fibrosis forms the substrate for reentry, and hemodynamic factors such as ventricular loading conditions, intracellular depletion of potassium or magnesium, heightened sympathetic tone, neurohormonal activation, and proarrhythmia from the use of diuretics, inotropic agents, or antiarrhythmic drugs all have been shown to be contributory.[104–106]

Identification of the patient at risk for sudden cardiac death in this substrate is a challenging task. There is no clear association between functional class or age and the risk of dying suddenly.[107] A history of syncope, however, is a significant prognostic factor for an increased risk of sudden death.[108] Although worsening hemodynamics and ventricular function are indicative of increasing mortality,[43,109] a distinction between sudden and nonarrhythmic death cannot be predicted. The standard electrocardiogram does not provide any predictive information, and the utility of the signal-averaged electrocardiogram in this regard has not been established.[110–112] The presence of complex ventricular ectopy is suggestive of an adverse outcome in idiopathic dilated cardiomyopathy, although discrimination between arrhythmic and nonarrhythmic death is difficult.[113] In contrast to patients with coronary artery disease, electrophysiological study–guided risk stratification and therapy in idiopathic dilated cardiomyopathy are hindered by significant limitations. Patients with clinical sustained ventricular tachycardia or cardiac arrest in this population face a significant risk of recurrence and sudden death.[114,115] Antiarrhythmic therapy in this subset is associated with a high mortality,[106] and hence, implantable cardioverter-defibrillator therapy is perhaps a better option, although this issue still remains unresolved.[116,117] In patients with asymptomatic complex ventricular ectopy who have poor ventricular function, the induction of sustained monomorphic ventricular tachycardia portends a higher risk of sudden cardiac death.[118] Currently, although supportive data for electrophysiological study–guided drug therapy and the use of the implantable cardioverter-defibrillator in this setting exist, the optimal approach is unclear. The use of empirical amiodarone in asymptomatic individuals with advanced ventricular dysfunction has been evaluated in two large trials.[36,37] Amiodarone was shown to be well tolerated and effective in suppression of ventricular ectopy, and both trials suggest that the drug may improve survival in patients with nonischemic cardiomyopathy.

Sudden Death in the Athlete

Sudden death during sporting activities has been reported as early as 490 BC with the dramatic, unexpected death of the Greek soldier Pheidippides after his run from Marathon to Athens to deliver the news of victory over the Persians. Such deaths among healthy, physically conditioned, and usually young athletes, although relatively uncommon, are totally unexpected and consequently have a devastating impact on the community. Sudden death in athletes usually occurs during or immediately after exertion, and most individuals have been asymptomatic during prior training and vigorous activities. In the majority of individuals, a variety of congenital cardiovascular diseases are responsible for this problem.[2,5,10] They are usually undetected and only recognized postmortem, and the pathophysiological mechanisms that trigger the event are largely unknown. The problem is compounded by the lack of effective screening tests and strategies for prevention.

Among the cardiovascular conditions alluded to previously, hypertrophic cardiomyopathy is perhaps the most common entity.[119] Included in the spectrum of this disease is idiopathic left ventricular concentric hypertrophy.[119-128] Congenital coronary arterial malformations can also be the cause of sudden death in young athletes.[126-129] The most common of these is anomalous origin of the left main coronary artery from the right sinus of Valsalva. Other entities in this category include coronary artery hypoplasia of the right, left, or circumflex coronary arteries; the origin of the left anterior descending artery or right coronary artery from the pulmonary trunk; myocardial bridging; or coronary arterial intussusception.[130] Aortic rupture due to underlying Marfan's syndrome is usually catastrophic and may occur in an individual without the classic physical evidence of the disease.[119,128]

Atherosclerotic coronary artery disease has also been responsible for sudden death in athletes and is usually the cause in those who are older.[119,131] Many of these individuals have been previously diagnosed or have experienced but ignored prodromal symptoms. Right ventricular cardiomyopathy is an unusual and perhaps unrecognized cause of sudden death in the young athlete.[121,123,132] Occult cardiac involvement by sarcoid granulomatous infiltration has also been reported as a finding in athletes who have died suddenly.[133] Although sarcoid may cause conduction abnormalities, atrioventricular conduction abnormalities unassociated with structural heart disease have also been reported to cause sudden death. Other arrhythmias, such as those seen in the Wolff-Parkinson-White syndrome[119,123] and the long-QT syndrome,[134] are important causes of sudden death in this population. The frequency of association of myocarditis or mitral valve prolapse with sudden death in the young athlete may have been overestimated, and currently, neither is believed to be an important cause.

Commotio cordis, or concussion of the heart, from nonpenetrating blunt trauma to the anterior chest wall can lead to a fatal cardiac arrest.[135,136] Typically, this results from a blow to the chest from a hockey puck or baseball, and it occurs in children with no underlying heart disease who engage in amateur sports. Usually, no demonstrable structural abnormalities can be identified despite careful evaluation to account for the sudden death. In these individuals, the cause remains speculative and may be due to transient functional or autonomic disturbances of the electrophysiological milieu that lead to arrhythmic death.

Sudden Death in the Wolff-Parkinson-White Syndrome

The Wolff-Parkinson-White syndrome is a rare cause of sudden cardiac death.[137,138] In the majority of individuals, the mechanism of this event is atrial fibrillation with a rapid ventricular response over the accessory pathway, which can lead to ventricular fibrillation. Most of these individuals have experienced symptomatic arrhythmias in the past, and only a minority have been truly asymptomatic before sudden cardiac death. The incidence of sudden cardiac death in the Wolff-Parkinson-White syndrome has been estimated to be up to 4%; however, it is probably no greater than 1 per 100 patient-years of follow-up in asymptomatic individuals.[139–141]

Electrophysiological assessment may be indicated in asymptomatic individuals with Wolff-Parkinson-White syndrome for whom even a small risk of ventricular fibrillation as the initial manifestation is unacceptable because of their high-risk occupation (athletes, pilots, etc). A greater risk is associated with the presence of posteroseptal accessory pathways, multiple accessory pathways, and a preexcited RR interval of <250 ms during atrial fibrillation. Although noninvasive testing can identify accessory pathways with a low potential risk for sudden cardiac death, it is an imperfect surrogate, and accurate assessment of this risk is possible only with an electrophysiological study.

Arrhythmogenic Right Ventricular Dysplasia

This condition is now increasingly recognized as an underlying cause of sudden cardiac death in young, usually male, individuals.[121,132,142,143] The spectrum of this disorder ranges widely both morphologically and in its electrophysiological manifestations. In its mildest form, it may be difficult to diagnose even at autopsy, and its most dramatic form is seen as extensive right ventricular dilatation with replacement of myocardium with fibrous tissue. Clinically, the disease may cause atrial arrhythmias, frequent ventricular ectopy, nonsustained or sustained ventricular tachycardia, or rarely ventricular fibrillation. Recognition of this condition may be possible by electrocardiographic signs during sinus rhythm and ventricular tachycardia or with imaging techniques such as echocardiography, radionuclide scan, or magnetic resonance imaging.[144,145] Histological diagnosis can be made with reasonable certainty by biopsy of the right ventricular free wall. Electrophysiological study–guided therapy is recommended for symptomatic individuals with serial drug testing with sotalol or amiodarone,[146] with catheter ablation, or with the implantable cardioverter-defibrillator when appropriate. In rare instances, recurrent disabling arrhythmias may require surgical isolation of the right ventricular free wall or cardiac transplantation.

The long-term outcome of patients treated with antiarrhythmic drugs is quite favorable if the manifestation is ventricular tachycardia. The prognosis is much worse if the clinical presentation is syncope or sudden cardiac death or if left ventricular involvement is also present.[147,148]

Sudden Cardiac Death in Hypertrophic Cardiomyopathy

Hypertrophic cardiomyopathy is a familial primary disorder of cardiac muscle with marked heterogeneity in morphology and natural history. Hypertensive hypertrophic cardiomyopathy is now recognized as a distinct subtype of this entity.[149] The disease is characterized by a marked increase in myocardial mass with heterogeneity in the amount of hypertrophy in different regions of the left ventricle and absence of left ventricular dilatation.[150] The characteristic abnormality is diastolic dysfunction that causes hemodynamic compromise. In most patients there is a disproportionate thickening of the interventricular septum and anterolateral wall compared with the posterior wall.[151] Pathological changes are notable for gross disorganization of the muscle bundles, fiber orientation, and cellular myofibril structure.[149] Alteration of the gap junction and increased connective tissue accumulation, in addition, can lead to abnormalities in intercellular communication. These structural and functional changes are therefore the substrate for the altered electrophysiological milieu in this disease.

Sudden cardiac death is a well-recognized complication of hypertrophic cardiomyopathy; in fact, it is the most common cause of sudden death in individuals <30 years old. Several mechanisms are implicated in the genesis of sudden cardiac death in these patients. Altered cellular electrophysiological function due to structural changes or abnormal calcium ion regulation, myocardial ischemia, left ventricular outflow tract obstruction, supraventricular tachycardias with rapid atrioventricular conduction, conduction disease, and neurohormonal dysfunction may contribute to the development of lethal arrhythmias. Natural history studies[40,152,153] have reported an annual mortality rate of 2% to 6% in patients with hypertrophic cardiomyopathy; however, these data may be an overestimate, since they are derived from hospital-based populations and are influenced by referral bias. In a population-based assessment of the natural history of this disease,[154] the annual risk of cardiac death was observed to be 0.7%, with comparable overall survival with age- and sex-matched populations, reflecting an outcome far more benign than previously reported. Factors associated with a poor outcome include New York Heart Association functional class, young age at presentation, atrial fibrillation, and myocardial infarction on the baseline electrocardiogram.[154] Cardiac mortality can be predicted by a history of atrial fibrillation, myocardial infarction, and mitral annular calcification; family history of sudden cardiac death; or prior cardiac arrest.[152]

The prognostic significance of nonsustained ventricular tachycardia of arrhythmic potential in hypertrophic cardiomyopathy has been the subject of considerable debate.[38-40,152] Although programmed electrical stimulation has been advocated for risk stratification,[155] its positive predictive accuracy for sudden cardiac death in those with inducible ventricular tachycardia is low.[155,156] A recent report suggested that the demonstration of early electrogram fractionation during ventricular extrastimulation, implying disparity in intramyocardial conduction, has been shown to correlate with sudden cardiac death.[157] Asymptomatic or minimally symptomatic patients with hypertrophic cardiomyopathy who have brief and infrequent nonsustained ventricular tachycardia on ambulatory monitoring have a low cardiac risk and need not be automatically treated with amiodarone, as they have been in the past, but rather may undergo more detailed characterization of risk to determine appropriate therapy.[38,158] Currently, no conclusive data support the notion that β-blockers, calcium blockers, permanent pacing, surgical myomectomy, or amiodarone prevents sudden cardiac death in hypertrophic cardiomyopathy.[151,159]

A minority of patients with chronic mild or moderate hypertension develop significant left ventricular hypertrophy as a seemingly inappropriate response. On the basis of epidemiological studies, left ventricular hypertrophy is not an asset but rather an ominous harbinger of cardiac mortality.[160] Asymptomatic ventricular arrhythmias appear more frequently in hypertensive patients with hypertrophy than in those without,[161] and regression of hypertrophy is associated with a decrease in ectopy.[162] Left ventricular hypertrophy documented by echocardiography confers an increased risk of sudden cardiac death when associated with asymptomatic ventricular ectopy.[163–165] At the present time, the mechanisms and therapeutic implications of this excess mortality remain unresolved.

Sudden Cardiac Death in Patients With Advanced Ventricular Dysfunction

In the United States, approximately 2 to 3 million patients suffer from heart failure, and this number is likely to increase.[166,167] Most of these individuals manifest frequent and complex ventricular ectopy, and the frequency and severity of the arrhythmia worsen with advancing ventricular dysfunction.[167] Survival of patients with advanced ventricular dysfunction is limited not only by progressive pump dysfunction but also by the risk of sudden cardiac death. The 1-year mortality risk exceeds 50% for patients with New York Heart Association functional class IV symptoms.[43,168,169] Recent advances in the medical management of heart failure have led to significant amelioration of symptoms, improved functional class, and prolonged survival.[41-45] The benefit extended by angiotensin-converting enzyme inhibitors in this regard has translated into a significant reduction in total mortality; however, a considerable risk of sudden cardiac death remains in 28% to 68% of these patients.[43,45,102] Although medical therapy has been shown to prolong survival in this population, cardiac transplantation remains the only long-term alternative for those who are suitable candidates. Unfortunately, it is estimated that up to 40% of patients awaiting cardiac transplantation will die suddenly.[8,9] Prevention of sudden cardiac death in this population may allow more patients to survive until hemodynamic and functional deterioration necessitates cardiac transplantation.

The principal mechanism of sudden cardiac death in this population remains arrhythmic, with ventricular tachycardia that degenerates into ventricular fibrillation being the most common arrhythmia.[4] As stated previously, bradyarrhythmic cardiac arrest and electromechanical dissociation are also well described and may be more common in idiopathic dilated cardiomyopathy.[4] Multiple factors are operative in the development of sudden cardiac death. Ventricular tachycardia due to reentry is the usual arrhythmia, although it may be modulated by a variety of triggers, such as alteration in myocardial wall stress from changing preload or afterload, myocardial ischemia, fluctuating neurohormonal tone, electrolyte abnormalities, and the proarrhythmic effect of antiarrhythmic drugs.[105,106,170–172]

Unfortunately, spontaneous ventricular ectopy and the degree of ventricular dysfunction do not reliably discriminate the excess risk of sudden cardiac death from overall cardiac mortality in patients with chronic heart failure.[29,72] Thus, identification of the person at risk for sudden cardiac death in this setting is a somewhat daunting task. Clearly, patients with reduced ventricular function who have been resuscitated from a cardiac arrest are at high risk for recurrence even if ventricular tachycardia is not inducible at electrophysiological study.[73,74] Those with inducible ventricular tachycardia have a 15% to 50% risk of recurrent arrest despite suppression of the inducible arrhythmia with antiarrhythmic drugs, including amiodarone.[73,75] It is also important to note that even if cardiac arrest in this population was attributed to a reversible cause, such as hypoxia or proarrhythmia, the risk of recurrence is reportedly 39% over the next year despite efforts to control the triggers.[76] Syncope in this population also carries an ominous prognosis, with an actuarial risk of sudden cardiac death of 45% over 1 year.[108,173] This risk was comparable even in those patients with advanced ventricular dysfunction in whom a cause for syncope could not be identified.

In patients with prior myocardial infarction and advanced heart failure, identification of late potentials by signal-averaged electrocardiography, decreased heart rate variability, and ventricular tachycardia induced by programmed electrical stimulation all predict an increased risk of sudden cardiac death.[87,89] These screening tests, however, do not have an equivalent negative predictive value. Also, their utility is limited in patients with nonischemic causes of heart failure. The treatment of these patients remains problematic; however, limited data suggest that the risk of sudden death may be reduced in this population with the use of amiodarone, although benefit was most evident in those with nonischemic cardiomyopathy.[36,37] The implantable cardioverter-defibrillator holds great promise when used as a "bridge" to cardiac transplantation,[174,175] although there is a somewhat higher occurrence of bradyarrhythmic deaths in those with advanced ventricular dysfunction, and the device is unlikely to benefit those individuals. Currently, it is not feasible to accurately identify those patients who are more likely to experience a tachyarrhythmic death than death from progressive pump dysfunction while awaiting transplantation.

Sudden Cardiac Death in Association With the Long-QT Syndrome

Primary QT-interval prolongation is an infrequently occurring disorder associated with a propensity to ventricular arrhythmias, syncope, and sudden cardiac death.[134,176-178] The condition is characterized by abnormal electrical repolarization of the myocardium and manifests electrocardiographically as prolongation of the QT interval and abnormalities of the T and U waves. A strong familial pattern of inheritance is associated with this condition,[179-181] and specific genetic defects have now been identified.[182-185] Consequently, an increased risk of cardiac events is observed in family members of the proband.[186]

It is believed, in a simplistic sense, that this genetic abnormality modulates the myocardial ionic channels,[184,185] increasing cellular susceptibility to autonomic influences, which can trigger polymorphic ventricular tachycardia and ventricular fibrillation. Clinically, this translates into bradycardia and prolonged repolarization as the substrate and sympathetic stimulation as a trigger, although the mechanism of this interaction is not well established. The usual presentation is syncope due to a self-limiting episode of torsade de pointes ventricular tachycardia. The diagnosis of long-QT syndrome may easily be overlooked, especially since these individuals are otherwise healthy, yet are at risk for recurrent events. Infrequently, sudden cardiac death is the first manifestation, or the disorder is noted incidentally on a screening electrocardiogram.

Both the individual and the family should be thoroughly evaluated to establish the diagnosis and determine risk of arrhythmic events.[186,187] A resting electrocardiogram is insufficient to exclude the diagnosis, because the repolarization abnormalities may be evanescent, and hence ambulatory Holter monitoring and an exercise test should be performed. The response of the QT interval to exercise in patients with a long-QT syndrome is either failure of shortening with tachycardia or an exaggerated prolongation in the recovery period.[188] High-resolution electrocardiography and invasive electrophysiological studies are unhelpful in diagnosis or management, although echocardiographic abnormality in the ventricular contraction pattern has been observed in symptomatic patients.[189]

An assessment of individual risk based on clinical and electrocardiographic criteria is then feasible. On one end of the spectrum is the high-risk individual who has experienced either an episode of cardiac arrest or syncope, especially if the event occurred at a young age. Included in this category are asymptomatic family members of probands with a virulent family history of syncope or sudden death spanning several generations. Asymptomatic individuals >30 years old who have never experienced syncope in the past appear to be at a very low risk for future events. This includes family members detected during pedigree evaluation and those detected incidentally. In those with borderline prolongation of the QT interval, close follow-up should be maintained to monitor electrocardiographic changes or the occurrence of symptoms. It is critical that patients with this condition avoid the use of medications, including over-the-counter drugs, that can potentially trigger lethal arrhythmias.

Conclusions

The magnitude of sudden cardiac death as an entity in industrialized nations overshadows the majority of publicized healthcare dilemmas. A variety of structural heart disease, most often coronary artery disease, may be the underlying substrate, and a complex influence of triggers is believed to incite the event. Ventricular tachyarrhythmias dominate as the fatal mechanism, and bradyarrhythmias account for a minority of deaths. Targeting secondary prevention of cardiac arrest alone is unlikely to have a significant impact, given the currently dismal outcome of cardiopulmonary resuscitation in the community, where a large attrition in survival occurs. Additionally, the larger population who remain at risk would be unaffected by this management strategy. Therefore, a multifaceted approach encompassing primary prevention of heart disease, substrate-oriented interventions, recognition of the individual at risk, and community awareness and education in cardiopulmonary resuscitation would most likely produce an optimal result.

References

1. DiMarco JP, Haines DE. Sudden cardiac death. *Curr Prob Cardiol.* 1990;15:183–232.
2. Myerburg RJ, Castellanos A. Cardiac arrest and sudden cardiac death. In: Braunwald E, ed. *Heart Disease. A Textbook of Cardiovascular Medicine.* 4th ed. Philadelphia, Pa: Saunders; 1992;756–789.
3. Bayes de Luna A, Coumel P, Leclercq JF. Ambulatory sudden cardiac death: mechanisms of production of fatal arrhythmia on the basis of data from 157 cases. *Am Heart J.* 1989;117:151–159.

4. Luu M, Stevenson LW, Brunken RC, et al. Diverse mechanisms of un-expected cardiac arrest in advanced heart failure. *Circulation.* 1989;80:1675–1680.
5. Myerburg RJ. Sudden cardiac death: epidemiology, causes, and mechanisms. *Cardiology.* 1987;74 (suppl 2):2–9.
6. Virmani R, Roberts WC. Sudden cardiac death. *Hum Pathol.* 1987;18:485–492.
7. Kreger BE, Cupples A, Kannel WB. The electrocardiogram in predic-tion of sudden death: the Framingham Study experience. *Am Heart J.* 1987;2:377–382.
8. DEFIBRILAT Study Group. Actuarial risk of sudden death while awaiting cardiac transplantation in patients with atherosclerotic heart disease. *Am J Cardiol.* 1991;68:545–546.
9. Stevenson WG, Stevenson LW, Weiss J, et al. Inducible ventricular ar-rhythmias and sudden death during vasodilator therapy of severe heart failure. *Am Heart J.* 1988;116:1447–1454.
10. Roberts WC. Sudden cardiac death: definitions and causes. *Am J Car-diol.* 1986;57:1410–1413.
11. Report of a WHO Scientific Group. Sudden cardiac death. *Who Tech Rep Ser.* 1985;726:5–25.
12. Greene HL, Richardson DW, Barker AH, et al. Classification of deaths after myocardial infarction as arrhythmic or nonarrhythmic (the Car-diac Arrhythmia Pilot Study). *Am J. Cardiol.* 1989;63:1–6.
13. Epstein AE. AVID necessity. *Pacing Clin Electrophysiol.* 1993;16:1773–1775.
14. Epstein AE, Carlson MD, Fogoros RN, et al. Classification of death in antiarrhythmia trials. *J Am Coll Cardiol.* 1996;27:433–442.
15. Kannel WB. Clinical misconceptions dispelled by epidemiological re-search. *Circulation.* 1995;92:3350–3360.
16. Demirovic J, Myerburg RJ. Epidemiology of sudden coronary death: an overview. *Prog Cardiovasc Dis.* 1994;37:39–48.
17. Schaffer WA, Cobb LA. Recurrent ventricular fibrillation and mode of death in survivors of out-of-hospital ventricular fibrillation. *N Engl J Med.* 1975;293:259–262.
18. Goldstein S, Landis JR, Leighton R, et al. Characteristics of the re-suscitated out-of-hospital cardiac arrest victim with coronary heart disease. *Circulation.* 1981;64:977–984.
19. Kannel WB, Schatzkin A. Sudden death: lessons from subsets in pop-ulation studies. *J Am Coll Cardiol.* 1985;5:141B–149B.
20. Albert CM, McGovern BA, Newell JB, et al. Sex differences in cardiac arrest survivors. *Circulation.* 1996;93:1170–1176.
21. Becker LB, Ostrander MP, Barrett J, et al. Outcome of CPR in a large metropolitan area: where are the survivors? *Ann Emerg Med.* 1991;20:355–361.
22. Lombardi G, Gallagher J, Gennis P. Outcome of out-of-hospital car-diac arrest in New York City. *JAMA.* 1994;271:678–683.
23. Cummins RO, Ornato JP, Thies WH, et al. Improving survival from sudden cardiac arrest: the "chain of survival" concept. A statement for health professionals from the Advanced Cardiac Life Support Subcommittee and the Emergency Cardiac Care Committee, Ameri-can Heart Association. *Circulation.* 1991;83:1832–1847.
24. Kuller LH, Perper JA, Dai WS, et al. Sudden death and the decline in coronary heart disease mortality. *J Chronic Dis.* 1986;39:1001–1019.

25. Goldberg RJ. Declining out-of-hospital sudden coronary death rates: additional pieces of the epidemiologic puzzle. *Circulation.* 1989;79: 1369–1373.
26. Levine G, Keaney JF Jr, Vita JA, et al. Cholesterol reduction in cardiovascular disease: clinical benefits and possible mechanisms. *N Engl J Med.* 1995;332:512–521.
27. SSSS Study Group. Randomized trial of cholesterol lowering in 4444 patients with coronary artery disease: the Scandinavian Simvastatin Survival Study. *Lancet.* 1994;344:1383–1389.
28. Shepherd J, Cobbe SM, Ford I, et al. Primary prevention of coronary heart disease with pravastatin in men with hypercholesterolemia. *N Engl J Med.* 1995;333:1301–1307.
29. Multicenter Postinfarction Research Group. Risk stratification and survival after myocardial infarction. *N Engl J Med.* 1983;309: 331–336.
30. Pfisterer M, Salamin P, Schwendener R, et al. Clinical risk assessment after first myocardial infarction: is additional noninvasive testing necessary? *Chest.* 1992;102:1499–1504.
31. β-Blocker Heart Attack Trial Research Group. A randomized trial of propranolol in patients with acute myocardial infarction. *JAMA.* 1982;247:1707–1714.
32. The Norwegian Multicenter Study Group. Timolol-induced reduction in mortality and reinfarction in patients surviving acute myocardial infarction. *N Engl J Med.* 1981;304:801–807.
33. Epstein AE, Hallstrom AP, Rogers WJ, et al. Mortality following ventricular arrhythmia suppression by encainide, flecainide, and moricizine after myocardial infarction. *JAMA.* 1993;270:2451–2455.
34. Burkart F, Pfisterer M, Kiowski W, et al. Effect of antiarrhytimic therapy on mortality in survivors of myocardial infarction with asymptomatic complex ventricular arrhythmias: Basal Antiarrhythmic Study of Infarct Survival (BASIS). *J Am Coll Cardiol.* 1990;16: 1711–1718.
35. Pfisterer ME, Kiowski, W, Brunner H, et al. Long-term benefit of 1-year amiodarone treatment for persistent complex ventricular arrhythmias after myocardial infarction. *Circulation.* 1993;87:309–311.
36. Singh SN, Fletcher RD, Gross Fisher S, et al. Amiodarone in patients with congestive heart failure and asymptomatic ventricular arrhythmia. *N Engl J Med.* 1995;333:77–82.
37. Doval HC, Nul DR, Grancelli HO, et al. Randomised trial of low-dose amiodarone in severe congestive heart failure. *Lancet.* 1994;344: 493–498.
38. Spirito P, Rapezzi C, Autore C, et al. Prognosis of asymptomatic patients with hypertrophic cardiomyopathy and nonsustained ventricular tachycardia. *Circulation.* 1994;90:2743–2747.
39. McKenna WJ, England D, Doi YL, et al. Arrhythmia in hypertrophic cardiomyopathy, 1: influence on prognosis. *Br Heart J.* 1981;46: 168–172.
40. Maron BJ, Savage DD, Wolfson JK, et al. Prognostic significance of 24 hour ambulatory electrocardiographic monitoring in patients with hypertrophic cardiomyopathy: a prospective study. *Am J Cardiol.* 1981;48:252–257.
41. Cohn JN, Archibald DG, Ziesche S, et al. Effect of vasodilator therapy on mortality in chronic congestive heart failure: results of a Veterans

Administration Cooperative Study. *N Engl J Med.* 1986;314: 1547–1552.

42. Cohn JN, Johnson G, Ziesche S, et al. A comparison of enalapril on mortality and the development of heart failure in asymptomatic patients with reduced left ventricular ejection fraction. *N Engl J Med.* 1992;327:685–691.

43. The CONSENSUS Trial Study Group. Effects of enalapril on mortality in severe congestive heart failure: results of the Cooperative North Scandinavian Enalapril Survival Study (CONSENSUS). *N Engl J Med.* 1987;316:1429–1435.

44. The SOLVD Investigators. Effect of enalapril on survival in patients with reduced left ventricular ejection fractions and congestive heart failure. *N Engl J Med.* 1991;325:293–302.

45. Fonorow GC, Chelimsky-Fallick C, Stevenson LW, et al. Effect of direct vasodilation vs angiotensin-converting enzyme inhibition on mortality in advanced heart failure: the Hy-C trial. *J Am Coll Cardiol.* 1992;19:842–850.

46. Holmes DR, Davis KB, Mock MB, et al. The effect of medical and surgical treatment on subsequent cardiac death in patients with coronary artery disease: a report from the Coronary Artery Surgery Study. *Circulation.* 1986;73:1254–1263.

47. Vatterott PJ, Hammill SC, Bailey KR, et al. Late potentials on signal-averaged electrocardiograms and patency of the infarct-related artery in survivors of acute myocardial infarction. *J Am Coll Cardiol.* 1991;17:330–337.

48. Saeger ST, Perlmutter RA, Rosenfeld LE, et al. Electrophysiologic effects of thrombolytic therapy in patients with a transmural anterior myocardial infarction complicated by left ventricular aneurysm formation. *J Am Coll Cardiol.* 1988;12:19–24.

49. Boehrer JD, Glamann B, Lange RA, et al. Effect of coronary angioplasty on late potentials one to two weeks after acture myocardial infarction. *Am J. Cardiol.* 1992;70:1515–1519.

50. Leor J, Hod H, Rotstein Z, et al. Effects of thrombolysis on the 12-lead signal-averaged ECG in the early post-infarction period. *Am Heart J.* 1990;120:495–502.

51. Moosvi AR, Goldstein S, Vandenburg MS, et al. Effect of empiric antiarrhythmic therapy in resuscitated out-of-hospital cardiac arrest victims with coronary artery disease. *Am J Cardiol.* 1990;65:1192–1197.

52. Siebels J, Kuck KH, CASH Investigators. Implantable cardioverter defibrillator compared with antiarrhythmic drug treatment in cardiac arrest survivors (the Cardiac Arrest Study Hamburg). *Am Heart J.* 1994;127:1139–1144.

53. CASCADE Investigators. Randomized antiarrhythmic drug therapy in survivors of cardiac arrest (the CASCADE Study). *Am J. Cardiol.* 1993;72:280–287.

54. Connolly SJ, Gent M, Roberts RS, et al. Canadian implantable defibrillator study (CIDS): study design and organization. *Am J Cardiol.* 1993;72:103F–108F.

55. Mason JW, the ESVEM Investigators. A comparison of seven antiarrhythmic drugs in patients with ventricular tachyarrhythmias. *N Engl J Med.* 1993;329:452–458.

56. Mason JW, the ESVEM Investigators. A comparison of electrophysiologic testing with Holter monitoring to predict antiarrhythmic drug

efficacy for ventricular tachyarrhythmias. *N Engl J Med.* 1993;329: 445–451.

57. Winkle RA, Mead RH, Ruder MA, et al. Long-term outcome with the automatic implantable cardioverter-defibrillator. *J Am Coll Cardiol.* 1989;13:1353–1361.

58. Nisam S, Mower M, Moser S. ICD clinical update: first decade, initial 10,000 patients. *Pacing Clin Electrophysiol.* 1991;14:255–262.

59. Akhtar M, Avitall B, Jazayeri M, et al. Role of implantable cardioverter defibrillator therapy in the management of high-risk patients. *Circulation.* 1992;85(suppl I):I–131. Abstract.

60. Farb A, Tang AL, Burke AP, et al. Sudden coronary death: frequency of active coronary lesions, inactive coronary lesions, and myocardial infarction. *Circulation.* 1995;92:1701–1709.

61. Davies MJ, Thomas AC. Plaque fissuring: the cause of acute myocardial infarction, sudden ischemic death, and crescendo angina. *Br Heart J.* 1985;53:363–373.

62. Little WC, Constantinescu M, Applegate RJ, et al. Can coronary angiography predict the site of a subsequent myocardial infarction in patients with mild-to-moderate coronary artery disease? *Circulation.* 1988;78:1157–1166.

63. Ambrose JA, Tannenbaum MA, Alexopoulos D, et al. Angiographic progression of coronary artery disease and the development of myocardial infarction. *J Am Coll Cardiol.* 1988;12:56–62.

64. Haerem JW. Mural platelet microthrombi and major acute lesions of main epicardial arteries in sudden coronary death. *Atherosclerosis.* 1974;19:529–541.

65. Baroldi G, Falzi G, Mariani F. Sudden coronary death: a post-mortem study in 208 selected cases compared to 97 "control" subjects. *Am Heart J.* 1979;98:20–31.

66. Reichenbach DD, Moss NS, Meyer E. Pathology of the heart in sudden cardiac death. *Am J Cardiol.* 1977;39:865–872.

67. Davies MJ. Anatomic features in victims of sudden coronary death: coronary artery pathology. *Circulation.* 1992;85(suppl I):I-19–I-24.

68. Stevenson WG, Linssen GC, Havenith MG, et al. The spectrum of death after myocardial infarction: a necropsy study. *Am Heart J.* 1989;118:1182–1188.

69. Moss AJ. Prognosis after myocardial infarction. *Am J Cardiol.* 1983; 52:667–669.

70. Brudada P, Smeet TJ, Mulleneer R, et al. The value of the clinical history to assess prognosis of patients with ventricular tachycardia or ventricular fibrillation after myocardial infarction. *Eur Heart J.* 1989;10:752–757.

71. Sanz G, Castaner A, Betriu A, et al. Determinants of prognosis in survivors of myocardial infarction: a prospective clinical angiographic study. *N Engl J Med.* 1982;306:1065–1070.

72. Bigger JT Jr, Fleiss JL, Kleiger R, et al. The relationship among ventricular arrhythmias, left ventricular dysfunction and mortality in the 2 years after myocardial infarction. *Circulation.* 1984;69:250–258.

73. Wilber DJ, Garan H, Finkelstein D, et al. Out-of-hospital cardiac arrest: use of electrophysiologic testing in the prediction of long-term outcome. *N Engl J Med.* 1988;318:19–24.

74. Sager PT, Choudhary R, Leon C, et al. The long-term prognosis of patients with out-of-hospital cardiac arrest but no inducible ventricular tachycardia. *Am Heart J.* 1990;120:1334–1342.

75. Weinberg BA, Miles WM, Klein LS, et al. Five-year follow-up of 589 patients treated with amiodarone. *Am Heart J.* 1993;125:109–120.
76. Stevenson, WG, Middlekauff HM, Stevenson LW, et al. Significance of aborted cardiac arrest and sustained ventricular tachycardia in patients referred for treatment therapy of advanced heart failure. *Am Heart J.* 1992;124:123–130.
77. Kuchar DL, Thorburn CW, Sammel NL. Prediction of serious arrhythmic events after myocardial infarction: signal-averaged electrocardiogram, Holter monitoring and radionuclide ventriculography. *J Am Coll Cardiol.* 1987;9:531–538.
78. Gomes JA, Winters SL, Martinson M, et al. The prognostic significance of quantitative signal-averaged variables relative to clinical variables, site of myocardial infarction, ejection fraction and ventricular beats: a prospective study. *J Am Coll Cardiol.* 1989;13:377–384.
79. Steinberg JS, Regan A, Sciacca RR, et al. Predicting arrhythmic events after acute myocardial infarction using the signal-averaged electrocardiogram. *Am J Cardiol.* 1992;69:13–21.
80. Schwartz, PJ, Priori SG. Sympathetic nervous system and cardiac arrhythmias. In: Zipes DP, Jalife J, eds. *Cardiac Electrophysiology: From Cell to Bedside.* Philadelphia, Pa: WB Saunders; 1990:330–343.
81. Schwartz PJ, Vanoli E. Cardiac arrhythmias elicited by interaction between acute myocardial ischemia and sympathetic hyperactivity: a new experimental model for the study of antiarrhythmic drugs. *Cardiovasc Pharmacol.* 1981;3:1251–1259.
82. Schwartz PJ, La Rovere MT, Vanoli E. Autonomic nervous system and sudden cardiac death. Experimental basis and clinical observations for post-myocardial infarction risk stratification. *Circulation.* 1992;85(suppl I):I-177–I-191.
83. Odemuyiwa O, Poloniecki J, Malik M, et al. Temporal influences on the prediction of postinfarction mortality by heart rate variability: a comparison with the left ventricular ejection fraction. *Br Heart J.* 1994;71:521–527.
84. Hohnloser SH, Klingenheben T, Loo A, et al. Reflex versus tonic vagal activity as a prognostic parameter in patients with sustained ventricular tachycardia or ventricular fibrillation. *Circulation.* 1994;89:1068–1073.
85. Rosenbaum DS, Jackson LE, Smith JM, et al. Electrical alternans and vulnerability to ventricular arrhythmias. *N Engl J Med.* 1994;330:235–241.
86. Bigger JT, Fleiss JL, Kleiger RE, et al. The relationships among ventricular arrhythmias, left ventricular dysfunction, and mortality in the 2 years after myocardial infarction. *Circulation.* 1984;69:250–258.
87. Farrell TG, Bashir Y, Cripps T, et al. Risk stratification for arrhythmic events in post-infarction patients based on heart rate variability, ambulatory electrocardiographic variables and the signal-averaged electrocardiogram. *J Am Coll Cardiol.* 1991;18:687–697.
88. Ruskin JN. Role of invasive electrophysiologic testing in the evaluation and treatment of patients at high risk for sudden cardiac death. *Circulation.* 1992; 85 (suppl I):I-152–I-159.
89. Bourke JP, Richards DAB, Ross DL, et al. Routine programmed electrical stimulation in survivors of acute myocardial infarction for prediction of spontaneous ventricular tachyarrhythmias during follow-up: results, optimal stimulation protocol and cost-effective screening. *J Am Coll Cardiol.* 1991;780–788.

90. Roy D, Marchand E, Theroux P, et al. Programmed ventricular stimulation in survivors of an acute myocardial infarction. *Circulation.* 1985;72:487–494.
91. Buxton AE, Fisher JD, Josephson ME, et al. Prevention of sudden death in patients with coronary disease: the Multicenter Unsustained Tachycardia Trial (MUSTT). *Prog Cardiovasc Dis.* 1993;36: 215–226.
92. MADIT Executive Committee. Multicenter Automatic Defibrillator Implantation Trial (MADIT): design and clinical protocol. *Pacing Clin Electrophysiol.* 1991;14:920–927.
93. The CABG Patch Trial Investigators and Coordinators. The coronary artery bypass graft (CABG) patch trial. *Prog Cardiovasc Dis.* 1993; 36:97–114.
94. Alderman EL, Fisher LD, Litwin P, et al. Results of coronary artery surgery in patients with poor left ventricular function (CASS). *Circulation.* 1983;68:785–795.
95. Bugiardini R, Borghi A, Pozzati A, et al. Relation of severity of symptoms in transient myocardial ischemia and prognosis in unstable angina. *J Am Coll Cardiol.* 1995;25:597–604.
96. Rogers WJ, Bourassa MG, Andrews TC, et al. Asymptomatic Cardiac Ischemia Pilot (ACIP) study: outcome at 1 year for patients with asymptomatic cardiac ischemia randomized to medical therapy or revascularization. *J Am Coll Cardiol.* 1995;26:594–605.
97. Gill JB, Cairns JA, Roberts RS, et al. Prognostic importance of myocardial ischemia detected by ambulatory monitoring early after acute myocardial infarction. *N Engl J Med.* 1996;334:65–70.
98. Fuster V, Gersh B, Giuliani ER, et al. The natural history of idiopathic dilated cardiomyopathy. *Am J Cardiol.* 1981;47:525–531.
99. Stevenson LW, Fowler MB, Schroeder JS, et al. Poor survival of patients with idiopathic cardiomyopathy considered too well for transplantation. *Am J Med.* 1987;83:871–876.
100. Tamburro P, Wilber D. Sudden death in idiopathic dilated cardiomyopathy. *Am Heart J.* 1992;124:1035–1045.
101. Stevenson WG, Stevenson LW, Middlekauff HR, et al. Sudden death prevention in patients with advanced ventricular dysfunction. *Circulation.* 1993;88:1953–1961.
102. Keogh AM, Baron DW, Hickie JB. Prognostic guides in patients with idiopathic or ischemic dilated cardiomyopathy assessed for cardiac transplantation. *Am J Cardiol.* 1990;65:903–908.
103. Kron J, Hart M, Schusl-Berke S, et al. Idiopathic dilated cardiomyopathy: role of programmed electrical stimulation and Holter monitoring in predicting those at risk of sudden death. *Chest.* 1988;93:85–90.
104. David S, Zaks JM. Arrhythmias associated with intermittent outpatient dobutamine infusion. *Angiology.* 1986;37:86–91.
105. Garan H, McGovern BA, Canzanello VJ, et al. The effect of potassium ion depletion on postinfarction canine cardiac arrhythmias. *Circulation.* 1988;77:696–704.
106. Roden DM. Drug therapy: risks and benefits of antiarrhythmic therapy. *N Engl J Med.* 1994;331:785–791.
107. Hofmann T, Melnertz T, Kasper W, et al. Mode of death in idiopathic dilated cardiomyopathy: a multivariate analysis of prognostic determinants. *Am Heart J.* 1988;116:1455–1469.

108. Tchou PJ, Krebs AC, Sra J, et al. Syncope: a warning sign in idiopathic dilated cardiomyopathy patients. *J Am Coll Cardiol.* 1991;7(suppl A):196A. Abstract.
109. Franciosa JA, Wilen, M, Ziesche S, et al. Survival in men with severe chronic left ventricular failure due to either coronary heart disease or idiopathic dilated cardiomyopathy. *Am J Cardiol.* 1983;51:831–836.
110. Hinkle LE, Thaler HT. Clinical classification of cardiac deaths. *Circulation.* 1982;65:457–464.
111. Middlekauff H, Stevenson WG, Woo M, et al. Comparison of frequency of late potentials in idiopathic dilated-cardiomyopathy and ischemic cardiomyopathy with advanced heart failure and their usefulness in predicting sudden death. *Am J Cardiol.* 1990;66:1113–1117.
112. Mancini DM, Wong KL, Simson MB. Prognostic value of an abnormal signal-averaged electrocardiogram in patients with nonischemic congestive cardiomyopathy. *Circulation.* 1993;87:1083–1092.
113. Romeo F, Pelliccia F, Cianfrocca C, et al. Predictors of sudden death in idiopathic dilated cardiomyopathy. *Am J Cardiol.* 1989;63:138–140.
114. Constantin L, Martins JR, Kienzle MG, et al. Induced sustained ventricular tachycardia in nonischemic dilated cardiomyopathy: dependence on clinical presentation and response to antiarrhythmic agents. *Pacing Clin Electrophysiol.* 1989;12:776–783.
115. Poll DS, Marchlinski FE, Buxton AE, et al. Usefulness of programmed stimulation in idiopathic dilated cardiomyopathy. *Am J Cardiol.* 1986;587:992–997.
116. Powell AC, Fuchs T, Finkelstein DM, et al. Influence of the implantable cardioverter-defibrillator on the long-term prognosis of survivors of out-of-hospital cardiac arrest. *Circulation.* 1993;88:1083–1092.
117. Akhtar M. Sudden cardiac death: management of high-risk patients. *Ann Intern Med.* 1991;114:499–512.
118. Gossinger HD, Jung M, Wagner L, et al. Prognostic role of inducible ventricular tachycardia in patients with dilated cardiomyopathy and asymptomatic nonsustained ventricular tachycardia. *Int J Cardiol.* 1990;29:215–220.
119. Maron BJ, Epstein SE, Roberts WC. Causes of sudden death in the competitive athlete. *J Am Coll Cardiol.* 1986;7:204–214.
120. Tsung SH, Huang TY, Chang MH. Sudden death in young athletes. *Arch Pathol Lab Med.* 1982;106:168–170.
121. Thiene G, Nava A, Corrado D, et al. Right ventricular cardiomyopathy and sudden death in young people. *N Engl J Med.* 1988;318:129–133.
122. Bharti S, Lev M. Congenital abnormalities of the conduction system in sudden death in young adults. *J Am Coll Cardiol.* 1986;8:1096–1104.
123. Corrado D, Thiene G, Nava A, et al. Sudden death in young competitive athletes: clinicopathologic correlations in 22 cases. *Am J Med.* 1990;898:588–596.
124. Northcote RJ, Ballantyne D. Sudden cardiac death in sport. *Br Med J.* 1983;287:1357–1379.
125. Goodin JC, Farb A, Smialek JE, et al. Right ventricular dysplasia associated with sudden death in young adults. *Mod Pathol.* 1991;4:702–706.

126. Kragel AH, Roberts WC: Anomalous origin of either the right or left main coronary artery from the aorta with subsequent coursing between aorta pulmonary trunk: analysis of 32 necropsy cases. *Am J Cardiol.* 1988;62:771–777.

127. Burke AP, Farb A, Virmani R. Causes of sudden death in athletes. *Cardiol Clin.* 1992;10:303–317.

128. Maron BJ, Roberts WC, McAllister HA, Rosing DR, Epstein SE. Sudden death in young athletes. *Circulation.* 1980;62:218–229.

129. Cheitlin MD, DeCastro CM, McAllister HA. Sudden death as a complication of anomalous left coronary origin from the anterior sinus of Valsalva. *Circulation.* 1974;50:780–787.

130. Roberts WC, Silver MA, Sapala JC. Intussusception of a coronary artery associated with sudden death in a college football player. *Am J Cardiol.* 1986;57:179–180.

131. Waller BF, Hawley DA, Clark MA, et al. Incidence of sudden athletic deaths between 1985 and 1990 in Marion County, Indiana. *Clin Cardiol.* 1992;15:851–858.

132. Marcus FI, Fontaine GH, Guiraudon G, et al. Right ventricular dysplasia: a report of 24 adult cases. *Circulation.* 1992;65:384–398.

133. Roberts WC, McAllister HA, Ferrans VJ: Sarcoidosis of the heart: a clinicopathologic study of 35 necropsy patients (group I) and review of 78 previously described necropsy patients (group II). *Am J Med.* 1977;63:86–108.

134. Moss AJ, Schwartz PJ, Compton RS, et al. The long QT syndrome: prospective longitudinal study of 328 families. *Circulation.* 1991;84:1136.

135. Maron BJ, Poliac LC, Kaplan J, et al. Blunt impact to the chest leading to sudden death from cardiac arrest during sports activities. *N Engl J Med.* 1995;333:337–342.

136. Abrunzo TJ. Commotio cordis: the single, most common cause of traumatic death in youth baseball. *Am J Dis Child.* 1991;145:1279–1282.

137. Klein GJ, Bashore TM, Sellers TD, et al. Ventricular fibrillation in the Wolff-Parkinson-White syndrome. *N Engl J Med.* 1979;301:1080–1085.

138. Waspe LE, Brodman R, Kim SG, et al. Susceptibility to atrial fibrillation and ventricular tachyarrhythmia in the Wolff-Parkinson-White syndrome: role of the accessory pathway. *Am Heart J.* 1986;112:1141–1152.

139. Leitch JW, Klein GJ, Yee R, et al. The prognostic value of electrophysiologic testing in asymptomatic patients with Wolff-Parkinson-White pattern. *Circulation.* 1990;82:1718–1723.

140. Beckman KJ, Gallastegui JL, Bauman JL, et al. The predictive value of electrophysiologic studies in untreated patients with Wolff-Parkinson-White syndrome. *J Am Coll Cardiol.* 1990;15:640–647.

141. Klein GJ, Prystowsky EN, Yee R, et al. Asymptomatic WPW: should we intervene? *Circulation.* 1989;80:1902–1905.

142. Marcus FI, Fontaine G, Guiraudon G, et al. Right ventricular dysplasia: a report of 24 cases. *Circulation.* 1982;65:384–399.

143. Corrado D, Thiene G. Sudden death in children and adolescents without apparent heart disease. *New Trends Arrhythmias.* 1991;7:209–219.

144. Scognamiglio R, Fasoli G, Nava A, et al. Relevance of subtle echocardiographic findings in early diagnosis of the concealed form of right ventricular dysplasia. *Eur Heart J.* 1989;10(suppl D):27–28.

145. Wichter T, Auffermann W, Borggrefe M, et al. Cine magnetic resonance imaging detects impairment of right ventricular diastolic relaxation in arrhythmogenic right ventricular dysplasia. *Pacing Clin Electrophysiol.* 1992;15(pt 2):596. Abstract.

146. Wichter T, Borggrefe M, Haverkamp W, et al. Efficacy of antiarrhythmic drugs in patients with arrhythmogenic right ventricular disease: results in patients with inducible and noninducible ventricular tachycardia. *Circulation.* 1992;86:29–37.

147. Marcus FI, Fontaine G, Frank R, et al. Long term follow-up in patients with arrhythmogenic right ventricular disease. *Eur Heart J.* 1989;10(suppl D):68–73.

148. Metzger J, Rodrigues LM, de Chillou C, et al. Can risk for sudden death and recurrent ventricular tachycardia be predicted in patients with arrhythmogenic right ventricular dysplasia? *Pacing Clin Electrophysiol.* 1993;16(pt 2):883. Abstract.

149. Topol EJ, Traill TA, Fortuin NJ. Hypertensive hypertrophic cardiomyopathy of the elderly. *N Engl J Med.* 1985;312:277–283.

150. Maron BJ, Bonow RO, Cannon RO, et al. Hypertrophic cardiomyopathy: interrelations of clinical manifestations, pathophysiology, and therapy. *N Engl J Med.* 1987;316:780–789, 844–852.

151. McKenna WJ. The natural history of hypertrophic cardiomyopathy, in cardiomyopathies: clinical presentation, differential diagnosis and management. *Cardiovasc Clin.* 1988;4:135–149.

152. McKenna W, Deanfield J, Faruqui A, et al. Prognosis in hypertrophic cardiomyopathy: role of age and clinical electrocardiographic and hemodynamic features. *Am J Cardiol.* 1981;47:532–538.

153. McKenna WJ, Deanfield JE. Hypertrophic cardiomyopathy: an important cause of sudden death. *Arch Dis Child.* 1984;59:971–979.

154. Cannan CR, Reeder GS, Bailey KR, et al. National history of hypertrophic cardiomyopathy. *Circulation.* 1995;92:2488–2495.

155. Fananapazir L, Chang AC, Epstein SE, et al. Prognostic determinants in hypertrophic cardiomyopathy: prospective evaluation of a therapeutic strategy based on clinical, Holter, hemodynamic, and electrophysiologic findings. *Circulation.* 1992;86:467–474.

156. Fananapazir L, Tracy CM, Leon MB, et al. Electrophysiologic abnormalities in patients with hypertrophic cardiomyopathy: a consecutive analysis in 155 patients. *Circulation.* 1989;80:1259–1268.

157. Saumarez RC, Camm AJ, Panagos A, et al. Ventricular fibrillation in hypertrophic cardiomyopathy is associated with increased fractionation of paced right ventricular electrograms. *Circulation.* 1992;86:467–474.

158. McKenna WJ, Sadoul N, Slade AKB, et al. The prognostic significance of nonsustained ventricular tachycardia in hypertrophic cardiomyopathy. *Circulation.* 1994;90:3115–3117.

159. DeRose JJ, Banas JS, Winters SL. Current perspectives on sudden cardiac death in hypertrophic cardiomyopathy. *Prog Cardiovasc Dis.* 1994;36:475–484.

160. Kannel WB, Cobb J. Left ventricular hypertrophy and mortality: results from the Framingham study. *Cardiology.* 1992;812:291–298.

161. Levy D, Anderson KM, Savage DD, et al. Risk of ventricular arrhythmias in left ventricular hypertrophy: the Framingham Heart Study. *Am J Cardiol.* 1987;60:560–565.

162. Gonzalez-Fernandez RA, Rivera M, Rodriguez PJ, et al. Prevalence of ectopic ventricular activity after left ventricular mass regression. *Am J Hypertens.* 1993;6(suppl):308–313.

163. Kannel WB. Prevalence and natural history of electrocardiographic left ventricular hypertrophy. *Am J Med.* 1983;75(suppl 3A):4–11.
164. Koren MJ, Devereux RB, Casale PN, et al. Relation of left ventricular mass and geometry to morbidity and mortality in uncomplicated essential hypertension. *Ann Intern Med.* 1991;114:345–352.
165. Bikkina M, Larson MG, Levy D. Asymptomatic ventricular arrhythmias and mortality risk in subjects with left ventricular hypertrophy. *J Am Coll Cardiol.* 1993;22:1111–1116.
166. Schocken DD, Arrieta MI, Leaverton PE, et al. Prevalence and mortality rate of congestive heart failure in the United States. *J Am Coll Cardiol.* 1991;20:301–306.
167. Greene HL. Clinical significance and management of arrhythmias in heart failure patients. *Clin Cardiol.* 1992;15(suppl I):I-13–I-21.
168. Kannel WB, Plehn JF, Cupples LA. Cardiac failure and sudden death in the Framingham Study. *Am Heart J.* 1988;115:869–874.
169. McKee PA, Castelli WP, McNamara M, et al. The natural history of congestive heart failure: the Framingham Study. *N Engl J Med.* 1971; 285:1141–1146.
170. Podrid PJ, Fogel RI, Fuchs TT. Ventricular arrhythmia in congestive heart failure. *Am J Cardiol.* 1992;69:82G–96G.
171. Castaigne A. Editorial overview. *Am J Cardiol.* 1990;65:39K–40K.
172. Cohn JN, Levine TB, Olivari MT. Plasma norepinephrine as a guide to prognosis in patients with congestive heart failure. *N Engl J Med.* 1984;311:819–823.
173. Middlekauff HM, Stevenson WG, Stevenson LW, et al. Syncope in advanced heart failure: high sudden death risk regardless of syncope etiology. *J Am Coll Cardiol.* 1993;21:110–116.
174. Bolling SF, Deeb GM, Morady F, et al. Automatic internal cardioverter defibrillator: a bridge to heart transplantation. *J Heart Lung Transplant.* 1991;10:562–566.
175. Klein H, Troster J, Haverich A. AICD as a bridge to transplant. *Rev Eur Technol Biomed.* 1990;12:110A. Abstract.
176. Levy D, Anderson KM, Savage DD, et al. Risk of ventricular arrhythmias in left ventricular hypertrophy: the Framingham Heart Study. *Am J Cardiol.* 1987;60:560–565.
177. McLenachan JM, Henderson E, Morris JI, et al. Ventricular arrhythmias in patients with hypersensitive left ventricular hypertrophy. *N Engl J Med.* 1987;317:787–792.
178. Siegel D, Cheitlin MD, Black DM, et al. Risk of ventricular arrhythmias in hypertensive men with left ventricular hypertrophy. *Am J Cardiol.* 1990;65:742–747.
179. James MA, Vann Jones J. Ventricular arrhythmia in untreated newly presenting hypertensive patients compared with a matched normal population. *J Hypertens.* 1989;7:409–415.
180. Ghali JK, Kadakia S, Cooper RS, Liao Y. Impact of left ventricular hypertrophy on ventricular arrhythmias in the absence of coronary artery disease. *J Am Coll Cardiol.* 1991;17:1277–1282.
181. Schmieder RE, Messerli FH. Determinants of ventricular ectopy in hypertensive cardiac hypertrophy. *Am Heart J.* 1992;123:89–95.
182. Keating MT, Dunn C, Atkinson D, et al. Consistent linkage of the long QT syndrome to the Harvey *ras*-1 locus on chromosome 11. *Am J Hum Genet.* 1991;49:1335–1339.

183. Jiang C, Atkinson JA, Towbin JA, et al. Two long QT syndrome loci map to chromosomes 3 and 7 with evidence for further heterogeneity. *Nat Genet.* 1994;8:141–147.
184. Curran ME, Splawski I, Timothy KW, et al. A molecular basis for cardiac arrhythmia: HERG mutations cause long QT syndrome. *Cell.* 1995;80:795–803.
185. Wang Q, Shen J, Splawski I, et al. SCN5A mutations associated with an inherited cardiac arrhythmia, long QT syndrome. *Cell.* 1995;80:805–811.
186. Zareba W, Moss A, LeCessie S, et al. Risk of cardiac events in family members of patients with long QT syndrome. *J Am Coll Cardiol.* 1995;26:1685–1691.
187. Moss A, Zareba W, Benhorin J, et al. ECG T-wave patterns in genetically distinct forms of the hereditary long QT syndrome. *Circulation.* 1995;92:2929–2934.
188. Benhorin J, Hewitt D, Moss A. Relationship between repolarization duration and cycle length during exercise testing in normals and long QT syndrome patients. *J Am Coll Cardiol.* 1991;17:60A. Abstract.
189. Nador F, Beria G, De Ferrari GM, et al. Unsuspected echocardiographic abnormality in the long QT syndrome: diagnosis, prognostic, and pathogenetic implications. *Circulation.* 1991;84:1530.

Chapter 2

Epidemiology of Sudden Cardiac Death:
Emerging Strategies for Risk Assessment and Control

Robert J. Myerburg, MD, Kenneth M. Kessler, MD, and Agustin Castellanos, MD

Sudden cardiac death (SCD), defined as unexpected death that occurs instantaneously or up to a maximum of 1 hour (if witnessed; 24 hours if not) after the onset of an abrupt change in clinical status,[1] accounts for ≈50% of all cardiac deaths.[1-4] This represents at least 250000 SCD events in the United States each year.[4,5] Despite the significant reduction in cardiovascular mortality during the past 20 to 30 years,[1,3,4] due at least in part to public and professional education and attention to control of risk factors for atherosclerosis and coronary artery disease, cardiovascular disease still remains the single largest categorical cause of natural death in the Western hemisphere. Moreover, the proportion of cardiac deaths that are sudden appears to have remained constant at 50%. The majority of SCDs are caused by acute fatal arrhythmias—ventricular tachycardia/ventricular fibrillation (VT/VF)[4]—and thus, to achieve an alteration in cardiovascular death rates attributable to a specific reduction in SCDs, the interactions between preventive epidemiology and the pathophysiology of VT/VF must be developed as a specific scientific and clinical discipline.[6]

The epidemiology of VT/VF and SCD must be explored from multiple perspectives, each of which provides important insights into the problem and no one of which exerts exclusive dominance for preventive strategies. These include (1) population dynamics derived from conventional epidemiological approaches; (2) time dependence

From: Dunbar SB, Ellenbogen KA, Epstein AE, (eds). *Sudden Cardiac Death: Past, Present, and Future.* Armonk, NY: Futura Publishing Company, Inc.; © 1997.

of risk; (3) conditioning risk factors that establish a probability of developing VT/VF when triggering conditions occur; (4) transient risk factors that are dynamic and exert adverse influences on cardiac electrophysiology at a specific point in time; and (5) "response risk," which refers to individual susceptibility to the adverse effects of longitudinal and/or dynamic risk factors. Major inroads into the SCD problem will require better understanding of each of these epidemiological/clinical/electrophysiological interactions. The disciplines range from epidemiology through clinical medicine to membrane channel physiology, genetic determinants, and molecular biology.

Population Dynamics and the Risk of Life-Threatening Arrhythmias

Among the epidemiological studies that provide information on the relative and absolute incidence of SCD, a 26-year follow-up of 5209 men and women in the Framingham, Mass, population who were 30 to 59 years old and free of identified heart disease at baseline observation demonstrated that SCD accounted for 46% of the coronary heart disease deaths among men and 34% among women.[7] The incidence of SCD increased with age, but the proportion of coronary heart disease deaths that were sudden and unexpected was greater in the younger age groups. Pooled data from Albany, NY, and Framingham, Mass, (4120 men) identified SCD as the initial and terminal manifestation of coronary heart disease in more than one half of all sudden death victims.[8] In the Tecumseh, Mich, study of 8641 subjects, 46% of all coronary heart disease deaths occurred within 1 hour of onset of acute symptoms,[9] and in the Yugoslavian cardiovascular disease study, involving 6614 men 35 to 62 years old and free of coronary disease at entry, 75% of all coronary deaths occurred suddenly, and 2 of every 3 victims had had no documented coronary events before death.[10]

When SCD is measured as the absolute number of events annually within defined subpopulations, it becomes evident that the highest-risk clinical subgroups most frequently cited, such as patients with low ejection fractions or a history of heart failure and survivors of out-of-hospital cardiac arrests, do not generate the majority of SCD events.[5] Thus, subgroups with the highest case-fatality rates have the lowest population-attributable risk. In contrast, the larger population subgroups, with much lower case-fatality rates, generate the largest absolute numbers of SCD events because of the size of the population pools from which the events emerge. The magnitude of risk, expressed as incidence, is compared with the total number of events annually under six different conditions in Figure 1. These estimates are based on published epidemiological and clinical data.[4,5,11] When the 300 000 SCDs that occur annually among an unselected adult population in the United States are expressed as a fraction of the total adult population, the overall incidence is 0.1% to 0.2% per year. When the more easily identified high-risk subgroups are removed from this total population base, the calculated incidence for the remaining population decreases and the identification of specific individuals at risk becomes more difficult. On the basis of these estimates, a preventive intervention designed for the general adult population would have to be applied to the 999 in 1000 people who will not have an event during the course of a year to reach and potentially influence the unidentified 1 in 1000 who will. A model of such limited efficiency prohibits the application of many active interventions and highlights the need for

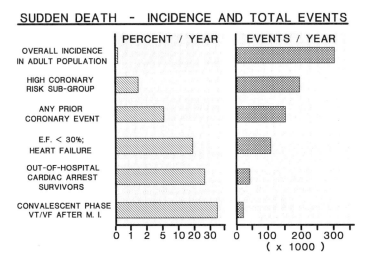

FIGURE 1. *Sudden cardiac deaths among population subgroups. Estimates of incidence (percent per year) and total number of sudden cardiac deaths per year are shown for the overall adult population in the United States and for higher-risk subgroups. The overall estimated incidence is 0.1% to 0.2% per year, totaling more than 300 000 deaths per year. Within subgroups identified by increasingly powerful risk factors, the increasing incidence is accompanied by progressively decreasing total numbers. Practical interventions for the larger subgroups will require identification of higher-risk clusters within the groups. EF indicates ejection fraction; MI, myocardial infarction. The horizontal axis for the incidence figures is nonlinear; see text for details. Reprinted with permission from Reference 19.*

new and specific markers of increased risk that can be applied to large segments of the general population.

The public health relevance of this point lies within the relationship between the size of the denominator in any population pool and the number of events occurring within that subgroup. For example, with escalation from high-coronary-risk subgroups without prior clinical events (risk=1% to 2% per year, see Figure 1) to those with prior coronary events, low ejection fraction, and heart failure or survival after out-of-hospital cardiac arrest, the probability of identifying individuals at higher risk becomes progressively greater, but the absolute number of individuals who can be identified for interventions decreases with each escalation. Thus, the major challenge resides not simply in the need to focus on the highest-risk clinical subgroups but rather to develop methods that will identify high-risk clusters within subgroups that have lower degrees of excess risk. Such strategies will provide better resolution of SCD risk and greater efficiency for preventive and therapeutic interventions. To approach this problem, it is necessary to know the total number of SCDs within a specified population, the fraction of deaths that are sudden, and total mortality. Diagnostic or screening procedures that are easily applied to larger populations and have specific implications for risk of VT/VF to or SCD are needed to resolve these population-based limitations. Examples of current interest are the clinical measures of the variability of autonomic influences on cardiac electrophysiology in groups at increased risk for ventricular tachyarrhythmias (VT/VF) or for SCD, such as the post–myocardial infarction patient[12,13] or the cardiac arrest survivor.[14] In the post–myocardial infarction patient, emerging data suggest that measures of heart rate variability provide information that can be obtained relatively easily on cardiac-autonomic interactions that may influence cardiac electrophysiology.[15,16] Added to other techniques for risk stratification, this is one among a number of evolving approaches that may help resolve higher-risk clusters within larger population bases.

Time Dependence of Risk

The risk of death after surviving a major change in cardiovascular status is not linear over time for most clinical circumstances.[17–20] Survival estimates for both total cardiac mortality and SCD demonstrate that the highest secondary death rates occur during the first 6 to 18 months after an index event. By 18 to 24 months, the slopes of survival curves begin to approach the configuration of those describing a similar population that has remained free of interposed cardiovascular events (Figure 2). The configura-

SURVIVAL AFTER MAJOR CARDIOVASCULAR EVENTS

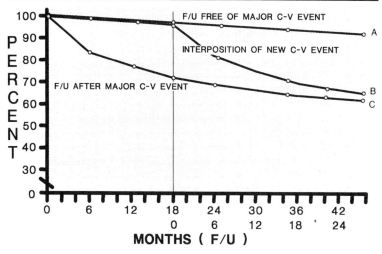

FIGURE 2. *Time dependence of risk after cardiovascular (C-V) events. Survival curves for hypothetical patients with known cardiovascular disease free of a major index event (curve A) and for patients surviving major cardiovascular events (curve C). Attrition is accelerated during the initial 6 to 24 months after the event. Curve B shows the dynamics of risk over time in low-risk patients with an interposed major event that is normalized to a time point (for example, 18 months). The subsequent attrition is accelerated for 6 to 24 months. F/U indicates follow-up. Reprinted with permission from Reference 5.*

tion of survival curves may also be influenced by the magnitude of increased risk after an index event. The data from the Cardiac Arrhythmia Suppression Trial (CAST)[21,22] demonstrate linear survival curves for the placebo population during long-term follow-up, whereas data from the multicenter postinfarction program[17,18] demonstrated that subgrouping post–myocardial infarction patients according to increasing risk on the basis of interactions between premature ventricular contraction (PVC) frequency and ejection fractions resulted in progressively higher risk as the number and power of risk factors increased. The added mortality in the higher-risk subgroups tended to be expressed early. Thus, among the higher-risk subgroups, time-dependent risk provides the greatest opportunity for effective intervention strategies in the early period after conditioning cardiovascular events. Mortality patterns having these characteristics have been observed among survivors of out-of-hospital cardiac arrest,[19] among patients with recent onset of heart failure, and those who have high-risk markers after myocardial infarction.[20] In contrast, data from one of the angiotensin-converting enzyme inhibitor trials (the Survival and Ventricular Enlargement Trial [SAVE]) suggested that benefit on subsequent mortality, as a result of limiting the delayed onset of cardiac enlargement, is expressed late after the index event.[23] Time as a dimension for estimating risk must be integrated into strategies designed for population interventions. Ignoring this characteristic of the clinical epidemiology of VT/VF and SCD may preselect study groups that are composed of lower-risk components. When merged into a population defined by high-risk characteristics, the predicted risk of the population is diluted by the time dynamics. For instance, studies that permit (or favor) the enrollment of patients more than 12 to 18 months after an index event will be characterized by lower-than-predicted event rates if late entrants are heavily represented in the study population. The greater the increase in early mortality related to the index event, the greater is the potential for distortion of event rates caused by late entrants.

Conditioning Risk Factors: The Structural Basis of Risk

In recent years, a distinction between structural preconditions for VT/VF (Figure 3) and acute functional events responsible for the initiation of potentially fatal arrhythmias (Figure 4) has emerged.[24] It is now axiomatic that (1) structural abnormalities provide the cardiac substrate for the genesis of VT/VF and SCD and (2) virtually all structural abnormalities can serve this function. Moreover, new knowledge of the genetic control of ion channel function in cardiac myocytes in patients with congenital long-QT-interval syndrome[25] now defines structural abnormalities at the molecular level.

Coronary atherosclerosis and its major structural consequences, acute and healed myocardial infarction, constitute the most common structural bases of SCD and initially received the greatest attention as structural risk factors. More recently, insights into other structural abnormalities, such as left ventricular hypertrophy and the cardiomyopathies, are emerging. The role of left ventricular hypertrophy as a risk factor for SCD has been recognized in epidemiological studies,[26,27] and clinical associations have been described.[28,29] New information on arrhythmogenic membrane channel and electrophysiological alterations of the hypertrophied myocardium is emerging,[30,31] providing insight into mechanisms by which this structural abnormality may contribute to the genesis of potentially fatal arrhythmias. The fact that regional hypertrophy is common af-

ETIOLOGICAL BASIS OF SUDDEN DEATH RISK

▷ **CORONARY HEART DISEASE**
- Acute ischemic events
- Chronic ischemic heart disease

▷ **CARDIOMYOPATHIES**
- Dilated cardiomyopathies
- Hypertrophic cardiomyopathies

▷ **INFLAMMATION / INFILTRATION**

▷ **SUBTLE, POORLY-DEFINED LESIONS**

▷ **LESIONS OF MOLECULAR STRUCTURE**

▷ **FUNCTIONAL ABNORMALITIES**

▷ **"NORMAL" HEARTS - IDIOPATHIC VF**

FIGURE 3. *Structural preconditions for potentially fatal arrhythmias. Structural heart disease establishes the long-term basis of risk for the best management of potentially fatal arrhythmias. It is the conditioning substrate that allows functional abnormalities to initiate a potentially fatal arrhythmia under specific conditions. Collectively, coronary artery disease and the myopathies account for 90% to 95% of the structural causes of sudden cardiac death in the United States. All of the remaining causes listed (including the absence of known or identifiable structural abnormalities—idiopathic ventricular fibrillation [VF]) account for the remainder. Genetically determined molecular abnormalities at an ion channel level of structure have recently been described as well.*

ter healing of myocardial infarction[32,33] carries further implications for the role of hypertrophy-related electrical disturbances in the generation of life-threatening arrhythmias.

Since coronary heart disease accounts for ≈80% of SCDs in Western societies,[4] most of the major studies of risk factors for SCD have focused on this etiologic category. Data from multiple studies have demonstrated a concordance between risk factors for coronary atherosclerosis, total cardiovascular mortality, and SCD.[1,2,11,34,35] In most studies, ≈50% of all deaths related to coronary heart disease are sudden and unexpected, although proportions of sudden to nonsudden deaths may vary as a function of the severity of left ventricular dysfunction and functional impairment.[36] Among patients

TRANSIENT RISK FACTORS

- ## Ischemia and Reperfusion
  - > Ischemic Ventricular Tachycardia/Fibrillation
  - > Initiation of Monomorphic VT by Ischemia
  - > Reperfusion Arrhythmias

- ## Systemic Inciting Factors
  - > Hemodynamic Dysfunction
  - > Hypoxemia, Acidosis
  - > Electrolyte Imbalance

- ## Neurophysiologic Interactions
  - > Central and Systemic Factors
  - > Local Cardiac Factors - Transmitters/Receptors

- ## Toxic Cardiac Effects
  - > Idiosyncratic Proarrhythmia
  - > Dose-dependent Proarrhythmia
  - > Transient Proarrhythmic Risk

FIGURE 4. *Functional triggering events for cardiac arrest. The four general categories listed encompass most of the functional factors responsible for initiating cardiac arrest. These factors may be responsible for both initiating and maintaining electrophysiological disturbances that interact with structural preconditions. VT indicates ventricular tachycardia.*

having cardiomyopathies, those with better-preserved functional capacity (New York Heart Association functional classes I and II) have lower total death rates, but the fraction of all deaths that are sudden and unexpected is higher; among class IV patients, total death rates are higher, but the fraction that are sudden is lower. There is a competing risk for sudden and nonsudden deaths, which implies, among other things, that the extent to which SCD mortality improvement will influence total mortality may be inherently limited by other mechanisms of death.[6,37,38]

For patients with coronary heart disease, the evolution of the structural abnormalities that condition risk is the physical expression of conventional coronary risk factors. The magnitude of risk relates well to the number of risk factors present. In the Framingham study,[7] there was a 14-fold increase in risk from the lowest-risk decile to the highest-risk decile, and in the Yugoslavian cardiovascular disease study, the probability of SCD was 11 times higher in the top quintile than in the bottom quintile of multivariate risk distribution.[10] Thus, risk factors such as age, family history, sex, cigarette smoking, the hypertension/hypertrophy complex, hyperlipidemias, and the other conventional coronary risk factors provide easily identifiable markers for risk of SCD. These markers are referred to as static because of their potential to be continuously present over time. Their limitation is that they identify primarily the risk of developing the underlying disease responsible for SCD rather than the pathophysiological event responsible for its expression. The ability of conventional risk factors to identify high-risk subgroups in epidemiological terms is unquestioned, and it is likely that for some of these risk factors, active preventive interventions (although difficult to apply) will influence risk and significantly alter the number of events occurring among the population. Because pathophysiological susceptibility does not necessarily equate with structural heart disease risk (see below), the ability of these long-term risk factors to identify specific individuals who will manifest VT/VF or SCD as an expression of the underlying disease is limited. Therefore, although conventional risk factors relate well to the anatomic basis for VT/VF and SCD and provide important preventive opportunities, they lack the specific focus required for efficient preventive strategies in large subgroups and in individual patients.

A higher power of risk prediction is provided by the presence of specific structural cardiac abnormalities. Once established, they constitute the substrate upon which triggering events can initiate unstable cardiac electrophysiological disturbances (Figure 5). The clinical recognition of structural disease defines individual risk much more specifically than do the conventional risk factors. At a different level of resolution, specific myocardial pathways that form the myocardial structural support for VT or VF (ie, potential reentrant circuits) have been well studied. These might provide a much more specific anatomic description of risk, but they lack direct clinical or epidemiological accessibility short of extensive and costly testing techniques.

Transient Risk Factors

When used in reference to the triggering VT/VF or SCD, transient risk indicates a time-limited and unpredictable event or state that has the potential to initiate or allow the initiation of an unstable electrophysiological condition (Figure 6). The term "unstable" is used to indicate an increased probability of transition from a normal or benign cardiac rhythm to a potentially fatal VT or VF. Historically, the relationship between PVCs and the initiation of VT/VF was the first use of the concept. The "PVC hypothesis" evolved as an expression of the premise that PVCs serve a primary triggering function for the initiation of VT/VF and presumed that

SUDDEN CARDIAC DEATH IN CORONARY HEART DISEASE:
Epidemiology / Pathophysiology

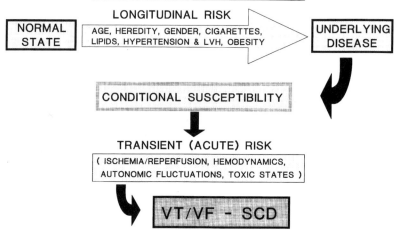

FIGURE 5. *Long-term risk factors versus transient risk. Longitudinal risk refers to those epidemiological risk factors that predict the evolution of the disease states predisposing to the event (ie, the conditioning factors). Transient or acute risk refers to those factors that are directly related to electrophysiological instability at a specific point in time. The latter may also be interpreted in terms of the individual susceptibility to the adverse influences of the transient risk factor. LVH indicates left ventricular hypertrophy; VT/VF, ventricular tachycardia/ventricular fibrillation; and SCD, sudden cardiac death. Reprinted with permission from Myerburg RJ, Kessler KM, Kimura S, Bassett AL, Cox MM, Castellanos A. Life threatening ventricular arrhythmias: the link between epidemiology and pathophysiology. In: Zipes DP, Jalife J, eds.* Cardiac Electrophysiology: From Cell to Bedside. *Philadelphia, Pa: WB Saunders; 1995:723–731.*

PVC suppression would protect against SCD by eliminating the electrophysiological triggers. Despite consistent data supporting chronic PVCs as a risk factor for SCD in patients with underlying heart disease,[17,39–41] special circumstances are required to demonstrate the initiation of life-threatening arrhythmias by PVCs. Ambulatory recordings of the spontaneous onset of cardiac arrest show a tendency to increases in sinus rate and PVC frequency before VF,[42–44] probably reflecting a change in sympathetic tone or hemodynamic status functioning as an intermediary in the PVC-VT/VF relationship. This supports the concept of a role for active transient influences in establishing the pathophysiological conditions for potentially fatal arrhythmias, as opposed to simple fortuitous relationships between chronic PVCs and steady-state

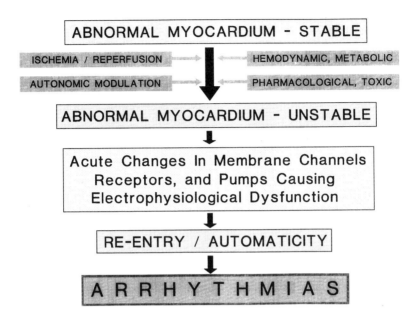

FIGURE 6. *Functional modulations responsible for destabilizing a structurally abnormal heart: an arrhythmic cascade. The abnormal heart has steady-state electrophysiological abnormalities that are stable until modifying influences cause changes that destabilize the myocardium. Acute or subacute changes in membrane channel receptors and pumps then cause electrical dysfunction leading to the genesis of arrhythmias. Reprinted with permission from Reference 61.*

structural abnormalities. Transient pathophysiological changes are proposed to be the factors that convert ventricular myocardium from a stable to an unstable state at a specific time, permitting the genesis of potentially fatal arrhythmias by a definable relationship between acute pathophysiological changes and chronic abnormalities (Figures 5 and 6). After recognizing that the PVC-VT/VF relationship generally required structural conditioning factors, clinical investigators and physiologists began to study the factors that are directly responsible for the initiation of fatal arrhythmias at a specific time. The transient nature of these events makes their prospective elucidation a difficult clinical and epidemiological chore.

The development of a base of experimental information on the role of myocardial ischemia in creating an electrophysiological risk of VT/VF first led to the concept of an initiating or transitional event in which the role of PVCs in the initiation of VT/VF could be defined by a predictable set of circumstances.[45] Subsequently, other functional perturbations received attention. Intense functional changes alone may destabilize this system in the absence of structural abnormalities, but the vast majority of cardiac arrests occur in hearts with preceding structural abnormalities. As shown in Figures 4 and 6, the major functional influences or categories of transient risk factors may be separated into four groups: (1) ischemia and reperfusion; (2) systemic abnormalities; (3) autonomic factors; and (4) cardiotoxic factors, including the general problem of proarrhythmia. Although each of these categories can be viewed as clinical events or pathophysiological influences, they are now starting to be modeled and applied as measurable epidemiological risk factors.[46,47]

Transient Ischemia and Reperfusion

Ischemia occurring at the onset and during the early phase of acute myocardial infarction has a clearly established clinical and experimental association with potentially fatal arrhythmias. However, the majority of SCD victims and survivors of out-of-hospital cardiac arrest do not have acute transmural myocardial infarctions.[48] Approximately 80% of SCDs caused by coronary heart disease are *not* associated with acute myocardial infarction,[49] and it is assumed that transient acute ischemia is one of the major triggering factors. However, its transient nature has precluded systematic clinical and epidemiological studies. Unstable angina pectoris and silent myocardial ischemia also appear to have the capability to initiate potentially fatal arrhythmias,[50-53] although there is only limited clinical documentation of such mechanisms.[54] Both are associated with a statistical increase in the risk of SCD when they accompany preexisting coronary artery disease.

Clinical and epidemiological data indicating associations between ischemia and potentially fatal arrhythmia are paralleled by experimental data that demonstrate adverse effects of ischemia, especially in the presence of a prior myocardial infarction. For example, a study in dogs with healed myocardial infarction was designed to determine the arrhythmogenic effects of graded reductions in blood flow through a non–infarct-related artery. The study demonstrated that smaller decreases in blood flow resulted in inducible VT or spontaneous VF in the presence of a prior myocardial infarction compared with controls without a prior infarction.[55] These and other[45] experimental data are providing insight into mechanisms responsible for ischemia-mediated arrhythmias. Techniques range from intact, in situ hearts to specific membrane channel characteristics studied in isolated myocytes and serve both as explanations for the deranged electrophysiology and as targets for treatment. In addition, the epidemiological impact of left ventricular hypertrophy, especially in the presence of coronary artery disease and prior myocardial infarction, is paralleled by observations of specific channel abnormalities in hypertrophied myocytes, some of which become manifest primarily during ischemia. These observations include differences in ATP-sensitive K^+ channels during ischemia in the hypertrophied myocardium compared with normal myocardium and between endocardium and epicardium in normal hearts,[56] as well as changes in Ca^{2+} and K^+ currents under conditions of metabolic inhibition as a surrogate for ischemia.[57] Thus, some of the epidemiological factors that increase risk of SCD are paralleled by abnormalities at the level of membrane channels, which could serve as an explanation for increased risk. Although the interaction between epidemiology and membrane physiology is only in its infancy, these relationships warrant further exploration.

Transient ischemia enhances susceptibility to sustained ventricular arrhythmias; in addition, the role of subsequent or concomitant reperfusion of ischemic muscle is beginning to be clarified. Reperfusion appears to induce electrical instability by several different mechanisms, both reentrant[57] and triggered activity.[31] The former is characterized by rapid electrical activity, which may be due to abrupt changes in refractoriness,[58] whereas the latter is due to generation of afterdepolarizations, which are experimentally sensitive to Ca^{2+} blockade.[59] Hypertrophied myocytes appear to be more prone to generate reperfusion-induced early afterdepolarizations and triggered activity than are normal myocytes, apparently because of depressed delayed rectifier current (I_K) in the hypertrophied myocyte.[31] In situ studies of the frequency of VF during ischemia and reperfusion in previously hypertrophied hearts supports the potential clinical relevance of such data.[60]

Systemic Factors in Transient Risk

Acute or subacute systemic abnormalities modulate chronic structural cardiac abnormalities, influencing electrophysiological stability and susceptibility to VT/VF and SCD.[61] Among the larger studies of survivors of out-of-hospital cardiac arrest, small subgroups have had recognizable reversible systemic abnormalities that contributed to the life-threatening arrhythmias. When transient systemic factors can be identified and predictably controlled, no other preventive interventions against recurrences are required.[49] Hypoxemia, acidosis, and electrolyte imbalances all may contribute to destabilization;[62–64] these factors are commonly clinically recognized and reversible with appropriate therapy. Clues regarding the mechanisms by which these forms of transient risk may influence electrophysiology are beginning to evolve. For instance, in myocytes from globally hypertrophied hearts, conductance through ATP-sensitive K^+ channels may be increased by a reduction of pH.[65] When a hypertrophied heart becomes regionally ischemic and acidotic, this characteristic may cause dispersion of electrophysiological properties, thereby predisposing to reentrant ventricular arrhythmias. Chronic electrolyte disturbances, most prominently hypokalemia associated with long-term use of diuretics, is associated with an increased risk of cardiovascular mortality.[63] Hypokalemia as a cause or contributor to the initiation of polymorphic VT and torsade de pointes is well recognized,[64,66] most commonly in patients with chronically abnormal hearts and in the presence of class I antiarrhythmic drugs and other proarrhythmic substances.

The most common systemic inciting factor, but one that is difficult to study clinically in a controlled manner, is the role of transient hemodynamic dysfunction in patients with abnormal hearts. Severe acute or subacute hemodynamic deterioration may cause a secondary cardiac arrest, which has long been known to carry a very high short-term mortality rate.[62,67] However, the less well-defined relationship between chronically impaired LV function, acute modulations in hemodynamic status, and predisposition to VT/VF is an important focus for the future. It has been shown experimentally that volume loading of isolated perfused canine left ventricles shortens refractory periods,[68,69] and regional disparity in hearts with prior myocardial infarction has been demonstrated.[69] Stretch-induced modulation of membrane channels may play a role in such changes. Clinical studies to define such mechanisms have been limited to date.

Autonomic Fluctuations and Transient Risk

Systemic, central nervous system, and local cardiac neurophysiological factors are receiving increasing attention as markers for identifying high-risk subgroups and for elucidating mechanisms of fatal arrhythmias.[70] At a local myocardial level, an increasing body of experimental information[70-76] and limited clinical data[12-16,77-80] suggest that prior myocardial infarction and other cardiac abnormalities predisposing to SCD are accompanied by changes in cardiac autonomic function. Several patterns of altered regional responses to sympathetic stimulation have been reported in different myocardial infarction models.[71,72,74] Regionally altered β-adrenergic receptor numbers and changes in coupling proteins and in adenylate cyclase activity have been observed in hearts with healed myocardial infarction.[76] Experimental and clinical imaging studies have also shown disruption of myocardial sympathetic innervation after acute myocardial infarction, with apparent reinnervation after convalescence.[71,73,74,77] Clinically, isoproterenol-dependent induction of sustained VT among cardiac arrest survivors and its prevention by β-adrenergic receptor–blocking drugs[78] suggest a role for autonomic stimuli in the genesis of potentially fatal arrhythmias.

At a systemic level, qualitative and quantitative estimates of neurophysiological alterations that may modulate cardiac activity have been proposed as a means of identifying subgroups at increased risk for SCD. Changes in heart rate variability or baroreceptor sensitivity have been studied in selected subgroups. Among myocardial infarction survivors[12,15] and survivors of out-of-hospital cardiac arrest,[14] altered heart rate variability has been suggested as a marker for SCD risk. Power spectrum analysis of heart rate variability in the frequency domain has suggested specific patterns that identify high-risk subgroups,[15] and short-term frequency-domain patterns differ before the onset of sustained VT compared with nonsustained VT.[16] A blunted baroreceptor response to phenylephrine infusion has also been suggested as a marker to identify subgroups at risk for SCD and VT after myocardial infarction.[13] An association between sinus node rate immediately after the onset of sustained VT and the electrophysiological and hemodynamic stability of the VT has been reported.[80] In patients with stable VT, sinus node rate during ventriculoatrial dissociation increases progressively during the first 30 seconds of VT. When VT is unstable, sinus node rate increases more rapidly during the initial 5 seconds of VT and then decreases abruptly. A role for autonomic dysfunction, as either a cause or a consequence of the arrhythmia pattern, has been suggested. These diverse observations provide strong arguments for abnormal patterns of autonomic function as a controlling factor in risk of VT/VF and SCD.

Effects of Toxic Substances on the Heart

The risk of VF during chloroform anesthesia was the first recognized relationship between a clinically used substance and potentially fatal arrhythmias.[81,82] Subsequently, relationships between antiarrhythmic drugs and proarrhythmic events, initially described in terms of the risk of torsade de pointes and VF during quinidine therapy,[83] identified a specific clinical circumstance in the ambulatory setting. It is now recognized that classic proarrhythmic responses of this type may occur with any of the class I-A antiarrhythmic drugs as well as the class III drugs. More subtle but possibly quite important is the emerging number of clinically used substances that are not used as antiarrhythmic drugs but are recognized to have induced similar proarrhythmic responses. These include such diverse categories of medications as erythromycin, pentamidine, a number of the psychotropic drugs, and terfenadine.[84] In addition, limited clinical data suggest an effect on QT interval and the risk of torsade de pointes in the susceptible individual for such diverse other substances as organic phosphate insecticides, cocaine,[85] and probucol.[86] For many of these substances, limited data at this time suggest that the offending substances prolong QT intervals by an effect on repolarizing currents, such as the delayed rectifier current, I_K (I_{KR}).[84,85] The combination of an inherent ability of a substance to prolong action potential duration and specific patterns of individual susceptibility to this effect may explain the sporadic occurrence of these responses. It follows that identification of an offending channel effect coupled with an ability to identify individual susceptibility might provide a method to identify risk prospectively. Unfortunately, since such events are more common in patients with underlying heart disease, the distinction between a proarrhythmic response and a confounding clinical arrhythmia caused by the underlying disease is difficult at the present time.

Response Variables: Identification of the Susceptible Individual

The concept of response risk is an attempt to introduce principles of epidemiology to the disciplines of cardiac electrophysiology and myocardial cell membrane function. It refers to the mechanism by which a specific individual who has a conditioning risk factor is susceptible to arrhythmogenesis when exposed to a transient functional risk influence. Based on the premises that the conditioning factors create a persistent substrate for arrhythmic risk and the transient functional factors serve an initiating role (see Figure 6), the epidemiological question focuses on the identification of those subjects whose inherent physiological characteristics make the initiation of electrophysiological instability more likely when these conditions are met. It requires clinically identifiable, genetically based or acquired individual differences in the responses of membrane channels, receptors, exchangers, and pumps in the susceptible individual. That such conditions exist in nature has been shown clinically in the long-QT-interval syndrome[25] and in the biological model of the *Drosophila* mutant that develops leg shaking when exposed to ether or environmental changes.[87] Specific membrane channel defects have been identified, one being an abnormal I_{KA} channel that is genetically determined to function abnormally on exposure to the inciting factor,[88] thereby identifying a population subgroup at risk for the abnormal response. Other variations have I_{Na} abnormalities.[87] Abnormalities of both potassium (I_{KR}) and sodium (I_{Na}) channels have been identified in genetic variants of long-QT-interval syndromes in humans.[25] A parallel concept not yet worked out genetically is the clinical model of "idiosyncratic" proarrhythmic responses to class I-A antiarrhythmic drugs, which is expressed as excessive prolongation of repolarization and generation of torsade de pointes. This response occurs in the 1% to 3% of the exposed population that appears to have the specific susceptibility. Exaggerated depression of I_{KR} may create individual susceptibility on exposure,[89] whereas the arrhythmia itself appears to be electrophysiologically mediated by $I_{Ca,L}$.[90] The ability to identify abnormal response characteristics of specific channels or receptors under a variety of pathophysiological conditions holds the promise of identifying individuals at risk for potentially fatal arrhythmias under conditions of specific substance exposures. This extends beyond proarrhythmic effects of antiarrhythmic drugs to include factors such as the response of specific channels to ischemia and reperfusion[30,89,90] and the response of previously conditioned hearts to other stimuli in the environment (eg, cocaine) that can influence specific ion channel function.[85]

In summary, therefore, the ability to identify specific individuals at risk for responding abnormally to a specific transient stimulus will provide increasing power for epidemiological approaches and yield greater resolution of risk within large population groups.

Summary and Conclusions

Classic epidemiology has provided a great deal of useful information regarding the risk of life-threatening ventricular arrhythmias and sudden cardiac death and possible approaches to their prevention. The additional emphasis on specific subgroup characteristics, the relationship between absolute numbers and relative risk, and the temporal modulation of risk all add power to available epidemiological information. Continued resolution of the problems of VT/VF and SCD and their control will require an interaction with other disciplines, both clinical and basic. Further study of clinical and experimental electrophysiology and acquisition of more information on membrane function in disease states are needed for better identification of individuals at risk.

References

1. *Report of the Working Group on Arteriosclerosis of the National Heart, Lung, and Blood Institute (Volume 2): Patient Oriented Research - Fundamental and Applied, Sudden Cardiac Death.* Washington, DC: US Dept of Health, Education, and Welfare publication NIH 83-2035;1981:114–122.
2. Epstein FH, Pisa Z. International comparisons in ischemic heart disease mortality. *Proceedings of the Conference on the Decline in Coronary Heart Disease Mortality.* Washington, DC: US Dept of Health, Education, and Welfare publication NIH 79-1610. US Government Printing Office. 1979:58–88.
3. Gillum RF. Sudden coronary deaths in the United States, 1980–1985. *Circulation.* 1989;79:756–765.
4. Myerburg RJ, Castellanos A. Cardiac arrest and sudden cardiac death. In: Braunwald E, ed. *Heart Disease: A Textbook of Cardiovascular Medicine.* 4th ed. Philadelphia, Pa: WB Saunders Publishing Co; 1992: chap 26.
5 Myerburg RJ, Kessler KM, Castellanos A. Sudden cardiac death: structure, function, and time-dependence of risk. *Circulation.* 1992;85(suppl I):I-2–I-10.
6. Myerburg RJ, Kessler KM, Castellanos A. Epidemiology of sudden cardiac death: population characteristics, conditioning risk factors, and dynamic risk factors. In: Spooner PM, Brown AM, Catterall WA, Kaczorowski GJ, Strauss HC, eds. *Ion Channels in the Cardiovascular System.* Armonk, NY: Futura Publishing Co; 1994:15–33.
7. Kannel WB, Thomas HE. Sudden coronary death: the Framingham study. *Ann NY Acad Sci.* 1982;382:3–21.
8. Doyle JT, Kannel WB, McNamara RM, Quikenton R, Gordon T. Factors related to suddenness of death from coronary heart disease: combined Albany-Framingham studies. *Am J Cardiol.* 1976;37:1073–1078.
9. Chiang BN, Perlman LV, Fulton M, Ostrander LD, Epstein FH. Predisposing factors in sudden cardiac death in Tecumseh, Michigan: a prospective study. *Circulation.* 1970;41:31–37.
10. Demirovic J. *Risk Factors in the Incidence of Sudden Cardiac Death and Possibilities for its Prevention.* Belgrade, Yugoslavia: University of Belgrade Press; 1985. Thesis.
11. Myerburg RJ, Demirovic J. Epidemiologic considerations in cardiac arrest and sudden cardiac death: etiology and prehospital and posthospital outcomes. In: Podrid RJ, Kowey PR, eds. *Cardiac Arrhythmia: Mechanisms, Diagnosis, and Management.* Baltimore, Md: Williams & Wilkins; 1995: chap. 44.
12. Kleiger RE, Miller JP, Bigger JT, Moss AJ, and the Multicenter Post-Infarction Research Group. Decreased heart rate variability and its association with increased mortality after acute myocardial infarction. *Am J Cardiol.* 1987;59:256–262.

13. Le Rovere MT, Specchia G, Mortara A, Schwartz PJ. Baroreflex sensitivity, clinical correlates and cardiovascular mortality among patients with first myocardial infarction: a prospective study. *Circulation.* 1988;78:816–824.

14. Huikuri HV, Linnaluoto MK, Seppanen T, et al. Heart rate variability and its circadian rhythm in survivors of cardiac arrest. *Am J Cardiol.* 1992;70:610–615.

15. Bigger JT, Fleiss JL, Steinman RC, Rolnitzky LM, Kleiger RE, Rottman JN. Frequency domain measures of heart period variability and mortality after myocardial infarction. *Circulation.* 1992;85:164–171.

16. Huikuri HV, Valkama JO, Airaksinen KEJ, et al. Frequency domain measures of heart rate variability before the onset of nonsustained and sustained ventricular tachycardia in patients with coronary artery disease. *Circulation.* 1993;87:1220–1228.

17. Bigger JT, Fleiss JL, Kleiger R, Miller JP, Rolnitzky LM, and the Multicenter Post-Infarction Research Group. The relationships among ventricular arrhythmias, left ventricular dysfunction, and mortality in the 2 years after myocardial infarction. *Circulation.* 1984;69:250–258.

18. Bigger JT. Antiarrhythmic therapy: an overview after myocardial infarction. *Am J Cardiol.* 1984;53:8B–16B.

19. Furukawa T, Rozanski JJ, Nogami A, Moroe K, Gosselin AJ, Lister JW. Time-dependent risk of and predictors for cardiac arrest recurrence in survivors of out-of-hospital cardiac arrest with chronic coronary artery disease. *Circulation.* 1989;80:599–608.

20. Schechtman KB, Bipone RJ, Kleiger RE, et al, and the Diltiazem Reinfarction Study Research Group. Risk stratification of patients with non-Q wave myocardial infarction. *Circulation.* 1989;80:1148–1158.

21. Echt DS, Liebson PR, Mitchell B, et al, and the CAST Investigators. Mortality and morbidity in patients receiving encainide, flecainide, or placebo: the Cardiac Arrhythmia Suppression Trial. *N Engl J Med.* 1991;324:781–788.

22. The Cardiac Arrhythmia Suppression Trial II Investigators. Effect of the antiarrhythmic agent moricizine on survival after myocardial infarctions. *New Engl J Med.* 1992;327:227–33.

23. Pfeffer MA, Braunwald E, Moye LA, et al, and the SAVE Investigators. The effect of captopril on mortality and morbidity in patients with left ventricular dysfunction after myocardial infarction: results of the Survival and Ventricular Enlargement trial. *N Engl J Med.* 1992;327:669–677.

24. Myerburg RJ, Kessler KM, Bassett AL, Castellanos A. A biological approach to sudden cardiac death: structure, function and cause. *Am J Cardiol.* 1989;63:1512–1516.

25. Roden DM, George AL, Bennett PB. Recent advances in understanding the molecular mechanisms of the long QT syndrome. *J Cardiol Electrophysiol.* 1995;6:1023–1031.

26. Kannel WB, Thomas HE. Sudden coronary death: the Framingham Study. *Ann NY Acad Sci.* 1982;38:3–21.

27. Cupples LA, Gagnon DR, Kannel WB. Long- and short-term risk of sudden coronary death. *Circulation.* 1992;85(suppl I):I-11–I-18.

28. Anderson KP. Sudden death, hypertension, and hypertrophy. *J Cardiovasc Pharmacol.* 1984;6(suppl III):S498–S503.

29. Messerli FH, Ventura HO, Elizardi DJ, Dunn FG, Frohlich ED. Hyper-

tension and sudden death: increased ventricular ectopic activity in left ventricular hypertrophy. *Am J Med.* 1984;77:18–22.

30. Furukawa T, Myerburg RJ, Furukawa N, Kimura S, Bassett AL. Ionic mechanism of increased susceptibility of hypertrophied feline myocytes to metabolic inhibition. *Circulation.* 1990;82(suppl III):III-522. Abstract.

31. Furukawa T, Bassett AL, Kimura S, Furukawa N, Myerburg RJ. The ionic mechanism of reperfusion-induced early after depolarizations in feline left ventricular hypertrophy. *J Clin Invest.* 1993;91:1521–1531.

32. Ginzton LE, Conant R, Rodrigues DM, Laks MM. Functional significance of hypertrophy of the non-infarcted myocardium after myocardial infarction in humans. *Circulation.* 1989;80:816–822.

33. Cox MM, Berman I, Myerburg RJ, Smets MJD, Kozlovskis PL. Morphometric mapping of regional myocyte diameters after healing of myocardial infarction in cats. *J Mol Cell Cardiol.* 1991;23:127–135.

34. Kannel WB, Doyle JT, McNamara PM, Quickenton P, Gordon T. Precursors of sudden coronary death: factors related to the incidence of sudden death. *Circulation.* 1979;51:606–613.

35. Kuller LH. Sudden death: definition and epidemiologic considerations. *Prog Cardiovasc Dis.* 1980;23:1–12.

36. Kjekshus J. Arrhythmias and mortality in congestive heart failure. *Am J Cardiol.* 1990;65:42-I–48-I.

37. Myerburg RJ, Kessler KM, Kimura S, Castellanos A. Sudden cardiac death: future approaches based on identification and control of transient risk factors. *J Cardiovasc Electrophysiol.* 1992;3:626–640.

38. Myerburg RJ, Castellanos A. Evolution, evaluation, and efficacy of implantable defibrillator technology. *Circulation.* 1992;86:691–693.

39. Vismara LA, Amsterdam BA, Mason DT. Relation of ventricular arrhythmias in the late-hospital phase of acute myocardial infarction to sudden death after hospital discharge. *Am J Med.* 1975;59:6–12.

40. Ruberman W, Weinblatt M, Goldberg JD, Frank CW, Chaudhary BS, Shapiro S. Ventricular premature complexes and sudden death after myocardial infarction. *Circulation.* 1981;64:297–305.

41. Schulze RA, Strauss HW, Pitt B. Sudden death in the year following myocardial infarction: relationship of ventricular premature contractions in the late hospital phase and left ventricular ejection fraction. *Am J Med.* 1977;62:192–199.

42. Nikolic G, Bishop RL, Singh JB. Sudden death recorded during Holter monitoring. *Circulation.* 1984;66:218–225.

43. Myerburg RJ, Kessler KM, Luceri RM, et al. Classification of ventricular arrhythmias based on parallel hierarchies of frequency and form. *Am J Cardiol.* 1984;54:1355–1358.

44. Leclercq JF, Coumel PH, Maisonblanche P, et al. Mise en évidence des mécanismes indéterminants de la morte subite: enquête cooperative portant sur 69 cas enregistrés par la méthode de Holter. *Arch Mal Coeur.* 1986;79:1024–1036.

45. Rosen MR, Janse MJ, Myerburg RJ. Arrhythmias induced by coronary artery occlusion: what are the electrophysiologic mechanisms? In: Hearse D, Manning A, Janse M, eds. *Life-Threatening Arrhythmias During Ischemia and Infarction.* New York, NY: Raven Press; 1987:chap 2.

46. Muller JE, Tofler GH, Stone PH. Circadian variation and triggers of onset of acute cardiovascular disease. *Circulation.* 1989;79:733–743.

47. Maclure M. The case-crossover design: a method for studying transient effects on the risk of acute events. *Am J Epidemiol.* 1991;133:144–153.

48. Baum RS, Alvarez H, Cobb LA. Survival after resuscitation from out-of-hospital ventricular fibrillation. *Circulation.* 1974;50:1231–1235.
49. Myerburg RJ, Kessler KM, Zaman L, Conde CA, Castellanos A. Survivors of prehospital cardiac arrest. *JAMA.* 1982;247:1485–1490.
50. Gottlieb SO, Weisfeldt MI, Ouyang P, Mellits ED, Gerstenblith G. Silent ischemia as a marker for early unfavorable outcomes in patients with unstable angina. *N Engl J Med.* 1986;314:1214.
51. Weintraub RM, Aroesty JM, Paulin S, et al. Medically refractory unstable angina pectoris, I: long-term follow-up of patients undergoing intra-aortic balloon counterpulsation and operation. *Am J Cardiol.* 1979;43:877.
52. Mulcahy R, Awadhi AHA, deBuitieor M, Tobin G, Johnson H, Contoy R. Natural history and prognosis of unstable angina. *Am Heart J.* 1985;109:753.
53. Nademanee K, Intarachot V, Josephson MA, Rieders D, Mody FV, Singh BN. Prognostic significance of silent myocardial ischemia in patients with unstable angina. *J Am Coll Cardiol.* 1987;1:1–9.
54. Myerburg RJ, Kessler KM, Mallon SM, et al. Potentially fatal arrhythmias in patients with silent myocardial ischemia due to coronary artery spasm. *N Engl J Med.* 1992;326:1451–1455.
55. Furukawa T, Moroe K, Mayrovitz HN, Sampsell R, Myerburg RJ. Arrhythmogenic effects of graded coronary blood flow reduction superimposed upon prior myocardial infarction in dogs. *Circulation.* 1991;84:368–377.
56. Furukawa T, Kimura S, Furukawa N, Bassett AL, Myerburg RJ. Role of cardiac ATP-regulated potassium channels in differential responses of endocardial and epicardial cells to ischemia. *Circ Res.* 1991;68: 1693–1702.
57. Coronel R, Wilms-Schopman FJG, Opthof T, Cinca J, Fiolet JWT, Janse MJ. Reperfusion arrhythmias in isolated perfused pig hearts: inhomogeneities in extracellular potassium, ST and TQ potentials, and transmembrane action potentials. *Circ Res.*1992;71:1131–1142.
58. Ideker RE, Klein GJ, Harrison L, et al. The transition to ventricular fibrillation induced by reperfusion after ischemia in the dog: a period of organized epicardial activation. *Circulation.* 1981;63:1371–1379.
59. Priori SG, Mantica M, Napolitano C, Schwartz PJ. Early afterdepolarization induced in vivo by reperfusion of ischemic myocardium. *Circulation.* 1990;81:1911–1920.
60. Koyha T, Kimura S, Myerburg RJ, Bassett AL. Susceptibility of hypertrophied rat hearts to ventricular fibrillation during acute ischemia. *J Mol Cell Cardiol.* 1988;20:159–168.
61. Myerburg RJ, Kessler KM, Castellanos A. Pathophysiology of sudden cardiac death. *Pacing Clin Electrophysiol.* 1991;14(pt 2):935–943.
62. Packer M. Sudden unexpected death in patients with congestive heart failure: a second frontier. *Circulation.* 1985;72:681–685.
63. Multiple Risk Factor Intervention Trial Research Group: Multiple-risk factor intervention trial: risk factor changes in mortality results. *JAMA.* 1982;248:1465–1477.
64. Gettes LS. Electrolyte abnormalities underlying lethal ventricular arrhythmias. *Circulation.* 1992;85(suppl I):I-70–I-76.
65. Kimura S, Bassett AL, Xi H, Tomita F, Myerburg RJ. Characteristics of ATP-sensitive K$^+$ channels in hypertrophied cells: effects of pH. *Circulation.* 1992;86(suppl I):I-92. Abstract.
66. Jackman WM, Friday KJ, Anderson JL, Aliot EM, Clark M, Lazzara

R. The long QT syndrome: a critical review, new clinical observations, and a unifying hypothesis. *Prog Cardiovasc Dis.* 1988;32: 115–172.

67. Robinson JS, Sloman G, Mathew TH, Goble AJ. Survival after resuscitation from cardiac arrest in acute myocardial infarction. *Am Heart J.* 1965;69:740–747.

68. Lab MJ. Contraction-excitation feedback in myocardium: physiologic basis and clinical relevance. *Circ Res.* 1982;50:757–766.

69. Calkins H, Maughan WL, Weissman HF, Sugiura S, Sagawa K, Levine JH. Effect of acute volume load on refractoriness and arrhythmia development in isolated chronically infarcted canine hearts. *Circulation.* 1989;79:687–697.

70. Schwartz PJ, La Rovere T, Vanoli E. Autonomic nervous system and sudden cardiac death: experimental basis and clinical observations for post–myocardial infarction risk stratification. *Circulation.* 1992; 85(suppl I):1-77–I-91.

71. Barber MJ, Mueller TM, Henry DF, Felton SJ, Zipes DP. Transmural myocardial infarction in the dog produces sympathectomy in noninfarcted myocardium. *Circulation.* 1982;67:787–796.

72. Gaide MS, Myerburg RJ, Kozlovskis PL, Bassett AL. Elevated sympathetic response of epicardium proximal to healed myocardial infarction. *Am J Physiol.* 1983;14:646–652.

73. Schwartz PJ, Billman GE, Stone HL. Autonomic mechanisms in ventricular fibrillation induced by myocardial ischemia during exercise in dogs with a healed myocardial infarction: an experimental preparation for sudden cardiac death. *Circulation.* 1984;69:780–790.

74. Kammerling JJ, Green FJ, Watanabe AM, et al. Denervation supersensitivity of refractoriness in non-infarcted areas apical to transmural myocardial infarction. *Circulation.* 1987;76:383–393.

75. Schwartz PJ, Vanoli E, Stramba-Badiale M, De Ferrari GM, Billman GE, Foreman RD. Autonomic mechanisms and sudden death: new insights from analysis of baroreceptor reflexes in conscious dogs with and without a myocardial infarction. *Circulation.* 1988;78:969–979.

76. Kozlovskis PL, Smets MJD, Duncan RC, Bailey BK, Bassett AL, Myerburg RJ. Regional beta-adrenergic receptors and adenylate cyclase activity after healing of myocardial infarction in cats. *J Mol Cell Cardiol.* 1990;22:311–322.

77. Tull M, Minardo J, Mock BH, et al. SPECT with high purity 1-123-MIBG after transmural myocardial infarction (TMI), demonstrating sympathetic denervation followed by reinnervation in a dog model. *J Nucl Med.* 1987;28:669.

78. Interian A, Fernandez P, Robinson E, et al. Long-term effect of propranolol in ventricular tachycardia/fibrillation patients with isoproterenol-dependent inducibility. *Circulation.* 1990;82(suppl III):435.

79. Huikuri HV, Cox M, Interian A Jr, Kessler KM, Castellanos A, Myerburg RJ. Efficacy of intravenous propranolol for suppression of inducibility of ventricular tachyarrhythmias with different electrophysiologic characteristics in coronary artery disease. *Am J Cardiol.* 1989;64:1305–1309.

80. Huikuri HV, Zaman L, Castellanos A, et al. Changes in spontaneous sinus node rate as an estimate of cardiac autonomic tone during stable and unstable ventricular tachycardia. *J Am Coll Cardiol.* 1989;13:646–652.

81. Hill IGW. Human heart in anaesthesia: electrocardiographic study. *Edinburgh Med J.* 1932;39:533–553.

82. Hill IGW. Cardiac irregularities during chloroform anaesthesia. *Lancet.* 1932;1:1139–1142.

83. Selzer A, Wray HW. Quinidine syncope: paroxysmal ventricular fibrillation occurring during treatment of chronic atrial arrhythmias. *Circulation.* 1964;30:17.

84. Woosley RL, Chen Y, Freiman JP, Gillis RA. Mechanism of cardiotoxic actions of terfenadine. *JAMA.* 1993;269:1532–1536.

85. Kimura S, Bassett AL, Xi H, Myerburg RJ. Early afterdepolarizations and triggered activity induced by cocaine: a possible mechanism of cocaine arrhythmogenesis. *Circulation.* 1992;85:2227–2235.

86. Gohn DC, Simmons TW. Polymorphic ventricular tachycardia (*torsades de pointes*) associated with the use of probucol. *N Engl J Med.* 1992;326:1435–1436.

87. Tanouye MA, Kamb CA, Iverson LE, Salkoff L. Genetic and molecular biology of ion channels in *Drosophila. Ann Rev Neurosci.* 1986;9: 255–276.

88. Iverson LE, Tanouye MA, Lester HA, Davidson N, Rudy B. A-type potassium channels expressed from Shaker locus cDNA. *Proc Natl Acad Sci USA.* 1988;85:5723–5727.

89. Roden DM, Bennett PB, Snyders DJ, Balser JR, Hondeghem LM. Quinidine delays I_k activation in guinea pig ventricular myocytes. *Circ Res.* 1988;62:1055–1058.

90. January CR, Riddle JM. Early afterdepolarizations: mechanisms of induction and block: a role for L-type Ca^{++} current. *Circ Res.* 1989; 64:977–990.

Chapter 3

Substrate-Trigger Interactions:
Role of Ventricular Repolarization

Steffen Behrens, MD, and
Michael R. Franz, MD, PhD

Sudden cardiac death is a leading cause of death in the United States, killing more than 300 000 people annually.[1] Most of these deaths are related to ventricular tachyarrhythmias.[2] Great effort is currently being made to identify patients at risk for sudden cardiac death, because new therapeutic options for high-risk patients have become available, such as the implantable cardioverter-defibrillator.[3] The detection of repolarization abnormalities as a potential risk factor for malignant tachyarrhythmias and sudden cardiac death has led to an increased interest in patients with various cardiac diseases.[4–7] Specifically, an increased dispersion of ventricular repolarization is believed to play an important role in the genesis of ventricular arrhythmias.[8–11] Dispersion of ventricular repolarization is defined as decreased synchronicity of ventricular repolarization (and refractoriness, because myocardial excitability usually follows the time course of repolarization[12]). Mapping studies have shown that desynchronized distribution of refractoriness facilitates the initiation of reentrant circuits within the myocardium by allowing areas of prolonged excitation to spread into areas repolarized prematurely.[13–15] Synchronized repolarization may therefore prevent reentry of activation wavefronts, whereas desynchronized repolarization (ie, increased dispersion of repolarization) may promote the occurrence of reentrant arrhythmias.

In the experimental setting, dispersion of repolarization has been determined from monophasic action potentials (MAPs) recorded from multiple sites in the ventricles.[9,16–20] In the clinical setting, body surface potential mapping[21–23] and the assessment of

From: Dunbar SB, Ellenbogen KA, Epstein AE, (eds). *Sudden Cardiac Death: Past, Present, and Future.* Armonk, NY: Futura Publishing Company, Inc.; © 1997.

QT dispersion from the 12-lead standard electrocardiogram (ECG)[10,11] have been proposed as measurements of dispersion of ventricular repolarization.

QT Dispersion

The QT dispersion is a simple and noninvasive ECG index widely used in patients as a measure of dispersion of ventricular repolarization and a potential predictor of ventricular tachyarrhythmias.[10] It is usually determined as the range between the longest and shortest QT intervals from the 12 leads of the surface ECG ($QT_{max} - QT_{min}$).[24]

QT dispersion has been studied in normal subjects[25] and in patients with coronary artery disease,[26–29] chronic heart failure,[30] left ventricular hypertrophy,[4,30] and the long-QT syndrome.[31–33] QT dispersion measurements have also been used to assess proarrhythmic and antiarrhythmic effects of antiarrhythmic drug therapy.[10,11,32–34] Hii et al[11] compared the effects of class Ia antiarrhythmic drugs and amiodarone on the QT dispersion in 38 patients, most of them (97%) with coronary artery disease. Nine of these patients had developed torsade de pointes (polymorphic ventricular tachycardia) during class Ia drug administration but not during subsequent amiodarone therapy. Figure 1 shows the effect on the mean QT interval and QT dispersion in patients with and without proarrhythmic class Ia drug effects. The data indicate that an increase in QT dispersion during class Ia drug therapy is associated with torsade de pointes and that chronic amiodarone therapy does not increase dispersion in these patients despite a comparable prolongation of the maximum QT interval. This suggests that antiarrhythmic drugs may prolong ventricular repolarization in both a homogeneous and nonhomogeneous fashion and that a nonhomogeneous repolarization prolongation may be associated with proarrhythmic effects. Cui et al,[34] who studied the effects of different class III antiarrhythmic drugs on repolarization dispersion, reported a significant decrease in QT dispersion only in those patients treated with amiodarone (Figure 2). Interestingly, amiodarone decreased QT dispersion in all patients with a history of myocardial infarction (in whom baseline QT dispersion was significantly greater than in patients without previous myocardial infarction), whereas sematilide and sotalol had various effects in these patients. QT dispersion has also been shown to be a useful tool to predict efficacy of antiadrenergic therapy in patients with long-QT syndrome.[32,33] For a cutoff value in QT dispersion of 100 ms, there is an 80% sensitivity

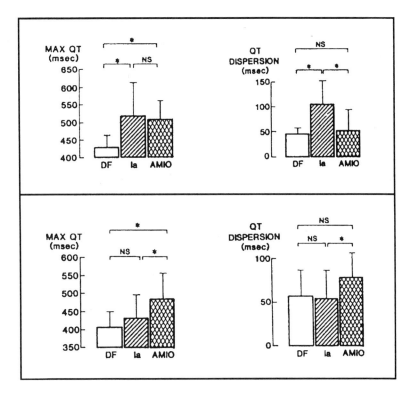

FIGURE 1. *Top, QT intervals and QT dispersion in patients who developed class Ia drug–induced proarrhythmic effects. Bottom, QT intervals and QT dispersion in patients without drug-induced proarrhythmic effects. DF indicates antiarrhythmic drug-free state (control); Ia, during class Ia drug administration; and AMIO, during chronic amiodarone treatment. *P <.05; NS, not statistically significant. Reprinted with permission from Reference 11.*

and 82% specificity in discriminating between patients with long-QT syndrome who are responders versus those who are nonresponders to β-blocker therapy.[32] There are also exercise-related effects on QT dispersion.[33] Zhao et al[33] demonstrated that during bicycle exercise, QT dispersion decreases in normal subjects but increases in patients with the long-QT syndrome (Figure 3). After β-blockade, there is an exercise-induced decrease of QT dispersion in both normal subjects and patients with the long-QT syndrome, indicating that the effects of exercise on QT dispersion might be a useful marker of therapeutic efficacy in these patients.

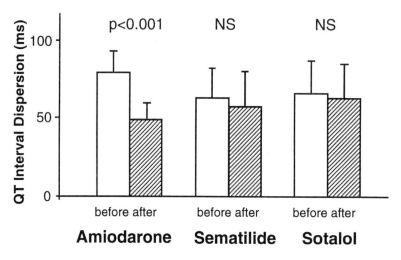

FIGURE 2. *QT dispersion in patients before and after different class III antiarrhythmic drugs. Reprinted with permission from Reference 34.*

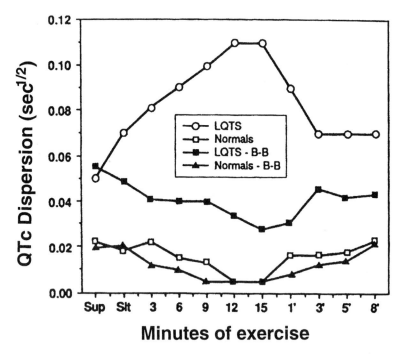

FIGURE 3. *Effect of exercise on the QT dispersion in normal subjects and in patients with long-QT syndrome (LQTS) before and after β-blocker therapy (B-B). Reprinted with permission from Reference 33.*

Although these data suggest that QT dispersion could be an important tool for risk stratification and monitoring of effects of antiarrhythmic therapy, a significant role for the method in clinical practice has yet not been established. There are methodological problems with manual QT dispersion measurements,[35] and a standardization of the method is still lacking.[36] Other important and more general questions are whether the 12-lead surface ECG allows the clinician to accurately and reliably assess the dispersion of ventricular repolarization and whether and how dispersion of ventricular repolarization is related to ventricular arrhythmia vulnerability.

We addressed these questions in a novel intact rabbit heart model in which we were able to simultaneously determine dispersion parameters from both a volume-conducted 12-lead ECG and multiple endocardial and epicardial MAP recordings. Electrical field stimuli were delivered as a tool to comprehensively describe ventricular arrhythmia vulnerability as an "area" of vulnerability (AOV). We then directly assessed the role of ventricular repolarization and its dispersion for ventricular arrhythmia vulnerability.

Validation of ECG Indexes of Dispersion of Ventricular Repolarization

For the widespread use of QT dispersion as a predictor of arrhythmias, it is important to know whether QT dispersion and other ECG indexes are appropriate and valid as a measure of dispersion of ventricular repolarization. This question was studied in isolated Langendorff-perfused rabbit hearts that were immersed into a tissue bath approximating the size of a rabbit thorax[20] (Figure 4). A 12-lead volume-conducted ECG (Figure 5) was recorded by means of silver-silver chloride electrodes positioned at the walls of the tissue bath in an approximate Einthoven and Wilson configuration. QT dispersion was defined as the maximal range of QT intervals ($QT_{max} - QT_{min}$). In addition, the T_{peak}-to-T_{end} interval (a measure of T-wave width) and the area under the curve between the J-point and T_{end} (total T-wave area) were determined as new ECG indexes of repolarization dispersion. Ventricular repolarization was measured directly at multiple widely spaced epicardial and endocardial sites of both ventricles by use of MAP recordings (two epicardial MAPs are shown in Figure 4). Dispersion of ventricular repolarization was defined as the range between the shortest and longest action potential durations (APD_{90}) or recovery time (RT_{90}), both measured at the 90% repolarization level.

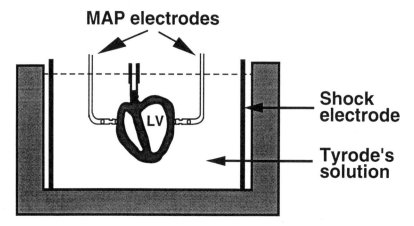

FIGURE 4. *Side view of the tissue bath in which the heart is immersed and which is filled with warm Tyrode's solution. MAPs are recorded from the epicardium (two MAPs shown) and the endocardium (not shown) of both ventricles. The tissue chamber is flanked by plate electrodes used to deliver electrical shocks to the heart. LV indicates left ventricle. See text for details.*

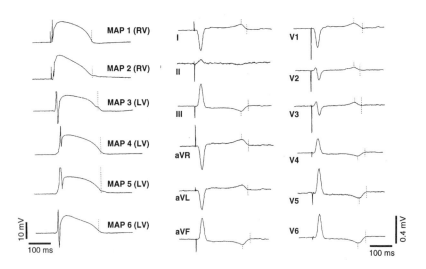

FIGURE 5. *Original recording of 6 MAPs and 12 ECG signals. Dashed lines indicate 90% repolarization for MAPs and the peak and the end of the T wave. ECG lead II was discarded from analysis. Modified with permission from Reference 20.*

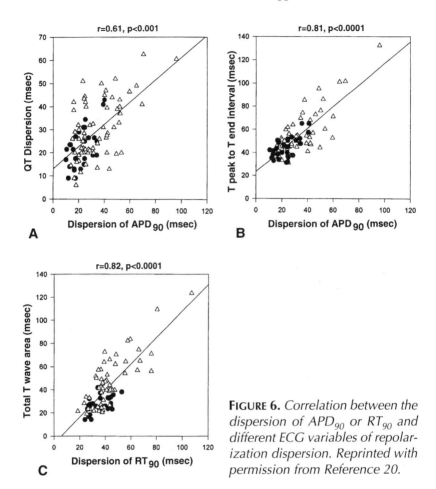

FIGURE 6. *Correlation between the dispersion of APD$_{90}$ or RT$_{90}$ and different ECG variables of repolarization dispersion. Reprinted with permission from Reference 20.*

The results are illustrated in Figure 6. QT dispersion and the dispersion of APD$_{90}$ are significantly correlated,[20] confirming the hypothesis that QT dispersion reflects the dispersion of ventricular repolarization with high and sufficient accuracy. However, the T$_{peak}$-to-T$_{end}$ interval and the total T-wave area show an even better correlation with the dispersion of APD$_{90}$ or RT$_{90}$. This suggests that these new and readily available ECG indexes might improve the ECG assessment of repolarization dispersion.

Area of Vulnerability

The electrophysiological conditions underlying arrhythmia susceptibility are incompletely understood. To determine the role of the dispersion of ventricular repolarization, it is essential to first characterize and define the precise borders of myocardial arrhythmia vulnerability. In the experimental setting, this can be accomplished by delivering electrical field stimuli (T-wave shocks) of various timings and intensities to the heart. Previous research has demonstrated that there is a minimal shock strength necessary to induce ventricular fibrillation (VF), known as the fibrillation threshold or lower limit of vulnerability (LLV),[37,38] a maximal shock strength (the upper limit of vulnerability [ULV]) above which VF is not inducible,[37,39–41] and a definitive time window of VF inducibility, called the vulnerable window, during which shocks can induce VF.[42,43] These bifunctional determinants of arrhythmia vulnerability (shock strength and shock coupling interval) mandate a two-dimensional representation of an AOV (Figure 7). It is important to know whether the ULV and LLV occur during a wide range of shock coupling intervals, indicating "indiscriminate" vulnerable windows, or whether these two extreme points of the AOV are "deterministic," ie, occurring within a narrow range of both shock strengths and shock coupling intervals. The characteristic shape of the AOV, its precise borders, and whether it is homogeneous in developing trigger-induced arrhythmias will be described in this section.[44]

To assess ventricular arrhythmia vulnerability, truncated exponential 5-ms monophasic shocks were delivered through two large shock-plate electrodes positioned at opposite sides of the tissue bath in which the rabbit heart was immersed (Figure 4). This shock elec-

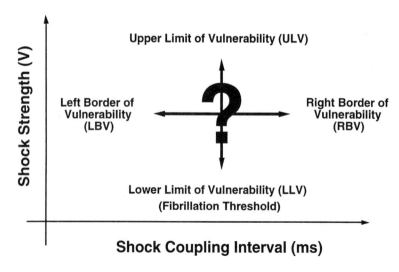

FIGURE 7. *The unknown AOV.*

trode configuration resulted in a highly uniform shock field in the center of the bath. ECG and MAP recordings were used to determine the arrhythmic response to the shocks, ie, whether VF, nonsustained arrhythmia, or no arrhythmia was induced. The horizontal boundaries of the AOV were determined as the longest and shortest shock coupling intervals that induced VF. The vertical AOV boundaries were defined as the LLV and ULV, respectively. The determination of these boundaries was executed randomly with a 5- to 10-ms accuracy for the horizontal borders and a 10-V accuracy for the LLV and ULV.

An example of the AOV is depicted in Figure 8. The AOV approximates the shape of a rhomboid and comprises more than 90% of all VF-inducing shocks. The AOV is surrounded by a transition zone in which nonsustained arrhythmias occur. Both the ULV and the LLV represent corners of the AOV, ie, they occur at single coupling intervals. The shock-induced arrhythmic responses at the ULV (Figure 9A) and LLV (Figure 9B) exceed 30 repetitive excitations, indicating a high probability of VF, whereas at coupling intervals 10 ms shorter or longer than the ULV or LLV, no or nonsustained arrhythmic responses occur. The shape of the AOV indicates that a definitive maximal or minimal arrhythmogenic shock strength exists that can be regarded as the "true" ULV or LLV. Thus, in an isolated heart model of relatively small mass conditioned by steady-state pacing and subjected to relatively uniform shock fields, the ULV and

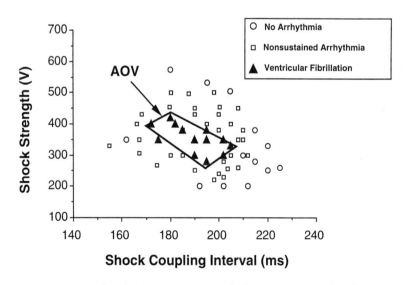

FIGURE 8. *Example of the AOV in a single heart. Reprinted with permission from Reference 44.*

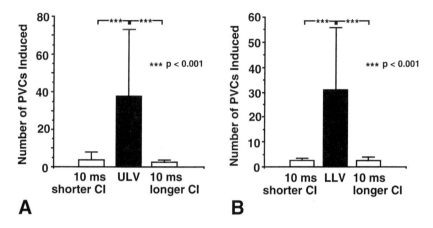

FIGURE 9. *Average number of shock-induced premature ventricular complexes (PVCs) at the ULV and at shock coupling intervals (CI) 10 ms shorter and longer than the CI at the ULV. Reprinted with permission from Reference 44.*

LLV are distinct and reproducible. This suggests that under controlled conditions, both the ULV and LLV may be deterministic rather than probabilistic variables. Under in-situ conditions, however, the ULV and LLV have been defined by a probability function.[45,46] Deale et al[47] previously suggested that probabilistic observations of the defibrillation threshold could be reproduced by complex deterministic models. In an earlier study, Fabiato et al[39] found fixed values for a 100% success rate in defibrillation and for equivalents of ULV and LLV within the same canine heart, whereas values between different dogs varied greatly. Probabilistic appearance of the ULV may therefore be due to instability of electrophysiological variables rather than to random changes in vulnerability.

The fact that >90% of all VF-inducing shocks are comprised within the boundaries of the AOV indicates that the AOV is homogeneous and provides a high degree of predictability for myocardial arrhythmia vulnerability.

Myocardial Vulnerability for Ventricular Fibrillation and Role of Ventricular Repolarization

The mechanism of VF induction by premature stimuli has been proposed to arise from the initiation of functional reentry within the ventricular myocardium.[14,48,49] Initiation of reentrant circuits requires unidirectional block of conduction[13] to allow a prematurely stimulated impulse to block in one direction while propagating in another direction, only to excite the previously refractory zone after a delay sufficient for its recovery.[48,49] Several years ago, a relation between VF induction and dispersion of ventricular repolarization was postulated on theoretical grounds. Figure 10 reproduces a hypothetical drawing by Watanabe and Dreifus,[50] who surmised that the differences in APDs between different regions of the heart, with their associated disparities in refractoriness, would allow an electrical stimulus to excite cells of earlier repolarization to become fully excited while causing only a graded response or no excitation at all in myocardium with longer repolarization. They further speculated that such derangement in ventricular excitation will lead to slowing of impulse propagation or functional conduction block in areas stimulated while they are partially or completely unexcitable.

Watanabe and Dreifus' hypothesis[50] was based on focal electrical stimulation, whose excitatory effects need to travel through the

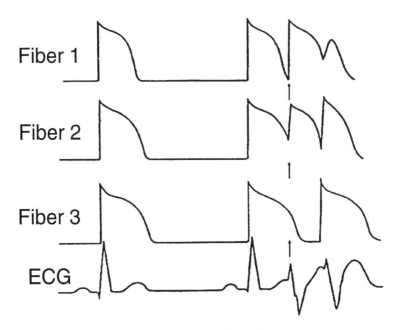

FIGURE 10. *Hypothetical drawing of the effect of a premature stimulus on the action potential response in three myocardial fibers with different APDs. Modified with permission from Reference 50.*

myocardium to encounter the disparity of ventricular repolarization and refractoriness in a sequential fashion. In contrast, global electrical field stimulation tends to alter the electrophysiological response of all myocardial cells simultaneously, suggesting that arrhythmia inducibility triggered by electrical shocks and its relation to the dispersion of ventricular repolarization could be studied more directly and without the influence of conduction delays.

The role of dispersion of ventricular repolarization for the induction of VF by field stimulation will be discussed in the following section. There are two different types of repolarization dispersion: (1) a preshock dispersion, representing the repolarization dispersion during normal or paced rhythm (ie, the dispersion before an intervention such as a T-wave shock), and (2) a postshock dispersion, representing the repolarization dispersion produced by a T-wave shock and thus present immediately after the shock.

Ventricular Fibrillation Inducibility and Preshock Dispersion

Previous studies have shown that the vulnerable window in response to electrical field shocks coincides with the ascending and to some extent the descending limb of the T wave of the surface ECG.[45,51,52] This agrees with the hypothesis that the vulnerable window is related to dispersion of ventricular repolarization.[53-55]

This hypothesis was tested in the isolated rabbit heart by assessment of the relation between VF inducibility by field stimulation (represented by the AOV) and the dispersion of ventricular repolarization present before shock application (preshock dispersion).[44] Preshock dispersion was defined as the range between the shortest and longest RTs measured at different repolarization levels. In Figure 11, the average AOV is depicted in relation to the preshock dispersion of the RT measured at the 50%, 70%, and 90% repolarization levels. The right and left borders of the AOV coincide with the shortest and longest RT at the 70% repolarization level. Interestingly, the same relation between the AOV width (ie, the maximal vulnerable window) and RT dispersion is present after a pharmacological intervention with a class III antiarrhythmic drug, d-sotalol.[56] d-Sotalol, an APD-prolonging drug,[57] shifts the vulnerable window and the RT dispersion to the right, toward longer repolarization times.[56] However, this affects neither the width of the vulnerable window and RT dispersion nor their relation as described above.

The facts that the vulnerable window falls within the dispersion of ventricular repolarization and that this correlation remains un-

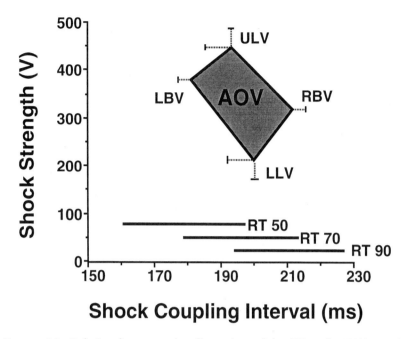

FIGURE 11. *Relation between the dispersion of the RT at the 50%, 70%, and 90% repolarization level (RT50, RT70, and RT90) and the AOV. The AOV is a rhomboid with four distinct corners: the ULV and LLV and the left and right borders of vulnerability (LBV and RBV). See text for details. Modified with permission from Reference 44.*

changed after administration of an APD-prolonging drug suggest a direct link between myocardial arrhythmia vulnerability and the present state of myocardial repolarization and further supports the hypothesis of a dispersion-related mechanism of arrhythmogenesis.

Ventricular Fibrillation Inducibility and Postshock Dispersion

In the previous section, we discussed the relation between the borders of the vulnerable window and repolarization dispersion present before the shock (preshock dispersion). However, Watanabe and Dreifus' hypothesis[50] also suggests that the dispersion produced by the stimulus and therefore present after a shock (postshock dispersion) may create the electrophysiological conditions for reentry to occur (Figure 10). This is consistent with data from mapping studies suggesting that electrical field stimuli of proper timing and strength may produce increased nonuniformity of refractoriness, thereby creating functional conduction block.[15,58,59] Several studies[60-67] have shown that electrical shocks may affect the APD (and thus the refractory period) by different degrees, depending on the instantaneous repolarization state and the voltage gradient produced by the shock. Thus, repolarization dispersion immediately after a field shock (postshock dispersion) should be affected by both shock coupling interval and shock strength.

To directly assess the influence of these two parameters (shock timing and strength) on postshock dispersion and to determine the role of postshock dispersion for myocardial arrhythmia vulnerability, truncated electrical field shocks were randomly delivered to the immersed rabbit heart over a wide range of shock coupling intervals and shock strengths.[68] The immediate postshock repolarization time was measured from the beginning of the shock artifact to the end of the repolarization phase in 10 MAPs that were simultaneously recorded from different ventricular sites of both ventricles. The postshock dispersion was defined as the range between the shortest and longest postshock repolarization time.

Figure 12 shows that shocks of moderate intensity that are delivered before (Figure 12A) or after (Figure 12C) the vulnerable window create only small differences in the postshock repolarization time at various ventricular sites, thus causing small postshock dispersion (indicated as the horizontal bars below the tracings in Figure 12). These shocks do not induce a tachyarrhythmic response. In contrast, shocks at coupling intervals within the vulnerable window create large differences between the postshock repolarization times, ranging from new action potentials (MAP 1 through 7 in Figure 12B) to short or "graded"[60] responses (MAP 8 through 10 in Figure 12B), thus resulting in large postshock dispersion and VF induction.

The postshock dispersions measured for various combinations of shock coupling intervals and shock strengths differ substantially (Figure 13). Postshock dispersion is small at coupling intervals early and late during the repolarization process (coupling intervals ≤160 and ≥200 ms in Figure 13), regardless of the shock strength. However, if shocks are delivered during the vulnerable window (coupling intervals >160 and <200 ms in Figure 13), the postshock dispersion is large at low shock strengths and progressively decreases toward higher shock intensities. The direct relation between VF inducibility for intermediate shock intensities and postshock dispersion is depicted in Figure 14. During the vulnerable window, postshock dispersion is large and decreases as shock coupling intervals move outside the borders of the vulnerable window where VF is no longer inducible. This supports the hypothesis

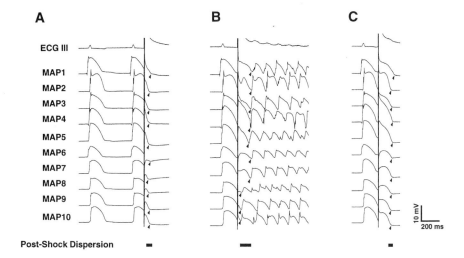

FIGURE 12. *Original recording of 10 MAP recordings and lead III of a volume-conducted ECG during the application of a field shock of intermediate strength. A, The shock was delivered before the vulnerable window (shock coupling interval, 160 ms). B, The shock was delivered within the vulnerable window and induced VF (shock coupling interval, 200 ms). C, The shock was delivered after the vulnerable window (shock coupling interval, 200 ms). The postshock dispersion of repolarization is indicated by black bars below the tracings. See text for details.*

that VF inducibility and postshock dispersion are directly related and that a certain amount of desynchronized repolarization is required for the induction of VF.

Postshock dispersion progressively decreases with increasing shock strengths (Figure 13), reaching its lowest values above the ULV, where VF is no longer inducible.[41,44,52] This suggests that repolarization synchronization may be a mechanism that explains the ULV. Below the LLV, however, where shocks are too weak to induce VF,[37,38] postshock dispersion remains large (Figure 13), probably because the repolarization extension produced by the shock is too small to create the functional conduction block necessary to initiate reentry.[13] The involved mechanisms for the ULV and LLV, therefore, appear to be different. Shocks above the ULV synchronize repolarization by producing large refractory period extension[69] and bidirectional block of conduction.[70] In contrast, shocks below the LLV, although they desynchronize repolarization, do not induce VF because repolarization is not sufficiently prolonged to create unidirectional block of conduction. Thus, shocks

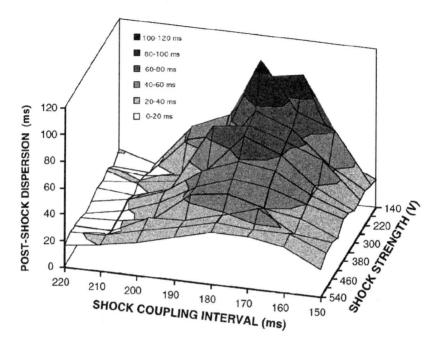

FIGURE 13. Three-dimensional graph of postshock dispersion of repolarization calculated for each combination of shock coupling intervals and shock strengths.

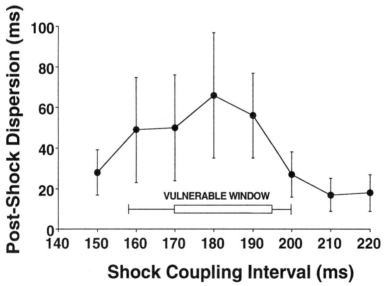

FIGURE 14. Relation between the postshock dispersion of repolarization and VF inducibility as a function of the shock coupling interval. VP inducibility was expressed as the range between the left and right borders (mean±SD) of the vulnerable window.

of various strengths result in VF if both desynchronized ventricular repolarization and a critical magnitude of repolarization extension are produced by the shock.

Summary

In this chapter, we reviewed selected aspects of dispersion of repolarization and its role for the interaction between the ventricular myocardium and electrical field stimuli. We discussed the potential usefulness of ECG indexes of repolarization dispersion as a measure to predict ventricular arrhythmias and to monitor antiarrhythmic or proarrhythmic drug effects. QT dispersion has been shown to reflect the dispersion of ventricular repolarization with high accuracy, but other ECG indexes may improve the ECG assessment of repolarization dispersion. Repolarization dispersion present before a shock (preshock dispersion) may be described as a conditioning factor for VF inducibility and repolarization dispersion produced by the shock (postshock dispersion) as a factor mediating the initiation of VF. Future studies should investigate whether and to what extent this relationship is influenced by cardiac diseases or pharmacological interventions.

Acknowledgments

The authors wish to thank Cuilan Li, PhD, Paulus Kirchhof, BS, Larissa Fabritz, BS, and Markus Zabel, MD, for their contributions in the study of ventricular repolarization dispersion and its role for myocardial arrhythmia vulnerability.

References

1. Gillum RF. Sudden coronary death in the United States. *Circulation.* 1989;79:756–765.
2. Bayes de Luna A, Coumel P, Leclercq JF. Ambulatory sudden cardiac death: mechanisms of production of fatal arrhythmia on the basis of data from 157 cases. *Am Heart J.* 1989;117:151–159.
3. Winkle RA, Mead RH, Ruder MA, et al. Long-term outcome with the automatic implantable cardioverter-defibrillator. *J Am Coll Cardiol.* 1989;13:1353–1361.
4. Linker NJ, Ward I, Griffith MJ. Repolarisation abnormalities in patients with hypertrophic cardiomyopathy and ventricular arrhythmias: are they important? *Br Heart J.* 1992;68:113–114.
5. Ahnve S. Is QT interval prolongation a strong or a weak predictor for cardiac death? *Circulation.* 1991;84:1862–1865.

6. Schwartz PJ, Wolf S. QT interval prolongation as a predictor of sudden death in patients with myocardial infarction. *Circulation.* 1978;57: 1074–1077.

7. Fei L, Statters DJ, Anderson MH, Katritsis D, Camm AJ. Is there an abnormal QT interval in sudden cardiac death survivors with a "normal" QTc? *Am Heart J.* 1994:73–76.

8. Vassallo JA, Cassidy DM, Kindwall KE, Marchlinski FE, Josephson ME. Nonuniform recovery of excitability in the left ventricle. *Circulation.* 1988;78:1365–1372.

9. Kuo CS, Munakata K, Reddy CP, Surawicz B. Characteristics and possible mechanism of ventricular arrhythmia dependent on the dispersion of action potential durations. *Circulation.* 1983;67:1356–1367.

10. Day CP, McComb JM, Campbell RW. QT dispersion: an indication of arrhythmia risk in patients with long QT intervals. *Br Heart J.* 1990;63: 342–344.

11. Hii JT, Wyse DG, Gillis AM, Duff HJ, Solylo MA, Mitchell LB. Precordial QT interval dispersion as a marker of torsade de pointes: disparate effects of class Ia antiarrhythmic drugs and amiodarone. *Circulation.* 1992;86:1376–1382.

12. Abildskov JA. The sequence of normal recovery of excitability in the dog heart. *Circulation.* 1975;52:442–446.

13. El-Sherif N. Reentrant mechanisms in ventricular arrhythmias. In: Zipes DP, Jalife J, eds. *Cardiac Electrophysiology: From Cell to Bedside.* Philadelphia, Pa: WB Saunders; 1995:567–582.

14. Shibata N, Chen PS, Dixon EG, et al. Epicardial activation after unsuccessful defibrillation shocks in dogs. *Am J Physiol.* 1988;255:H902–H909.

15. Allessie MA, Bonke FI, Schopman FJ. Circus movement in rabbit atrial muscle as a mechanism of tachycardia; II: the role of nonuniform recovery of excitability in the occurrence of unidirectional block, as studied with multiple microelectrodes. *Circ Res.* 1976;39:168–177.

16. Bonatti V, Rolli A, Botti G. Recording of monophasic action potentials of the right ventricle in long QT syndromes complicated by severe ventricular arrhythmias. *Eur Heart J.* 1983;4:168–179.

17. Kuo CS, Amlie JP, Munakata K, Reddy CP, Surawicz B. Dispersion of monophasic action potential durations and activation times during atrial pacing, ventricular pacing, and ventricular premature stimulation in canine ventricles. *Cardiovasc Res.* 1983;17:152–161.

18. Kurz RW, Ren XL, Franz MR. Dispersion and delay of electrical restitution in the globally ischaemic heart. *Eur Heart J.* 1994;15:547–554.

19. Franz MR. Bridging the gap between basic and clinical electrophysiology: what can be learned from monophasic action potential recordings? *J Cardiovasc Electrophysiol.* 1994;5:699–710.

20. Zabel M, Portnoy S, Franz MR. Electrocardiographic indexes of dispersion of ventricular repolarization: an isolated heart validation study. *J Am Coll Cardiol.* 1995;25:746–752.

21. De Ambroggi L, Negroni MS, Monza E, Bertoni T, Schwartz PJ. Dispersion of ventricular repolarization in the long QT syndrome. *Am J Cardiol.* 1991;68:614–620.

22. Abildskov JA, Green LS. The recognition of arrhythmia vulnerability by body surface potential mapping. *Circulation.* 1987;75(suppl III):III-79–III-83.

23. Flowers NC, Horan LG. Body surface potential mapping. In: Zipes DP, Jalife J, eds. *Cardiac Electrophysiology: From Cell to Bedside.* Philadelphia, Pa: WB Saunders: 1995:1049–1067.

24. Higham PD, Campbell RWF. QT dispersion. *Br Heart J.* 1994;71:508–510.
25. Day CP, McComb JM, Campbell RW. QT dispersion in sinus beats and ventricular extrasystoles in normal hearts. *Br Heart J.* 1992;67:39–41.
26. Mirvis DM. Spatial variation of QT intervals in normal persons and patients with acute myocardial infarction. *J Am Coll Cardiol.* 1985;3:625–631.
27. Day CP, McComb JM, Matthews J, Campbell RW. Reduction in QT dispersion by sotalol following myocardial infarction. *Eur Heart J.* 1991;12:423–427.
28. Higham PD, Campbell RWF. QT dispersion in ischaemia and infarction. *Eur Heart J.* 1992;14:448. Abstract.
29. Glancy JM, Garratt CJ, Woods KL, de Bono DP. QT dispersion and mortality after myocardial infarction. *Lancet.* 1995;345:945–948.
30. Davey PP, Bateman J, Mulligan IP, Forfar C, Barlow C, Hart G. QT interval dispersion in chronic heart failure and left ventricular hypertrophy: relation to autonomic nervous system and Holter tape abnormalities. *Br Heart J.* 1994;71:268–273.
31. Linker NJ, Colonna P, Kekwick CA, Till J, Camm AJ, Ward DE. Assessment of QT dispersion in symptomatic patients with congenital long QT syndromes. *Am J Cardiol.* 1992;69:634–638.
32. Priori S, Napolitano C, Diehl L, Schwartz PJ. Dispersion of the QT interval: a marker of therapeutic efficacy in the idiopathic long QT syndrome. *Circulation.* 1994;89:1681–1689.
33. Zhao F, Timothy K, Fox J, Vincent M. Beta-blockers markedly affect QT dispersion during exercise in long QT syndrome patients. *J Am Coll Cardiol.* 1993;21:93A. Abstract.
34. Cui G, Sen L, Sager P, Uppal P, Singh B. Effects of amiodarone, sematilide, and sotalol on QT dispersion. *Am J Cardiol.* 1994;74:896–900.
35. Murray A, McLaughlin NB, Bourke JP, Doig JC, Furniss SS, Campbell RWF. Errors in manual measurements of QT intervals. *Br Heart J.* 1994;71:386–390.
36. Statters DJ, Malik M, Ward DE, Camm AJ. QT-dispersion: problems of methodology and clinical significance. *J Cardiovasc Electrophysiol.* 1994;5:672–685.
37. Lesigne C, Levy B, Saumont R, Birkul P, Bardou A, Rubin B. An energy-time analysis of ventricular fibrillation and defibrillation thresholds with internal electrodes. *Med Biol Eng.* 1976;14:617–622.
38. Wharton JM, Richard VJ, Murry CE, et al. Electrophysiological effects of monophasic and biphasic stimuli in normal and infarcted dogs. *Pacing Clin Electrophysiol.* 1990;13:1158–1172.
39. Fabiato A, Coumel P, Gourgon R, Saumont R. The threshold of synchronous response of the myocardial fibers: application to the experimental comparison of the efficacy of different forms of electroshock defibrillation [in French; author's translation]. Le seuil de réponse synchrone des fibres myocardiques: application à la comparaison expérimentale de l'efficacité des différentes choc électriques de défibrillation. *Arch Mal Coeur Vaiss.* 1967;60:527–544.
40. Chen PS, Shibata N, Dixon EG, Martin RO, Ideker RE. Comparison of the defibrillation threshold and the upper limit of ventricular vulnerability. *Circulation.* 1986;73:1022–1028.
41. Shibata N, Chen PS, Dixon EG, et al. Influence of shock strength and timing on induction of ventricular arrhythmias in dogs. *Am J Physiol.* 1988;255:H891–H901.

42. Wiggers CJ. The mechanism and nature of ventricular fibrillation. *Am Heart J.* 1940;20:399–412.
43. Hoffman BF, Gorin EF, Wax FF, Siebens AA, Brooks CM. Vulnerability to fibrillation and the ventricular excitability curve. *Am J Physiol.* 1951;167:88–94.
44. Fabritz CL, Kirchhof PF, Behrens S, Zabel M, Franz MR. Myocardial vulnerability to T wave shocks: relation to shock strength, shock coupling interval, and dispersion of ventricular repolarization. *J Cardiovasc Electrophysiol.* 1996;7:231–242.
45. Malkin RA, Idriss SF, Walker RG, Ideker RE. Effect of rapid pacing and T-wave scanning on the relation between the defibrillation and upper-limit-of-vulnerability dose-response curves. *Circulation.* 1995; 92:1291–1299.
46. Cha YM, Peters BB, Birgersdotter-Green U, Chen PS. A reappraisal of ventricular fibrillation threshold testing. *Am J Physiol.* 1993;264: H1005–H1010.
47. Deale OC, Wesley R Jr, Morgan D, Lerman BB. Nature of defibrillation: determinism versus probabilism. *Am J Physiol.* 1990;259:H1544–H1550.
48. Frazier DW, Wolf PD, Wharton JM, Tang AS, Smith WM, Ideker RE. Stimulus-induced critical point: mechanism for electrical initiation of reentry in normal canine myocardium. *J Clin Invest.* 1989;83:1039–1052.
49. Chen PS, Wolf PD, Dixon EG, et al. Mechanism of ventricular vulnerability to single premature stimuli in open-chest dogs. *Circ Res.* 1988;62:1191–1209.
50. Watanabe Y, Dreifus LS. *Cardiac Arrhythmias: Electrophysiological Basis for Clinical Interpretation.* Orlando, Fla: Grune & Stratton Inc; 1977.
51. Chen PS, Feld GK, Kriett JM, et al. Relation between upper limit of vulnerability and defibrillation threshold in humans. *Circulation.* 1993;88:186–192.
52. Hwang C, Swerdlow C, Kass R, et al. Upper limit of vulnerability reliably predicts the defibrillation threshold in humans. *Circulation.* 1994;90:2308–2314.
53. Surawicz B, Gettes LS, Ponce ZA. Relation of vulnerability to ECG and action potential characteristics of premature beats. *Am J Physiol.* 1967;212:1519–1528.
54. Burgess MJ. Relation of ventricular repolarization to electrocardiographic T wave-form and arrhythmia vulnerability. *Am J Physiol.* 1979;236:402.
55. Zipes DP. Electrophysiological mechanisms involved in ventricular fibrillation. *Circulation.* 1975;52:120–130.
56. Kirchhof PF, Fabritz CL, Zabel M, Franz MR. The vulnerable period for low and high energy T wave shocks: role of dispersion of repolarization and sotalol. *J Cardiovasc Res.* In press.
57. Hohnloser SH, Woosley RL. Sotalol. *N Engl J Med.* 1994;331:31–38.
58. Restivo M, Gough WB, El-Sherif N. Ventricular arrhythmias in the subacute myocardial infarction period: high-resolution activation and refractory patterns of reentrant rhythms. *Circ Res.* 1990;66:1310–1327.
59. Knisley SB, Hill BC. Optical recordings of the effect of electrical stimulation on action potential repolarization and the induction of reentry in two-dimensional perfused rabbit epicardium. *Circulation.* 1993; 88:2402–2414.

60. Kao CY, Hoffman BF. Graded and decremental response in heart muscle fibers. *Am J Physiol.* 1958;194:187–196.
61. Knisley SB, Smith WM, Ideker RE. Effect of field stimulation on cellular repolarization in rabbit myocardium: implications for reentry induction. *Circ Res.* 1992;70:707–715.
62. Zhou XH, Knisley SB, Wolf PD, Rollins DL, Smith WM, Ideker RE. Prolongation of repolarization time by electric field stimulation with monophasic and biphasic shocks in open-chest dogs. *Circ Res.* 1991; 68:1761–1767.
63. Jones JL, Jones RE. Effects of monophasic defibrillator waveform intensity on graded response duration in a computer simulation of the action potential. *Proc Annu Int Conf IEEE Eng Med Biol Soc.* 1991;13: 598–599.
64. Jones JL, Jones RE, Milne KB. Refractory period prolongation by biphasic defibrillator waveforms is associated with enhanced sodium current in a computer model of the ventricular action potential. *IEEE Trans Biomed Eng.* 1994;41:60–68.
65. Dillon SM. Optical recordings in the rabbit heart show that defibrillation strength shocks prolong the duration of depolarization and the refractory period. *Circ Res.* 1991;69:842–856.
66. Swartz JF, Jones JL, Jones RE, Fletcher R. Conditioning prepulse of biphasic defibrillator waveforms enhances refractoriness to fibrillation wavefronts. *Circ Res.* 1991;68:438–449.
67. Tovar O, Bransford P, Moubarak J, Milne K, Amanna A, Jones J. Correlation between shock induced response duration and success of defibrillation. *IEEE Trans Biomed Eng.* 1994;21–22.
68. Behrens S, Li C, Kirchhof P, Fabritz FL, Franz MR. Reduced arrhythmogenicity of biphasic versus monophasic T wave shocks: implications for defibrillation efficacy. *Circulation.* In press.
69. Sweeney RJ, Gill RM, Reid PR. Characterization of refractory period extension by transcardiac shock. *Circulation.* 1991;83:2057–2066.
70. Gotoh M. Chen PS, Fishbein MC, Mandel WJ, Karagueuzian HS. Cellular mechanism of the upper limit of vulnerability during electrical induction of reentry in vitro. *Pacing Clin Electrophysiol.* 1994;17:839. Abstract.

Chapter 4

Drug and Metabolic Factors in Sudden Death

Milou-Daniel Drici, MD, PhD,
David A. Flockhart, MD, PhD, and
Raymond L. Woosley, MD, PhD

Drug-induced arrhythmia is an often unrecognized cause of sudden death. The Cardiac Arrhythmia Suppression Trial[1] (CAST) and the Survival With Oral *d*-Sotalol[2] (SWORD) Trial clearly demonstrated that thousands of patients may die annually from the effects of sodium and potassium channel blocking drugs and subsequently led to a more conservative approach to the prescription of such drugs. However, many medications other than antiarrhythmic drugs can block sodium or potassium channels, raising the possibility that a large proportion of the population may be exposed to the risk of sudden death.

In addition to cardiac drugs, commonly prescribed drugs such as the antibiotic erythromycin, the antihistamines terfenadine (Seldane) and astemizole (Hismanal), the lipid-lowering agent probucol (Lorelco), the antihypertensive agent indapamide (Lozol), the neuroleptic drug haloperidol (Haldol), or the gastrointestinal motility enhancer cisapride (Propulsid), among others, can prolong cardiac repolarization through potassium channel blockade at the cellular level.[3] It has also become clear that these drugs can cause a polymorphic ventricular arrhythmia known as torsades de pointes that can lead to sudden death. Makkar et al[4] reviewed reports of torsades de pointes with quinidine, procainamide, disopyramide, sotalol, bepridil, prenylamine, and amiodarone and found an excessive incidence in women after correction for other risk factors, such as hypokalemia, hypo-

From: Dunbar SB, Ellenbogen KA, Epstein AE, (eds). *Sudden Cardiac Death: Past, Present, and Future.* Armonk, NY: Futura Publishing Company, Inc.; © 1997.

magnesemia, digoxin administration, or baseline-corrected QT. The most common feature of these drugs is that they block the rapid component of the delayed rectifier K^+ current, which is of utmost importance in repolarizing cardiac tissue, leading to prolongation of the action potential. In most cases, the drugs have a direct blocking effect on the channel. In other cases, one or several of their metabolites are the active agents. Drug interactions or alterations of physiological function, such as renal failure or hepatic disease, can facilitate the emergence of drug-induced arrhythmias. Understanding the actions of these drugs, their kinetic and dynamic interactions with other drugs, and the importance of sex, electrolyte disorders, and metabolic pathways are essential for preventing drug-induced arrhythmias and sudden death.

Determinants of Repolarization

The cardiac action potential is the result of variation of the membrane voltage as a function of time and is determined by differential flow of ions that form currents across the membrane (Fig. 1). Outward currents carried by K^+ ions are the major determinant of repolarization.[5] Activated by voltages that are reached during the upstroke and the plateau of the action potential, the transient outward current (I_{to}) causes the earliest repolarization of the cell (phase 1) to voltages that subsequently activate the delayed rectifier K^+ channels (phase 2) and allow more potassium to leave the cell (phase 3). Near the end of the action potential, the outward conductance of potassium by the inward rectifier current (I_{K1}) brings the membrane voltage close to the resting potential. Other potassium channels contribute to the particular shape and duration of the action potential, such as currents regulated by adenosine triphosphate (I_{KATP}) or acetylcholine (I_{KAch}). However, I_{to} and I_K are considered to be the major determinants of ventricular repolarization.[6]

The delayed rectifier K^+ current has three components, I_{Ks}, I_{Kr}, and I_{Kur}, that have been identified.[7,8] I_{Ks} activates very slowly, I_{Kr} more rapidly, and I_{Kur} ultrarapidly. I_{Kr} is the target of a number of antiarrhythmic drugs (quinidine, dofetilide, *d*-sotalol, etc) and other compounds (pimozide, astemizole, terfenadine, etc) that prolong repolarization. It now appears that many of the drugs that cause torsades de pointes also block I_{Kr}[9] and induce prolongation of the action potential and the QT interval.[10]

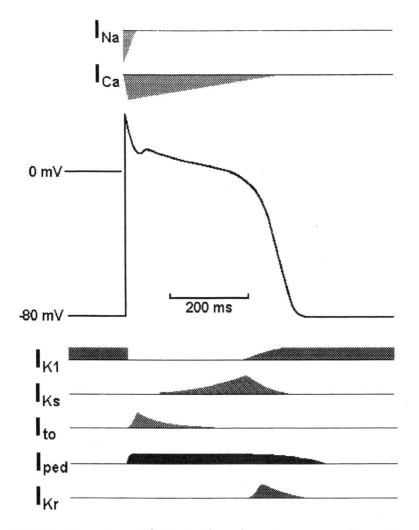

FIGURE 1. *Currents contributing to the voltage-time course of a cardiac action potential.*

Action Potential and QT-Interval Lengthening as Underlying Conditions for the Occurrence of Torsades de Pointes

Many class III antiarrhythmic drugs prolong the action potential duration and therefore the QT interval on the electrocardiogram. QT prolongation can reflect a global delay in repolarization or regional changes associated with inhomogeneity in the repolarization process.

Uniform delay in repolarization does not appear to be arrhythmogenic, but inhomogeneous repolarization is thought to be a basic cause of arrhythmias.[6] The mechanism by which prolonged repolarization induces torsades de pointes is still uncertain, but early afterdepolarizations are considered to be the triggering mechanism.[11] Early afterdepolarizations are due to slow inward Na^+ and Ca^{2+} currents that interrupt the repolarization process early during phase 3 of prolonged action potentials.

Pharmacological, Physiopathological, and Clinical Implications

A large number of drugs and their metabolites are capable of lengthening the QT interval in proportion to the dose administered or the resulting concentration. However, the link between the degree of QT prolongation and the plasma drug concentration is not always complete—eg, for quinidine, for which some patients have a marked QT-interval prolongation at very low plasma concentrations.[12]

The drugs capable of prolonging the QT interval, blocking the delayed rectifier potassium current, or inducing torsades de pointes are numerous and belong to broadly different classes[4,11,13–15] (Table 1).

Whether a QT-interval prolongation results from a direct action of a drug or the action of its metabolite on the channels involved, any pathophysiological or pharmacological interference in metabolism that raises the plasma concentration of the drug or enhances its potency may then have dangerous consequences for the patient.

Many different factors may alter the pharmacological activity of drugs. Most drugs that prolong repolarization undergo hepatic or intestinal metabolism after gastrointestinal absorption and are excreted in the urine or in the feces either unchanged or as metabolites. Drug interactions or changes in pharmacokinetic parameters due to kidney or liver disease or cardiovascular or metabolic conditions can decrease the elimination of drugs and potentiate their activity, thus facilitating the emergence of torsades de pointes. The clinical consequences of such interactions between the drug and the pharmacological environment may be of great importance. Even though clear warnings have been placed in the labeling for most of the drugs that can interact and cause torsades de pointes, it is clear that coprescription continues.[16] A recent survey of a prescription database found that 2.5% of prescriptions for terfenadine were filled at a time coincident with prescriptions for drugs capa-

TABLE 1

Drugs That May Contribute to Cardiac Arrhythmias

Antiarrhythmic drugs	Amiodarone, dofetilide, disopyramide, d-sotalol, procainamide, quinidine
Antihistamines	Astemizole, diphenhydramine, terfenadine
Antimalarials	Chloroquine, halofantrine
Tricyclic antidepressants	Amitriptyline, nortriptyline
Lipid-lowering agents	Probucol
Neuroleptics	Haloperidol, pimozide, resperidone, thioridazine
Antibiotics	Erythromycin, pentamidine, trimethoprim-sulfamethoxazole
Antifungals	Ketoconazole, itraconazole

ble of interacting with it and blocking its metabolism.[16] When two prescriptions for interacting drugs capable of causing torsades de pointes (terfenadine and erythromycin) were presented simultaneously to pharmacists, one third were filled without any warning.[16] This failure emphasizes the importance for physicians to be aware of potential drug interactions.

Drug Interactions

Pharmacokinetic Interactions

Terfenadine blocks the delayed rectifier K^+ channel in vitro, prolongs the QT interval, and induces torsades de pointes. Plasma levels of terfenadine are usually extremely low, because it is converted by cytochrome P450 3A[17] principally into the carboxylate metabolite fexofenadine, which is devoid of potassium channel blocking properties. Any drug capable of inhibiting this particular family of cytochromes, eg, erythromycin, ketoconazole, or itraconazole,[18] that is coprescribed with terfenadine inhibits terfenadine metabolism. Plasma terfenadine then accumulates, resulting in prolongation of the QT interval and occurrence of torsades de pointes ventricular arrhythmias.[19]

Sometimes the parent drug does not produce any harmful effect, but its metabolite lengthens the duration of the QT interval. This is the case with procainamide and its metabolite N-acetylprocainamide and with the widely used drug for AIDS patients pentamidine. In theory, agents that induce formation of N-hydroxypentamidine, eg, rifampin, could increase the risk of torsades de pointes.

Pharmacodynamic Interactions

In some cases, a pharmacodynamic interaction is involved: this can be the case in metabolic interactions due to ketoconazole or erythromycin that not only inhibit the cytochrome P450 system but also have I_{Kr} blocking properties that prolong QT per se and can cause torsades de pointes. Diuretic-induced hypokalemia also potentiates the blockade exerted on the delayed rectifier I_{Kr} by these compounds.[20]

Pathological Conditions

Renal or hepatic failure can lead to the accumulation of drugs to harmful concentrations.[19] Certain diseases may predispose to the occurrence of torsades de pointes, such as congenital long-QT syndrome, which can be caused either by defective Na^+ channel inactivation[21] or by a defect in a K^+ channel.[22] Hypokalemia (eg, resulting from combined diuretic and corticosteroid treatment) and bradyarrhythmia can lengthen and potentiate the arrhythmogenic effect of drugs.[12,15,20] Hypothyroidism and severe coronary artery disease with abnormally prolonged QT duration usually contraindicates the use of these drugs.

Physiological Conditions

Pharmacogenetics

The actions of a drug are determined by complex interrelationships between a subject's pharmacokinetics, pharmacogenetics, and environment. More than the environmental factors that may induce (eg, smoking or ingestion of charcoaled beef) or inhibit (eg, broccoli, grapefruit juice) hepatic enzymes, inherited differences in expression of the metabolic pathways of drugs can account for larger interindividual variability in response to those drugs. Genetic polymorphism in hepatic metabolic enzymes, notably N-acetyltransferase (procainamide) or cytochrome P450 2 D6 (amitriptyline, nortriptyline, desipramine, etc), may predispose individual patients to drug-induced prolongation of the QT and subsequently torsades de points.[23]

Sex Differences

In addition to the known sex differences in the pharmacokinetics of drugs,[24] it has been shown that the occurrence of torsades de pointes in the acquired long-QT syndrome displays a strong sex difference, with 30% of the cases in men compared with 70% in women.[4] It has also long been known that the QT duration is different in women and in men, but only recently has this difference been attributed to a possible role of androgen in shortening the QT interval after puberty in men.[25] Studies in an animal model have found that androgen treatment can decrease the responsiveness of cardiac tissue to K^+ channel blocking drugs[26] (Figure 2). It was also found that the QT duration, longer in female rabbits, was associated with a lower amplitude of outward repolarizing K^+ currents in cardiac myocytes[27] (Figure 3).

Conclusions

It is clear that the incidence of torsades de pointes arrhythmias and sudden death is greater among patients in whom the QT interval is prolonged by drugs. A cardiac predisposition to prolongation of the QT in the form of bradycardia or congenital prolongation of the QT is easily screened for. At present, we have no reliable means of predicting which patients taking medicines known to prolong QT will in fact experience dangerous arrhythmias. Such predictions are

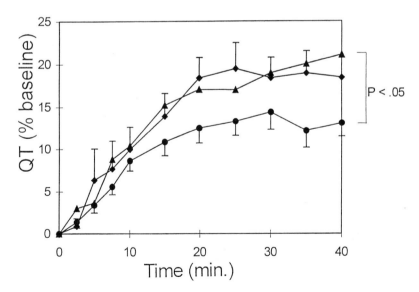

FIGURE 2. *Changes in QT interval after quinidine infusion (3 μm/L) in isolated hearts from ovariectomized rabbits treated with estradiol (▲,n=6), dihydrotestosterone) (●, n=6), or placebo (◆,n=4).*

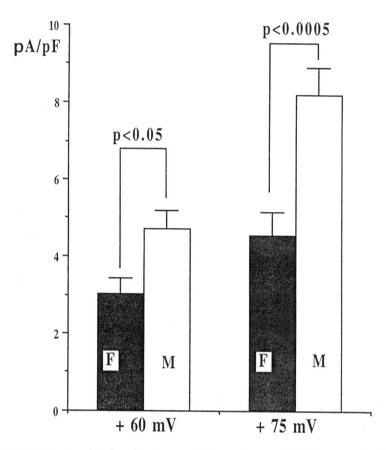

FIGURE 3. *Amplitude of I_{to} in a rabbit cardiac ventricular myocyte from male (open bars, n=20 cells) and female (solid bars, n=19 cells) animals.*

enhanced by recent research showing that women are more vulnerable to prolongation of the QT by drugs and that inhibition of drug metabolism increases concentrations of drugs and thereby increases the risk for arrhythmias.

References

1. Greene HL, Roden DM, Katz RJ, et al. The Cardiac Arrhythmia Suppression Trial: first CAST . . . then CAST-II. *J Am Coll Cardiol.* 1992;19:894–898.
2. Waldo AL, Camm AJ, deRuyter H, et al. Effect of d-sotalol in patients with left ventricular dysfunction after recent and remote myocardial infarction: (the SWORD trial). *Am J Cardiol.* 1996;348:7–12.

3. Napolitano C, Priori SG, Schwartz PJ. Torsades de pointes: mechanisms and management. *Drugs.* 1994;47:51–65.
4. Makkar RR, Fromm BS, Steinman RT, et al. Female gender as a risk factor for torsades de pointes associated with cardiovascular drugs. *JAMA.* 1993;270:2590–2597.
5. Colatsky TJ. Voltage-clamp measurements of sodium channel properties in rabbit cardiac Purkinje fibers. *J Physiol.* 1980;395:215–234.
6 Rosen MR, Jeck CD, Steiberg SF. Autonomic modulation of cellular repolarization and of the electrocardiographic QT interval. *J Cardiovasc Electrophysiol.* 1992;3:487–499.
7. Fedida D, Wible B, Wang Z, et al. Identity of a novel delayed rectifier current from human heart with a cloned K$^+$ channel current. *Circ Res.* 1993;73:210–216.
8. Sanguinetti MC, Jurkiewicz NK. Two components of cardiac delayed rectifier K$^+$ current: differential sensitivity to block by class III antiarrhythmic agents. *J Gen Physiol.* 1990;96:195–215.
9. Roden DM. Early after depolarizations and torsades de pointes: implications for the control of cardiac arrhythmias by controlling repolarization. *Eur Heart J.* 1993;14H:56–61.
10. Zehender M. Hohnloser SH, Just H. QT-interval prolonging drugs: mechanisms and clinical relevance of their arrhythmogenic hazards. *Cardiovasc Drug Ther.* 1991;5:515–530.
11. January CT, Riddle JM, Salata JJ. A model for early afterdepolarization: induction with the CA^{2+} channel agonist Bay K 8644. *Circ Res.* 1988;62:563–571.
12. Roden DM, Woosley RL, Primm RK. Incidence and clinical features of the quinidine-associated long QT syndrome: implications for patient care. *Am Heart J.* 1986;111:1088–1093.
13. Hohnloser SH, Arendts W, Quart B. Incidence, type, and dose-dependence of proarrhythmic events during sotalol therapy in patients treated for sustained VT/VF. *Pacing Clin Electrophysiol.* 1992;15:551.
14. Ahmed I, Dagincourt PG, Miller LG, et al. Possible interaction between fluoxetine and pimozide causing sinus bradycardia. *Can J Psychiatry.* 1993;38:62–63.
15. Jackman WM, Friday KJ, Anderson JL, et al. The long QT syndromes: a critical review, new clinical observations and a unifying hypothesis. *Prog Cardiovasc Dis.* 1988;31:115–172.
16. Cavuto NJ, Woosley RL, Sale ME. Pharmacies and prevention of potentially fatal drug interactions. *JAMA.* 1996;275:1086.
17. Yun C, Okerholm RA, Guengerich FP. Oxidation of the antihistaminic drug terfenadine in human liver microsomes: role of cytochrome P450 3A4 in N-dealkylation and C-hydroxylation. *Drug Metab Dispos.* 1993; 21:403–409.
18. Honig PK, Wortham DC, Hull R, et al. Itraconazole affects single-dose terfenadine pharmacokinetics and cardiac repolarization pharmacodynamics. *J Clin Pharmacol.* 1993;33:1201–1206.
19. Woosley RL, Chen Y, Freiman JP, et al. Mechanism of the cardiotoxic actions of terfenadine. *JAMA.* 1993;269:1532–1536.
20. Yang T, Roden DM. Extracellular potassium modulation of drug block of I$_{Kr}$: implications for torsades de pointes and reverse use-dependence. *Circulation.* 1996;93:407–411.
21. Wang Q, Shen J, Splawski I, et al. SCN5A mutations associated with an inherited cardiac arrhythmia, long QT syndrome. *Cell.* 1995;80:805–811.

22. Curran ME, Splawski I, Timothy KW, et al. A molecular basis for cardiac arrhythmia: HERG mutations cause long QT syndrome. *Cell.* 1995;80:795–803.
23. Ketter TA, Flockhart DA, Post RM, et al. Cytochrome P450 3A in psychopharmacology. *J Clin Psychopharmacol.* 1995;15:387–398.
24. Harris RZ, Benet LZ, Schwartz JB. Gender effects in pharmacokinetics and pharmacodynamics. *Drugs.* 1995;50:222–239.
25. Rautaharju PM, Zhou SH, Wong S, et al. Sex differences in the evolution of the electrocardiographic QT interval with age. *Can J Cardiol.* 1992;8:690–695.
26. Drici M-D, Burklow TR, Haridasse V, et al. Sex steroid hormones prolong the QT interval and downregulate potassium channel expression in the rabbit heart. *Circulation.* 1996;94:1472–1475.
27. Drici M-D, Ducic I, Morad M, et al. Inward rectifier K$^+$ current and transient outward current have lower expression in female rabbits. *FASEB J.* 1996;10:A428. Abstract.

Chapter 5

The Nature of Activation During Ventricular Fibrillation

Gregory P. Walcott, MD, Xiaohong Zhou, MD,
Bruce H. KenKnight, MS, and
Raymond E. Ideker, MD, PhD

Sudden cardiac death is a major cause of mortality in the United States.[1] Most cases of sudden cardiac death are caused by ventricular fibrillation, frequently preceded by ventricular tachycardia.[2] For this reason, ventricular fibrillation has been studied extensively.[3,4] A better understanding of ventricular fibrillation and how the rhythm changes over time will potentially lead to better drug and device therapy for patients suffering from this arrhythmia.[5,6] Ventricular fibrillation is primarily a problem with the electrical system of the heart, including how the electrical impulse is produced by the myocardial cells (the action potential) and how the impulse is conducted from one cell to the next (the activation sequence). This chapter will briefly discuss the nature of the action potential and activation sequences during ventricular fibrillation.

Action Potentials During Ventricular Fibrillation

Until recently, little was known about the nature of action potentials during ventricular fibrillation. Action potentials have traditionally been studied in small pieces of myocardial tissue that are superfused in a tissue bath. A critical mass of myocardium, $\approx 25\%$ of the ventricular mass in the dog,[7] is required for ventricular fibrillation to continue without stopping spontaneously. Although an

Supported in part by the National Institutes of Health Research Grant HL-28429 and the National Science Foundation Engineering Research Center Grant CDR-8622201.

From: Dunbar SB, Ellenbogen KA, Epstein AE, (eds). Sudden Cardiac Death: Past, Present, and Future. Armonk, NY: Futura Publishing Company, Inc.; © 1997.

artificial type of fibrillation can be induced in isolated cells by poisoning with drugs,[8] realistic ventricular fibrillation cannot be induced in a small piece of myocardium in a tissue bath. In the past few years, however, methods have been developed to record action potentials in whole hearts, either in vivo or in isolated, perfused hearts. These techniques include monophasic action potential recordings,[9] floating microelectrodes,[10,11] closely spaced arrays of extracellular electrodes to estimate transmembrane current,[12] and optical recordings from potentiometric fluorescent dyes.[13] These techniques have greatly increased our knowledge of the nature of the action potential during ventricular fibrillation.

Action potentials recorded during ventricular fibrillation indicate that discrete action potentials do occur during ventricular fibrillation (Figures 1, 2, and 3). The activation rate during the first few seconds of fibrillation is quite rapid, with a cycle length of 90 to 120 ms in dogs[14] and a mean cycle length of 213 ± 27 ms in patients undergoing defibrillator implantation.[9] Because of this rapid activation rate, diastolic intervals are rarely seen during early fibrillation. The upstroke of most action potentials occurs before the transmembrane potential has returned to baseline from the previous action potential (Figure 1).

The action potential occurs because of membrane channels that differentially allow ions to flow either into or out of the cell. Both fast channel activity, which allows Na^+ into the cell, and slow channel ac-

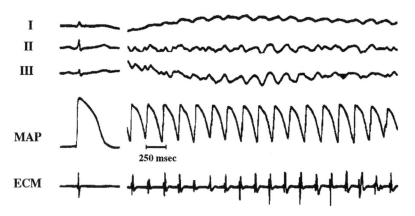

FIGURE 1. *Recording taken during ventricular fibrillation in a human. Leads I, II, and III are body surface electrocardiograms. MAP indicates right ventricular monophasic action potentials; ECM, local bipolar electrogram. Note that there is no period of diastole between action potentials. Modified with permission from Reference 9.*

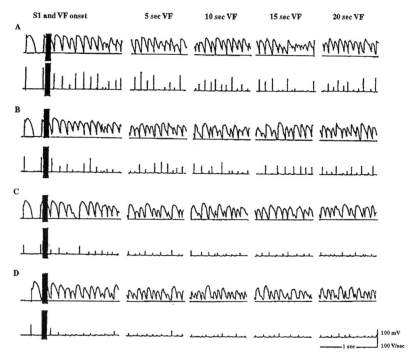

FIGURE 2. *Tracing of action potentials and dV/dt of the action potential during ventricular fibrillation (VF). A, Recordings made before drug. B, Low-dose tetrodotoxin fibrillation. C, High-dose tetrodotoxin fibrillation. D, Fibrillation after both local tetrodotoxin and verapamil and intravenous verapamil. Recordings were made with a floating microelectrode in a dog heart. The first action potential was recorded during paced rhythm, which was followed by action potentials at the onset of fibrillation and after 5, 10, 15, and 20 seconds of fibrillation. The horizonal line beneath each tracing represents the resting potential level for the corresponding records. The height of the spikes in the dV/dt trace below the action potentials indicates the magnitude of the maximum upstroke rate of depolarization. Reprinted with permission from Reference 11.*

tivity, which allows both Na^+ and Ca^{2+} into the cell, appear to be present during the first few seconds of ventricular fibrillation.[11] The presence of fast channel activity is indicated by the rapid upstroke of the action potential during fibrillation and by the decrease in the maximum derivative of the upstrokes (dV/dt_{max}) after the administration of tetrodotoxin, a Na^+ channel blocker (Figure 2). Without tetrodotoxin, dV/dt_{max} of the action potentials decreases with time during fibrillation. In dogs, it decreases from 104 ± 14 V/s in paced

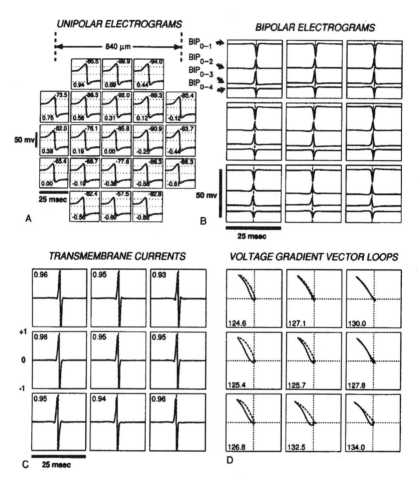

FIGURE 3. *Propagating epicardial activation during ventricular fibrillation. A, Unipolar electrograms from each of 21 electrodes of a recording array shown with individual minimal dV/dt deflections indicated by vertical dashed lines (somewhat obscured by intrinsic deflections). The time of the minimal dV/dt deflection (in milliseconds) relative to the deflection timing at the central electrode of the 21-element array (0.00 ms) is given in the lower left corner of each box; the value of the dV/dt (in V/s) is found in electrodes that form a 3×3 matrix of subarrays, with each subarray formed by five electrodes. Calculated bipolar electrograms are formed from the five-electrode subarray in each of the nine regions, with center-to-center bipolar distances of 210 μm. The central recording site of the five-element subarray is designated as site 0, with site 1 located above it at 210 μm, and other sites proceed clockwise to sites 2, 3, and 4. B, Bipolar electrograms BIP$_{0-1}$ to BIP$_{0-4}$ are shown from top to bottom, where BIP$_{0-1}$ is the bipolar signal formed by subtracting the unipolar signal at*

rhythm to 55±32 V/s at the beginning of ventricular fibrillation and to 37±23 V/s after 20 seconds of fibrillation.[11] With low-dose tetrodotoxin (2.8×10^{-5}mol/L), it decreases from 86±15 V/s in paced rhythm to 39±20 V/s at the beginning of ventricular fibrillation to 18±11 V/s after 20 seconds of fibrillation. With high-dose tetrodotoxin (1×10^{-4}mol/L), the effects are even more striking. The maximum derivative of the upstroke decreased from 55±14 V/s in paced rhythm to 18±12 V/s at the beginning of fibrillation to 12±7 V/s after 20 seconds of fibrillation. After 1 to 5 minutes of fibrillation, action potential upstrokes are even slower and are insensitive to tetrodotoxin, suggesting that the action potentials at this time are caused primarily by slow channel activity.[10]

Changes in Activation Patterns With Time During Ventricular Fibrillation

Wiggers[15] used high-speed cinematography of fibrillating dog hearts to show that ventricular fibrillation passes through four stages. The first stage, called the undulatory or tachysystolic stage, lasts for only 1 or 2 seconds (Figure 4). This stage consists of three to six undulatory contractions similar to a series of closely timed premature systoles. Each contraction appears to involve the sequential contraction of large areas of myocardium. The second stage, called convulsive incoordination, lasts from 15 to 40 seconds. During this stage, more frequent waves of contraction sweep over smaller portions of the ventricles than during the first stage. Since the contractions in each region are not in phase with the contrac-

---

(**FIGURE 3 *Continued.***) *recording site 1 from that at site 0. The vertical dashed line in the bipolar signals indicates the location of the intrinsic deflection at the central recording site of the five-element subarray. C, Calculated transmembrane current (I_m) curves for each of the nine regions, with corresponding values for the ratio of the negative to positive area under $I_m(-/+I_m$ area) as shown in the upper left corner for each of the nine regions. Each I_m waveform is normalized to its own peak positive or negative value. As in the bipolar displays, the vertical dashed line in the I_m waveforms indicates the location of the intrinsic deflection at the central recording site of the five-element array, with the solid lines representing the 5 ms after this event. D, The angle of the voltage gradient at the time located by the intrinsic deflection at the central recording site of the five-element subarray is given in degrees in the lower left corner for each of the nine regions. Reprinted with permission from Reference 12.*

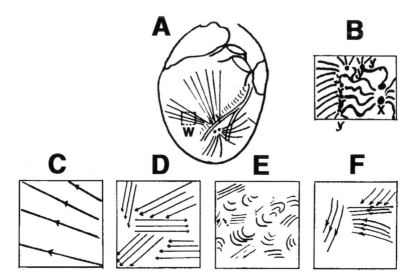

FIGURE 4. *Diagrams indicating the spread of waves observed in analysis of moving pictures during the four stages of fibrillation described by Wiggers. A, Spread of wave front during initial, undulatory stage. B, Theoretical passage of impulses from point x to form a wave front at y. C through F, Appearance of contraction waves in small rectangular area W, magnified: C, undulatory stage; D, convulsive stage; E, tremulous stage; and F, atonic stage. Reprinted with permission from Reference 15.*

tions in the other regions, the ventricles are pulled about in a convulsive manner. The third stage, called tremulous incoordination, lasts 2 to 3 minutes. During this third stage, the ventricular surface is broken up into progressively smaller independently contracting areas, which give the heart a tremulous appearance. The fourth stage, called atonic fibrillation, develops within 2 to 5 minutes after the onset of fibrillation. It is characterized by the slow passage of feeble contraction wavelets over short distances along the ventricular surface. With time, more and more areas become quiescent. During the first two stages, activation is rapid throughout the myocardium (Figure 5). During the last two stages, the activation rate progressively slows as fibrillation progresses, with greater slowing in the epicardial portion of the ventricular wall than in the endocardial portion (Figure 5). This slowing of the activation rate is probably caused by ischemia. Perfusing the coronary arteries with oxygenated blood during fibrillation keeps stages three and four from occurring.[14,16]

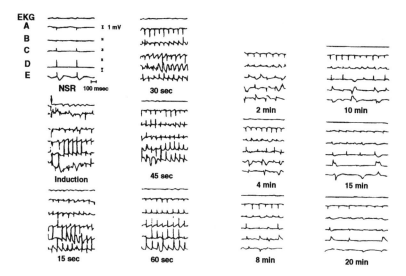

FIGURE 5. *Activation patterns during the first 20 minutes of electrically induced fibrillation in the dog. The upper tracing in each panel is the body surface electrocardiogram (EKG). Tracings A through E are bipolar recordings from plunge electrodes. A is near the endocardium; E is near the epicardium. NSR indicates normal sinus rhythm. Electrograms show how ventricular fibrillation changes through Wiggers' four stages of fibrillation. Reprinted with permission from Reference 14.*

The slowing of the activation rate over time has been used to estimate the duration of ventricular fibrillation in patients in whom the onset of fibrillation was not observed. An indirect technique to estimate the activation rate is frequency analysis of the body surface recordings.[17,18] There is usually a clear, dominant frequency with a narrow bandwidth during ventricular fibrillation. This dominant frequency is related to the activation frequency during fibrillation, and like the activation frequency, the dominant frequency slows as the duration of fibrillation increases during Wiggers' stages three and four of fibrillation.[19] Dzwonczyk et al[20] developed a method to estimate the duration of fibrillation from frequency analysis of electrocardiogram recordings as an aid to help decide when to stop cardiopulmonary resuscitation (Figure 6). Since the success rate of cardiopulmonary resuscitation decreases with increasing time that the patient has been in ventricular fibrillation,[21] it has been proposed that this dominant frequency can be used to determine when resuscitation attempts should be terminated.

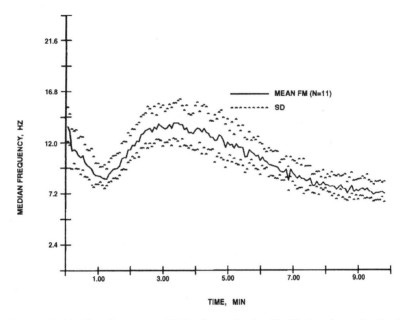

FIGURE 6. *Median frequency (FM) of ventricular fibrillation from the body surface electrocardiogram as a function of the duration of fibrillation. Average data from 11 dogs are shown. SD indicates standard deviation. Note how the activation rate slows (frequency gets slower) as fibrillation continues longer than 3 minutes. Reprinted with permission from Reference 21.*

Activation Sequences During Ventricular Fibrillation

The activation sequence describes the path that the electrical signal takes to excite the myocardium. Activation patterns can be divided into two groups: (1) focal, in which activation arises de novo from a region of tissue and propagates to the surrounding tissue, and (2) reentrant, in which activation travels continuously from one region of the heart to the next. Although activation arising from a focus has been reported to play a role during the initiation of ventricular fibrillation[22,23] and occasionally during its maintenance (Figure 7), several studies suggest that fibrillation is

FIGURE 7. *A focal activation pattern during ventricular fibrillation in a dog. A through C, Three consecutive cycles of a fibrillation episode in the dog in which activation fronts in the upper right side of the mapped region appear to originate from a focus for the first two cycles. The three maps from left to right in each panel represent endocardial, myocardial,*

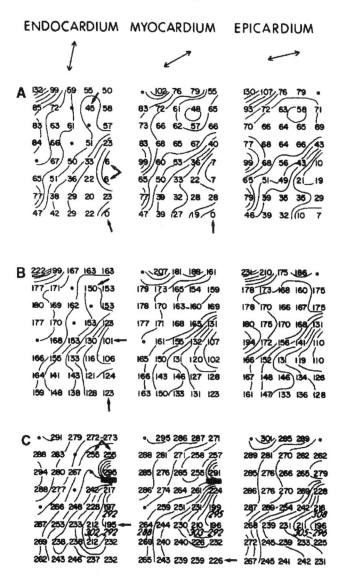

(**FIGURE 7 Continued**) *and epicardial layers of recording electrodes. Each number gives the activation time at an electrode site in milliseconds. Small circles indicate bad recording electrodes. Isochronal lines are 10 ms apart. Double activations were observed occasionally in some electrode recordings, probably representing two activation fronts activating or electronically influencing either the same region or adjacent regions near the recording site. Arrows indicate sites of early activation for each activation front. The mean direction of fiber orientation at each layer is parallel to the double-headed arrows above panel A. Reprinted with permission from Reference 25.*

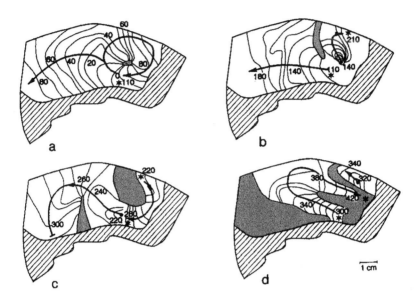

FIGURE 8. *Epicardial activation patterns during 420 ms of ventricular fibrillation in a dog heart that has previously undergone cryoablation of the endocardial portion of the left ventricle. Note the presence of one, or at most two, different wandering reentrant waves for each beat. The wave fronts follow constantly changing pathways from one beat to the next. Each panel shows a later time interval. The ruled areas have been frozen and are electrically inactive. Areas of block are stippled, numbers are in milliseconds, and time zero is chosen arbitrarily. Asterisks indicate reexcitation. Reprinted with permission from Reference 31.*

maintained by reentry. In most cases, reentry appears to be caused by "wandering wavelets" of activation, in which activation fronts follow continually changing pathways from cycle to cycle (Figure 8).[24] In some studies, though, activation sequences appear moderately repeatable from cycle to cycle, following approximately the same pathway (Figure 9).[25,26]

During the first minute of fibrillation, activation sequences become more repeatable as fibrillation continues.[27] Occasionally, a spiraling pattern of functional reentry emanates from the same region for several cycles (Figure 10). Sometimes, the central core of these spirals can meander across the heart (Figure 11).[13] At other times, new reentrant activation fronts are generated when one front interacts with another during its vulnerable period (Figure 12).[26]

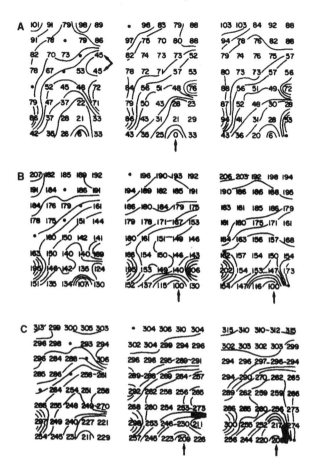

FIGURE 9. *Three successive cycles of fibrillation in a dog illustrating moderate repeatability in activation sequences during ventricular fibrillation. The thick line in the lower right corner of the mapped region indicates conduction block. See Figure 7 for further explanation. Reprinted with permission from Reference 25.*

Existence of an Excitable Gap During Ventricular Fibrillation

The term "excitable gap" refers to the idea that there is a time after the upstroke of an action potential but before the beginning of the next action potential during which myocardial tissue can be electrically stimulated. Until recently, most investigators thought

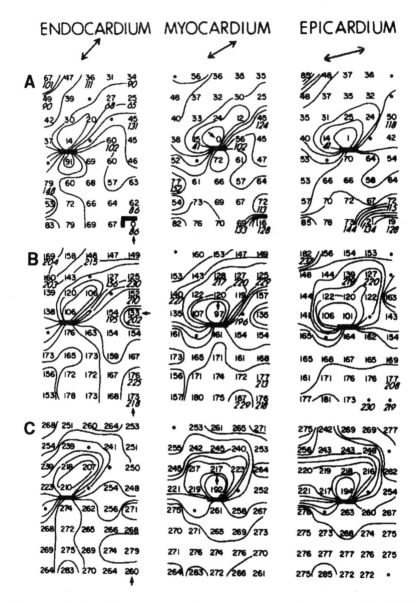

FIGURE 10. *A stable reentrant activation pattern during ventricular fibrillation in a dog. The thick line in the center of the mapped region does not indicate block but rather is a frame line representing the jump from one map to the next and is required because each static isochronal map can show only a single cycle of a continuous dynamic reentrant circuit. See Figures 7 and 9 for further explanation. Reprinted with permission from Reference 25.*

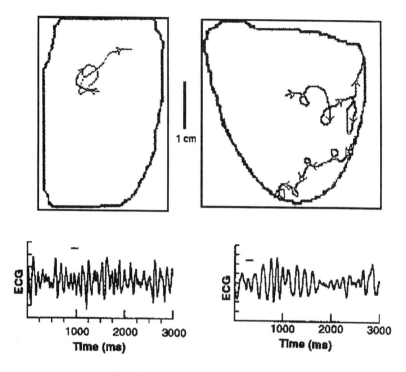

FIGURE 11. *Ventricular fibrillation sometimes follows a spiral pattern of functional reentry called rotors. This figure plots the centers of rapidly moving rotors. Left, Experiment in isolated sheep heart. Right, Computer simulation. Portions of the paths of the organizing centers (cores) of the nonstationary rotors are depicted during fibrillation. Trajectories of the rotor cores were calculated from the surface recordings by use of time-space plots. These rapidly moving cores resulted in irregular electrocardiograms that are characteristic of fibrillation as shown in the bottom two graphs. Reprinted with permission from Reference 13.*

that there was no excitable gap during ventricular fibrillation because the myocardium appeared to be excited as soon as it passed out of its refractory period. Allessie et al[28] recently showed that there is an excitable gap in fibrillating atrial tissue. Evidence now suggests that an excitable gap is present during ventricular fibrillation as well. One piece of evidence is that the refractory period of ventricular muscle to a monophasic electrical stimulus lasting 5 ms with an electrical field strength of 5 V/cm is much shorter than the cycle length during ventricular fibrillation in small dogs. These data suggest that fibrillating myocardium can be field-stimulated well

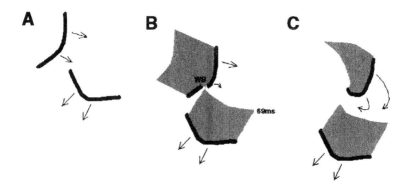

FIGURE 12. *Schematic of the mechanism of spontaneous initiation of reentrant wave fronts. A, Two wave fronts are propagating at roughly right angles to each other. B, One wave front interacts with the tail of the second wave front. The shaded areas represent refractory tissue. Because only part of the wave front encounters refractory tissue, there is a wave break (WB) above which the wave front encounters excitable tissue and thus continues to propagate. The wave break then sets the stage for reentrant excitation (C). Reprinted with permission from Reference 26.*

FIGURE 13. *Fibrillating myocardium can be entrained by use of properly timed electrical stimuli. A, Typical extracellular electrogram from a plaque electrode while pacing during ventricular fibrillation in a pig. The position of this electrode is indicated by the symbol in the upper left frame in B. A 4-second interval of data is shown beginning about 8 seconds after ventricular fibrillation was electrically induced. Periodic vertical lines indicate artifacts from pacing stimuli. The pacing cycle length was 125 ms. Rapid negative deflections indicate depolarization of the myocardium beneath the sensing electrode. At the asterisk, the electrogram morphology changes and activations abruptly become 1:1 phase-locked to the stimulus artifact with repeatable latency, suggesting capture of the tissue around this recording electrode. B, The activation state of fibrillating myocardium beneath the plaque at 10-ms intervals before pacing, during the time interval B in panel A. The frames read from left to right, top row then bottom row. The frame boundary represents the outside border of the 22×23 array of electrodes within the plaque. Areas shaded black within each frame indicate the locations of those electrodes in which the derivative of the potential recording at that instant was more negative than −0.5 V/s, a commonly used threshold value for activation during ventricular fibrillation. In the first frame, an activation front enters at top right and crosses the mapped region over the next several frames. Later activation fronts traverse the mapped region in patterns that change*

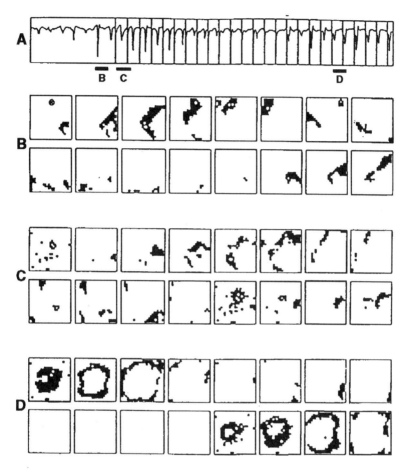

(FIGURE 13 *Continued*) *from cycle to cycle. Activation is present throughout the 150-ms interval represented by the 16 frames. C, Activation sequences during pacing that did not capture the tissue during the time interval C in panel A. Pacing stimuli were applied near the center of the mapped region a few milliseconds before frames 1 and 3. The stippled pattern in the center of these two frames is a result of the pacing artifacts. Activation fronts move across the mapped region unaffected by the pacing stimuli. In the second frame, an activation enters the top of the mapped region and moves from the upper myocardium during the time interval D in panel A. Again, pacing stimuli were applied just before frames 1 and 13. In this case, however, the pacing stimuli directly activate tissue immediately adjacent to the pacing electrodes. Resultant capture occurs until pacing is terminated. This pattern strongly suggests that the tissue was directly excited by the pacing stimulus that gave rise to the propagated activation wave front. A long period of complete electrical quiescence was present in the mapped area during each cycle, as seen in frames 9 through 12. Reprinted with permission from Reference 30.*

before the next action potential would normally occur.[29] The ability to field-stimulate fibrillating myocardium may play an important role in how an electric shock defibrillates the heart.

The second piece of evidence is the demonstration in pigs that it is possible to capture at least 5 cm^2 of ventricular epicardium by rapid pacing during ventricular fibrillation.[30] When pacing stimuli captured the tissue, striking differences in activation patterns were observed compared with either fibrillation without pacing or fibrillation with pacing that did not capture the tissue (Figure 13).

Summary

An understanding of ventricular fibrillation may lead to better drug and device therapies to stop this catastrophic arrhythmia. For instance, knowing which membrane channels are involved in ventricular fibrillation may lead to the development of drugs that are more effective in halting this arrhythmia. Knowledge of how ventricular fibrillation changes over time may be important for developing different therapies for hearts that have been fibrillating for a long time versus hearts that have been fibrillating for only a short time. Likewise, knowledge of the cardiac activation sequence during ventricular fibrillation and how it changes with drugs may lead to therapies that cause the activation sequence to become more amenable to defibrillation. Finally, demonstration that there is an excitable gap during ventricular fibrillation and definition of that excitable gap may lead to device therapies that are more effective and less invasive than current therapies.

References

1. Gillum RF. Sudden coronary death in the United States. *Circulation.* 1989;79:756–765.
2. Bayes de Luna A, Coumel P, Leclercq JF. Ambulatory sudden cardiac death: Mechanisms of production of fatal arrhythmia on the basis of data from 157 cases. *Am Heart J.* 1989;117:151–159.
3. Surawicz B. Ventricular fibrillation, II: progress report since 1971. *Clin Prog Electrophysiol Pacing.* 1984;2:395–419.
4. Jones JL. Ventricular fibrillation. In: Singer I, ed. *Implantable Cardioverter Defibrillator.* Armonk, NY: Futura Publishing Co. Inc; 1994: 43–67.
5. Jones JL, Swartz JF, Jones RE, Fletcher R. Increasing fibrillation duration enhances relative asymmetrical biphasic versus monophasic defibrillator waveform efficacy. *Circ Res.* 1990;67:376–384.
6. Brown CG, Dzwonczyk R, Martin DR. Physiologic measurement of the

ventricular fibrillation ECG signal: estimating the duration of ventricular fibrillation. *Ann Emerg Med.* 1993;22:70–74.

7. Garrey WE. The nature of fibrillatory contractions of the heart: its relation to tissue mass and form. *Am J Physiol.* 1914;33:397–414.

8. Sano T, Sawanobori T. Mechanism initiating ventricular fibrillation demonstrated in cultured ventricular muscle tissue. *Circ Res.* 1970; 26:201–210.

9. Swartz JF, Jones JL, Fletcher RD. Characterization of ventricular fibrillation based on monophasic action potential morphology in the human heart. *Circulation.* 1993;87:1907–1914.

10. Akiyama T. Intracellular recording of in situ ventricular cells during ventricular fibrillation. *Am J Physiol.* 1981;240:H465–H471.

11. Zhou X, Knisley SB, Guse PA, et al. Existence of both fast and slow channel activity during the early stage of ventricular fibrillation. *Circ Res.* 1992;70:773–786.

12. Witkowski FX, Plonsey R, Penkoske PA, Kavanagh KM. Significance of inwardly directed transmembrane current in determination of local myocardial electrical activation during ventricular fibrillation. *Circ Res.* 1994;74:507–524.

13. Gray RA, Jalife J, Panfilov AV, et al. Mechanisms of cardiac fibrillation. *Science.* 1995;270:1222–1223.

14. Worley SJ, Swain JL, Colavita PG, Smith WM, Ideker RE. Development of an endocardial-epicardial gradient of activation rate during electrically induced, sustained ventricular fibrillation in the dog. *Am J Cardiol.* 1985;55:813–820.

15. Wiggers CJ. Studies of ventricular fibrillation caused by electric shock: cinematographic and electrocardiographic observations of the natural process in the dog's heart: its inhibition by potassium and the revival of coordinated beats by calcium. *Am Heart J.* 1930;5: 351–365.

16. Opthof T, Ramdat Misier AR, Coronel R, Vermeulen JT, Verberne HJ, Frank RGJ, Moulijn AC, van Capelle FJL, Janse MJ. Dispersion of refractoriness in canine ventricular myocardium: effects of sympathetic stimulation. *Circ Res.* 1991;68:1204–1215.

17. Herbschleb JN, Heethaar RM, Tweel L, Meijler RL. Frequency analysis of the ECG before and during ventricular fibrillation. 1980;365–368. Abstract.

18. Carlisle EJF, Allen JD, Bailey A, et al. Fourier analysis of ventricular fibrillation and synchronization of DC countershocks in defibrillation. *J Electrocardiol.* 1988;21:337–343.

19. Carlisle EJF, Allen JD, Kernohan WG, Anderson J, Adgey AAJ. Fourier analysis of ventricular fibrillation of varied aetiology. *Eur Heart J.* 1990;11:173–181.

20. Dzwonczyk R, Brown CG, Werman HA. The median frequency of the ECG during ventricular fibrillation: its use in an algorithm for estimating the duration of cardiac arrest. *IEEE Trans Biomed Eng.* 1990;37:640–646.

21. Yakaitis RW, Ewy GA, Otto CW, Taren DL, Moon TE. Influence of time and therapy on ventricular defibrillation in dogs. *Crit Care Med.* 1980;8:157–163.

22. Janse MJ, van Capelle FJL, Morsink H, et al. Flow of "injury" current and patterns of excitation during early ventricular arrhythmias in acute regional myocardial ischemia in isolated porcine and canine

hearts: evidence for two different arrhythmogenic mechanisms. *Circ Res.* 1980;47:151–165.

23. Pogwizd SM, Corr PB. Mechanisms underlying the development of ventricular fibrillation during early myocardial ischemia. *Circ Res.* 1990;66:672–695.

24. Moe GK, Rheinboldt WC, Abildskov JA. A computer model of atrial fibrillation. *Am Heart J.* 1964;67:200–220.

25. Chen P-S, Wolf PD, Melnick SB, Danieley ND, Smith WM, Ideker RE. Comparison of activation during ventricular fibrillation and following unsuccessful defibrillation shocks in open chest dogs. *Circ Res.* 1990; 66:1544–1560.

26. Lee JJ, Kamjoo K, Hough D, et al. Reentrant wavefronts in Wiggers' stage II ventricular fibrillation. *Circ Res.* 1996;78:660–675.

27. Bayly PV, Johnson EE, Wolf PD, Smith WM, Ideker RE. Predicting patterns of epicardial potentials during ventricular fibrillation. *IEEE Trans Biomed Eng.* 1995;42:898–907.

28. Allessie M, Kirchhof C, Scheffer GJ, Chorro F, Brugada J. Regional control of atrial fibrillation by rapid pacing in conscious dogs. *Circulation.* 1991;84:1689–1697.

29. Zhou X, Wolf PD, Rollins DL, Afework Y, Smith WM, Ideker RE. Effects of monophasic and biphasic shocks on action potentials during ventricular fibrillation in dogs. *Circ Res.* 1993;73:325–334.

30. KenKnight BH, Bayly PV, Gerstle RJ, et al. Regional capture of fibrillating ventricular myocardium: evidence of an excitable gap. *Circ Res.* 1995;77;849–855.

31. Janse MJ, Wilms-Schopman FJG, Coronel R. Ventricular fibrillation is not always due to multiple wavelet reentry. *J Cardiovasc Electrophysiol.* 1996;6:512–521.

Chapter 6

Temporal Patterns of Ventricular Tachyarrhythmias:
Insights from the Implantable Cardioverter-Defibrillator

Mark A. Wood, MD, Pippa M. Simpson, PhD,
Larry S. Liebovitch, PhD,
Angelo T. Todorov, PhD, and
Kenneth A. Ellenbogen, MD

The implantable cardioverter-defibrillator (ICD) has revolutionized the management of patients with recurrent life-threatening ventricular arrhythmias by preventing sudden death, as shown in many studies.[1,2] The incorporation of data storage capacity into ICD's has greatly advanced our understanding of the function of these devices and has provided valuable insights into the many clinical aspects of spontaneous ventricular arrhythmias.[3,4] By continuously monitoring heart rate and recording the time and date of ventricular tachyarrhythmia (VT) events, these devices provide an unprecedented source of data for the analysis of the temporal patterns of ventricular arrhythmias. Knowledge of these long-term temporal patterns can have important implications for the management of these arrhythmias. This chapter describes our current understanding of the temporal patterns of ventricular arrhythmias as made possible by the ICD and describes the many clinical implications of this knowledge.

Data Logging by ICDs

The ICD continuously monitors the ventricular heart rate through epicardial or endocardial pacing/sensing leads and re-

From: Dunbar SB, Ellenbogen KA, Epstein AE, (eds). *Sudden Cardiac Death: Past, Present, and Future.* Armonk, NY: Futura Publishing Company, Inc.; © 1997.

sponds by delivering antitachycardia therapies when programmable heart rate and duration criteria are met for tachycardia detection. The time, date, tachycardia rate, delivered therapy, and response to therapy can be stored in clearable electronic memory for 1 to >100 tachycardia detections, depending on the features of the ICD. These data are retrieved by use of the ICD programmer, with the time and date of the arrhythmic events generated by reference to the programmer's internal clock (Figure 1). Regular device interrogation can provide accurate temporal records of all arrhythmic events fulfilling detection criteria over years of follow-up in individual patients.[5] The continuous long-term nature of this follow-up by ICDs represents a major technological advance in chronological research. The previously relied-upon patient interviews, hospital records, and limited ambulatory electrocardiographic (Holter) monitoring to establish the times of arrhythmic events all suffer from the shortcomings of inherent inaccuracy or very limited periods of observation.[6,7] For chronobiological studies, continuous monitoring over prolonged durations is optimal.[8] In ICD studies, the confirmation of each detection as due to VT and not supraventricular arrhythmias or noise is crucial to the accuracy

```
** PATIENT THERAPY HISTORY **

        Date : 05/15/1993    Episode - 15    Attempt - 1   of 1

        Time of detection      - 21:26:43
        Device State           - Monitor + Therapy
        Pre-attempt R-R mean   -  375 msec.  160 BPM
        Detection criteria met - Duration
        Zone of Therapy        - 1
        Therapy used           - Defib Shock #1 @   5 joules
        Conversion successful  - Yes
        Therapy aborted        - No
        Arrhythmia accelerated - No
        Post-attempt monitoring- 11 cycles
        Post-attempt R-R mean  -  750 msec.   80 BPM

        Pre and Post Episode R-R intervals
Pre :  344, 336, 375, 375, 375, 367, 359, 363, 367, 398, 344, 398 msec.
Post:  148, 883,1172,1031, 914, 828, 781, 773, 758, 750, 750, 742 msec.
```

FIGURE 1. Data printout for a spontaneous VT event recorded by a CPI PRx defibrillator. The time and date of the detections are shown, as well as the tachycardia cycle length, therapy delivered (5-J cardioversion), and response to therapy. The 12 RR intervals before and immediately after therapy are shown.

of the study. The analysis of stored electrograms and RR intervals during arrhythmia detections can accurately discriminate between spurious and appropriate detections.[3,9]

Circadian Patterns of Ventricular Arrhythmias

To date, five published studies have documented a circadian periodicity to the occurrence of VT detections by ICDs.[5,10-13] The salient features of these studies are summarized in Table 1. In the study by Wood et al,[5] the times of detection of 830 sustained or nonsustained VTs from 43 patients with ischemic and nonischemic heart disease were fit to a single harmonic sine curve model with 24-hour periodicity. The single harmonic model best fit the data in Loess curve analysis. Detection in each individual patient was weighted according to the total number of detections in that patient during follow-up to give all patients equal representation in the analysis. Mean follow-up duration was 226 ± 179 days. In this study, the distribution of all 830 detections fit the sine curve model, with 95% confidence intervals for the peak frequency from 1:13 to 4:13 PM ($r=0.75$, $P<0.05$) (Figure 2). Similar circadian distributions were found in analysis of only those detections resulting in shock or antitachycardia pacing therapy, shock, spontaneous termination, detections from only those patients with coronary artery disease (81% of the study group), or patients taking no antiarrhythmic medication during follow-up (all $r=0.53$ to 0.73; all $P<0.05$). The 95% confidence intervals for the peak frequencies for these subgroups were from 11:38 AM to 5:44 PM. The nadir occurred 12 hours before peak frequencies in all analyses. Notably, no circadian pattern was discernable in 15 patients receiving antiarrhythmic drug therapy continuously during follow-up (70% of these patients took either amiodarone or propafenone). A similar blunting of the circadian pattern for ventricular ectopy has also been described for patients receiving β-blockers or sotalol.[14,15]

Lampert et al[10] reported a distinct circadian pattern to 2558 sustained VT detections recorded from 32 patients with coronary artery disease. In that study, only tachyarrhythmias with rates <240 bpm were analyzed, so as to exclude ventricular fibrillation events. Follow-up averaged 14 ± 7 months. For all events, the 24-hour distribution fit a fourth-order harmonic regression model with primary peak between 6 AM and noon (first harmonic peak, 9:18 AM) and a secondary peak between noon and 6 PM ($R^2=0.91$; both $P<0.05$). These data were then weighted for each patient by

TABLE 1

Summary of Five Published Studies Using Implantable Defibrillators to Document Circadian Patterns to Ventricular Tachycardia Recurrences.

Study (Reference)	No. of Patients	Disease	No. of Events	Statistical Methodology	Primary Peak	Secondary Peak	Nadir	Comments
Wood et al (5)	43	CAD NI	830	Loess curve Single harmonic model	2:43 PM (1:13 to 4:13 PM)*	None	2:43 AM	Weighted analysis No circadian pattern on AAD therapy
Lampert et al (10)	32	CAD	2558	ANOVA Single harmonic regression	6 AM to noon	Noon to 6 PM	Not specified	Weighted and unweighted analyses No effect of AAD
Tofler et al (11)	483	CAD NI	10483	X^2 goodness-of-fit	9 AM to noon	Noon	3 to 6 AM	Unweighted analysis Same results for fast and slow VT analysis
Mallavarapu et al (12)	390	CAD	2692	Sinusoidal density function	10 to 11 AM	None	2 to 3 AM	Unweighted analysis 81% of known events not analyzed
Behrens et al (13)	39	CAD NI	207	X^2 goodness-of-fit	7 to 11 AM	4 to 8 PM	Not specified	83% of known events not analyzed

CAD indicates coronary artery disease; NI, nonischemic heart disease; and AAD, antiarrhythmic drug therapy.
*95% confidence intervals.

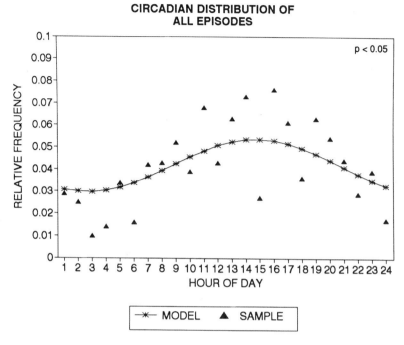

FIGURE 2. *Circadian distribution of 830 ICD detections recorded from 43 patients. The data are represented in weighted hourly totals for events to give each patient equal representation in the analysis regardless of the absolute number of detections during follow-up. The peak frequency of detections occurs at 2:43 PM (95% confidence interval, 1:13 to 4:13 PM).*

counting only a single episode in any hour on a given day to reduce skewing of the data by patients with frequent repetitive events. The weighted analysis fit a third-order harmonic regression curve with a peak between 6 AM and noon ($P<0.001$). A secondary peak was evident between noon and 6 PM. The presence or absence of circadian pattern in individual patients was not predicted by left ventricular ejection fraction, total frequency of detections, presenting arrhythmia, or use of β-blockers or antiarrhythmic drugs.

Tofler et al[11] used X^2 goodness-of-fit analysis to study data from 483 patients with 9266 episodes of VT ≤250 bpm and 1217 episodes of VT >250 bpm. Both "fast" and "slow" VT detections showed maximal frequencies in the period of 9 AM to noon (both, $P < 0.001$). In this study, patients with lower ejection fractions and NYHA class IV heart failure demonstrated blunted 6 AM to noon peaks and an attenuated nighttime fall in arrhythmia frequency.

In this study, detections occurring ≤1 minute apart were counted as a single event; however, no other weighting of patient data was included. Mallavarapu et al[12] found a peak in ventricular arrhythmia frequency between 10 and 11 AM in 390 patients with 2692 detections. This pattern was not influenced by left ventricular ejection fraction or detection cycle length. The findings of Behrens et al[13] also describe a peak frequency between 6 AM and noon and a secondary peak between 4 and 6 PM. In both the studies by Mallavarapu et al and Behrens et al, only 17% of all recorded tachycardia detections could be analyzed because of characteristics of the ICDs used.

Direct comparisons of these studies as published is made difficult by differing patient populations, selection of events for analysis, and statistical methodologies. Particularly different are the methods (if any) used to correct for grossly unequal numbers of recorded events for each patient and choice of a temporal model for data fitting in these studies. In an effort to compare these studies, the published data on the hourly frequencies of events from Wood et al, Lampert et al, Tofler et al, and Mallavarapu et al were each subjected to Loess curve analysis (Figure 3). This iterative curve-fitting analysis involves no a priori assumptions about the data distribution. When published, the weighted data sets were used in this analysis. Under this uniform method of analysis, the data from these four studies show striking similarity in circadian periodicities for the arrhythmic events. Each data set fit a single harmonic model (all $P<0.05$). Importantly, there is overlap in the calculated 95% confidence intervals for the time of peak frequency in all four studies between 1:18 and 1:48 PM. This convergence of findings suggests a common circadian pattern to ICD detections; however, the description of this pattern is influenced by statistical approaches and possibly by individual patient data in unweighted studies. Other potential sources of discrepancy between studies include nonuniform antiarrhythmic drug use, differing study criteria for exclusion of spurious tachycardia detections, and the unanalyzed influences of sleep-wake cycles in the ICD patient population.

In general, these studies agree with the primary morning peak in the occurrence of sudden cardiac death described in several large epidemiological studies.[16-18] The primary or secondary afternoon peaks for ICD detections in two studies may reflect the secondary peak described in the occurrence of sudden death. The lack of uniformity in afternoon ICD detection peaks between studies may represent somewhat different patient populations and differing statistical techniques, as described above. Primary afternoon peaks in ventricular arrhythmia frequency have been described in Holter

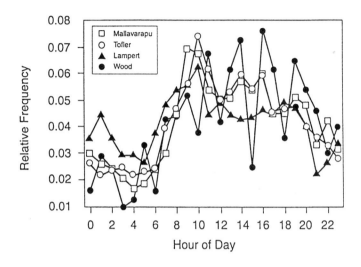

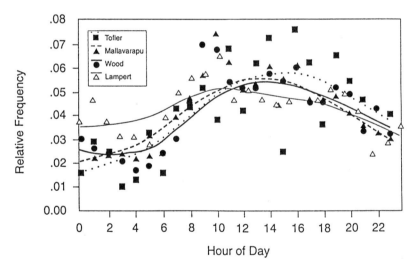

FIGURE 3. *Top, Combined graph showing circadian distribution of ICD detections from four published studies (Wood et al, Lampert et al, Tofler et al, and Mallavarapu et al). This graph shows the distribution of detections as published in each study. Bottom, Combined graph showing data from each of the four studies at top after each study was subjected to Loess curve-fitting analysis. Each study data set fit a sine curve model (all P<0.05). The 95% confidence intervals for the peaks of each study in the analysis overlapped between 1:18 and 1:48 PM.*

studies of postinfarction patients, however.[14,19] Although a similar pattern for both sudden cardiac death and ICD detections may seem logical, it need not necessarily follow that peak ICD detection coincides precisely with epidemiologically derived times of sudden death. Possibly, the mechanisms responsible for these events differ; ie, morning sudden death may result more frequently from acute ischemia and afternoon ventricular arrhythmias from electrical, autonomic, or metabolic factors. A significant percentage of sudden deaths also result from bradyarrhythmias and nonarrhythmic deaths, which are not reflected by ICD detections.[20] Also, differing hemodynamic tolerance of arrhythmias at different times of day could result in a higher proportion of sudden death in the early morning, despite a lower absolute morning VT frequency. Notably, Johns et al[21] found a reduced ICD first-shock efficiency to terminate ventricular arrhythmia occurring between 6 and 9 AM compared with all other times of day.[21] This suggests a more compromised electrophysiological substrate in the morning hours. Finally, it is interesting to speculate that recurrent arrhythmic events in ICD patients represent highly nonphysiological situations in that survival of the first episode of sudden death by definition does not occur in nature. The temporal patterns of subsequent "fatal" events may differ from the first.

Infradian Patterns of Ventricular Arrhythmias

Infradian (>28-hour) periodicity as well as circadian periodicity has been described for the occurrence of ventricular arrhythmias. Analysis of the data on circadian patterns for 830 ICD detections in 43 patients reveals a significant weekly pattern to these events, with peak frequencies occurring Monday through Tuesday and the nadir on Sunday. These findings are in agreement with the findings of Arntz et al[22] in describing peak incidence of sudden death on Mondays in 24061 patients. That study found a similar primary morning and secondary afternoon peak to sudden death occurrence on each weekday and also a seasonal variation, with lowest incidence in summer (May through July) and highest incidence in winter (November through January). Mittleman et al[23] also described a winter peak in ICD detections of ventricular arrhythmias in 194 patients.

We have undertaken a more detailed characterization of the long-term temporal patterns to ventricular arrhythmias. In a study of 31 patients with ICDs, the observed distribution of interdetection intervals was compared with a model for the expected random distribution of these events over the follow-up duration in each patient.[24] The average number of detections was 23±35 per patient (range, 3 to 101), and mean follow-up was 227±183 days. In 28 of 31 patients, the observed distribution of these events over time differed significantly from the expected random distribution because of a propensity of interdetection intervals that were shorter than predicted by the random models in all patients (Figure 4). This pattern denotes a

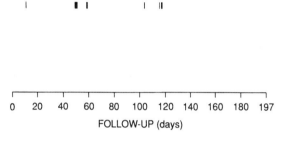

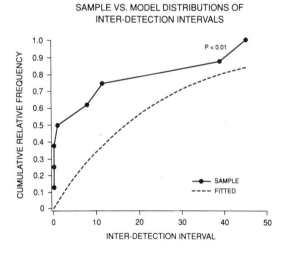

FIGURE 4. *Top, Distribution of 11 tachycardia detections during 197 days of follow-up in a 57-year-old man. Multiple closely timed detections are represented by the width of the graph markers. One detection occurred on day 11, 4 on day 50, 2 on day 58, 1 on day 104, 1 on day 116, and 2 on day 117. Bottom, Line graph showing cumulative relative frequency vs interdetection interval for the observed distribution of events in the top and the same patient's model for expected random distribution of these events. The difference between these lines (P<0.01) results from a higher frequency of shorter interdetection intervals than is predicted by the model of random distribution.*

temporal clustering of tachycardia detections, with 55% of all inter-detection intervals ≤1 hour and 69% ≤24 hours. This clustering of events was not altered by the presence or absence of antiarrhythmic drugs, tachycardia cycle length, indication for ICD implant, nature of heart disease, or exclusion of nonsustained arrhythmias. This study demonstrates that the occurrences of ICD detections are non-randomly distributed over time because of temporal clustering and has important implications for the management of ventricular arrhythmias (see below).

Determinants of Temporal Patterns

The circadian pattern to sudden death has been closely associated with the known circadian pattern of myocardial ischemia, as evidenced by morning peaks in the frequencies of myocardial infarction, silent ischemia, and provocable ischemia.[25-27] Because most patients in the ICD studies presented here had underlying coronary artery disease, morning ischemia is a likely factor contributing to the circadian pattern of ICD detections. The ischemia, in turn, results from enhanced morning platelet aggregability, elevated serum catecholamine levels, increased coronary artery resistance and systolic blood pressure, increased heart rate, and elevated ventricular wall stress.[28] The attenuation of circadian patterns of both myocardial ischemia and ventricular ectopy by β-blocker therapy appears to support the role of sympathetic activation and/or enhanced myocardial oxygen demands in these events.[14,29]

A variety of metabolic changes, for example, in serum potassium, cortisol, and catecholamines, also follow circadian variations that may influence the temporal patterns of arrhythmic events.[28,30] The occurrence of circadian distribution in patients not taking drugs excludes waning drug effects as a cause.[9]

Circadian patterns in electrophysiological properties of the heart may be influential. Kocovic et al[31] demonstrated correlation between ventricular ectopic activity and diurnal QT shortening. Ventricular refractoriness begins to shorten about 9 AM after maximal values from midnight to early morning.[32] Heart rate variability is minimal during the hours from 8 AM to noon in sudden death survivors.[33] Several studies have documented late morning and afternoon peaks in the frequency of isolated premature ventricular beats and nonsustained ventricular ectopy, which may serve as triggers for sustained arrhythmias.[34,35]

At present, the precise factors or interplay of factors that determine the temporal patterns of ventricular arrhythmias remain undefined. Undoubtedly, myocardial ischemia plays a role; however, the clustering of arrhythmic events into hours and days suggests more long-lasting influences, such as persistent metabolic or autonomic states. The electrophysiological influences of a primary arrhythmic event facilitating subsequent episodes by changes in dispersion of repolarization may also explain clustering of events. The mechanistic explanation for these temporal patterns is a fertile area for research.

Clinical Implications

The recognition of the temporal patterns of ventricular arrhythmias has far-reaching implications for the understanding and management of these events. First, the circadian and temporal patterns provide clues to the triggers of and influences on the occurrence of ventricular arrhythmias, as described above.

Second, characterization of such chronological patterns may provide prognostic information about individual patients. Previous studies have demonstrated that an amplified and phase-shifted circadian pattern of ventricular ectopy can differentiate those patients who die of sudden death from those surviving in the 5 years after myocardial infarction.[8] In this study, comparison of mean and variance of the frequency of ventricular ectopy failed to separate these two patient groups. Conceivably, demonstration of "atypical" temporal patterns to ventricular arrhythmia recurrences may also identify patients with poor prognosis.

Third, understanding temporal patterns appears to identify, in some measure, periods of vulnerability for arrhythmia occurrence. On the basis of the current literature, mornings and/or early afternoons, Mondays, and winter months are statistically the times of greatest risk. Also, the clustering of events suggests that the hours and days after a single ICD tachycardia detection is perhaps a better-defined time of risk. This knowledge may allow for preemptive drug or electrical therapies during these periods.

Finally, description of nonrandom, systematic, long-term patterns to ventricular arrhythmias as presented above may force a reevaluation of the current practice of directing antiarrhythmic drug therapy on the basis of serial short-term electrocardiographic monitoring. This approach assumes that the frequencies of ventricular arrhythmic events during serial short-term electrocardiographic monitoring can be characterized and compared by conventional statistical parameters, such as mean and variance. Reduction or exacerbation of arrhythmia frequency beyond statistical limits on repeated observations is commonly used to evaluate the safety and efficiency of pharmacological therapies, although the day-to-day baseline variations in arrhythmia frequency is recognized as large.[36] The demonstration that recurrent ICD detections are nonrandomly distributed over time necessitates that some systematic pattern is present. To characterize this systematic pattern, the authors examined the relationship between the value of the ICD interdetection interval and relative frequency for that interval for 28 patients with 800 recorded ICD detections. In Figure 5, the linear re-

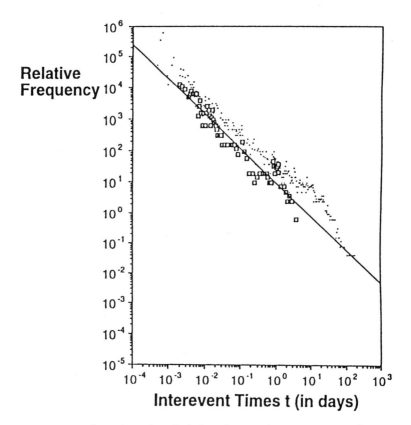

FIGURE 5. *Log-log plot of probability density function P(t) (ordinate), vs interdetection interval (abscissa) for a single patient recording 196 detections over 90 days of follow-up (large markers). The distribution fits a power-law distribution P(t) = t⁻ᵃ, with α = 1.09). This distribution is consistent with a self-affine (fractal) time distribution for these events. The small markers represent the power-law distribution of 800 detections recorded by 23 patients. The value of α for these pooled data is 0.98, again consistent with a self-affine pattern.*

lationship between these variables in the log-log plot follows the power law distribution $P(t)=t^{-\alpha}$, where $P(t)$ is the probability density function of the number of detections and t is the interdetection time interval. The value of α for this data sample is 0.98. Such a distribution is said to be scale invariant, fractal, or more correctly, self-affine up to intervals of 10 days.[37] This means that the temporal distribution is statistically similar over a wide range of time scales or periods of observation. This pattern is also evident in an individual patient (not included in the group analysis) with frequent detections (Figure 5). This patient had 196 detections over 90 days of follow-up. The value of α for this relationship was 1.09.

The significance of the self-affine pattern is that the concepts of mean and variance do not apply for the frequency of these events. Because of the time scale invariance, any derivation of mean and variance of arrhythmia frequency is an artifact of the duration of observation. With progressively longer periods of observation, the values of mean and variance increase as well without approaching a single finite value. Without valid estimates of mean and variance, the practice of suppressing arrhythmia recurrence to statistical limits on the basis of these calculations may be in question. These findings are based on relatively sustained arrhythmic events meeting detection criteria of ICDs and require validation for the distribution of isolated ventricular ectopic events, which are the predominant form analyzed on electrocardiographic monitoring. Stein et al,[38] however, demonstrated a fractal character to isolated ventricular ectopy recurrence over very short periods of observation.

Conclusions

The data storage capacity of ICDs has demonstrated daily, weekly, and seasonal variations in tachycardia recurrences. At this time, long-term temporal patterns of ventricular arrhythmias are characterized as nonrandom and possibly self-affine over different time scales. The mechanisms during these temporal patterns are unknown and require further investigation. Knowledge of these temporal patterns will advance our understanding of the arrhythmias and may dramatically influence our current practice of assigning drug therapy.

References

1. Kelly PA, Cannon DS, Garan H, et al. The automatic implantable cardioverter-defibrillator: efficacy, complications and survival in

patients with malignant ventricular arrhythmias. *J Am Coll Cardiol.* 1988;11:1278–1286.

2. Fogoros R. The effect of the implantable cardioverter-defibrillator on sudden death and on total survival. *Pacing Clin Electrophysiol.* 1993;16: 506–510.

3. Hurwitz JL, Hook BG, Flores BT, Marchlinski FE. Importance of abortive shock capability and electrogram storage in cardioverter-defibrillator devices. *J Am Coll Cardiol.* 1993;21:895–900.

4. Wood MA, Stambler BS, Damiano RJ, Greenway P, Ellenbogen KA. Lessons learned from data logging in a multicenter clinical trial using a late-generation implantable cardioverter-defibrillator. *J Am Coll Cardiol.* 1994;24:1692–1699.

5. Wood MA, Simpson PM, London WB, et al. Circadian pattern of ventricular tachyarrhythmias in patients with implantable cardioverter-defibrillators. *J Am Coll Cardiol.* 1995;25:901–907.

6. Twisdale N, Taylor S, Heddle WF, Ayres BF, Tonkin AM. Morning increase in the time of onset of sustained ventricular tachycardia. *Am J Cardiol.* 1989;64:1204–1206.

7. Raeder EA, Hohnloser SH, Graboys TB, Podrid PJ, Lambert S, Lown B. Spontaneous variability and circadian distribution of ectopic activity in patients with malignant ventricular arrhythmia. *J Am Coll Cardiol.* 1988;12:656–661.

8. Cornelissen G, Bokken E, Delmore P, et al. From various kinds of heart rate variability to chronocardiology. *Am J Cardiol.* 1990;66:863–868.

9. Wang PJ, Mandalakas N, Clyne C, et al. Accuracy of rhythm classification using a data log system in implantable cardioverter defibrillators. *Pacing Clin Electrophysiol.* 1991;14:1911–1916.

10. Lampert R, Rosenfeld L, Batsford W, Lee F, McPherson C. Circadian variation of sustained ventricular tachycardia in patients with coronary artery disease and implantable cardioverter defibrillators. *Circulation.* 1994;90:241–247.

11. Tofler GH, Gebara OCE, Mittleman MA, et al. Morning peak in ventricular tachyarrhythmias detected by time of implantable cardioverter/defibrillator therapy. *Circulation.* 1995;92:1203–1208.

12. Mallavarapu C, Pancholy S, Swartzman D, et al. Circadian variation of ventricular arrhythmia recurrences after cardioverter-defibrillator implantation in patients with healed myocardial infarction. *Am J Cardiol.* 1995;75:1140–1144.

13. Behrens S, Galecka M, Bruggeman T, et al. Circadian variation of sustained ventricular tachyarrhythmias terminated by appropriate shocks in patients with an implantable cardioverter defibrillator. *Am Heart J.* 1995;130:79–84.

14. Gillis AM, Peters RW, Mitchell LB, Duff HJ, MacDonald M, Wyse DG. Effects of left ventricular dysfunction on the circadian variation of ventricular premature complexes in healed myocardial infarction. *Am J Cardiol.* 1992;69:1009–1014.

15. Hohnloser SH, Zabel M, Just H, Ralder EA. Relation of diurnal variation of ventricular repolarization to ventricular ectopic activity and modification by sotalol. *Am J Cardiol.* 1993;71:475–478.

16. Muller JE, Ludmer PL, Willich RN, et al. Circadian variation in the frequency of sudden cardiac death. *Circulation.* 1987;75:131–138.

17. Willich SN, Levy D, Rocco MB, Tofler GH, Stone PH, Muller JE. Circadian variation in the incidence of sudden cardiac death in the Framingham heart study population. *Am J Cardiol.* 1987;60:801–806.

18. Arntz HR, Willich SN, Oeff M, et al. Circadian variation of sudden cardiac death reflects age-related variability in ventricular fibrillation. *Circulation.* 1993;88:2284–2289.
19. Zehender M, Meinertz T, Hohnloser S, et al. Prevalence of circadian variations in spontaneous variability of cardiac disorders and ECG changes suggestive of myocardial ischemia in systemic arterial hypertension. *Circulation.* 1992;85:1808–1815.
20. Bayes de Luna AB, Coumel P, Leclercq JF. Ambulatory sudden cardiac death: mechanisms of production of fatal arrhythmias. *Am Heart J.* 1989;117:151–159.
21. Johns RM, Martin DT, Vendetti FJ. Circadian variation in first shock efficacy of an ICD system. *J Am Coll Cardiol.* 1996;27:98A. Abstract.
22. Arntz HR, Willich RN, Brüggeman T, et al. Seasonal and weekly variations in risk of sudden death. *J Am Coll Cardiol.* 1996;27:107A. Abstract.
23. Mittleman RS, Zhang X, Stanlk EJ, et al. Ventricular tachyarrhythmias occur more frequently in winter and less frequently in spring than in other seasons: report from a multicenter implantable cardioverter defibrillator (ICD) database. *J Am Coll Cardiol.* 1996;27:97A. Abstract.
24. Wood MA, Simpson PM, Stambler BS, Herre JM, Bernstein RC, Ellenbogen KA. Long-term temporal patterns of ventricular tachyarrhythmias. *Circulation.* 1995;91:2371–2377.
25. Muller JE, Stone PH, Turi ZG, et al. Circadian variation in the frequency of onset of acute myocardial infarction. *N Engl J Med.* 1985;313:1315–1322.
26. Rocco MB, Barry J, Campbell S, et al. Circadian variation of transient myocardial ischemia in patients with coronary artery disease. *Circulation.* 1987;75:395–400.
27. Quyyumi AA. Circadian rhythms in cardiovascular disease. *Am Heart J.* 1990;120:726–733.
28. Rocco MB. Timing and triggers of transient myocardial ischemia. *Am J Cardiol.* 1990;66:18G–21G.
29. Imperi GA, Lambert CR, Coy K, Lopez C, Pepine LJ. Effects of titrated beta blockade (metoprolol) on silent myocardial ischemia in ambulatory patients with coronary artery disease. *Am J Cardiol.* 1987;60:519–524.
30. Soloman R, Weinberg MS, Dubey A. The diurnal rhythm of plasma potassium: relationship to diuretic therapy. *J Cardiovasc Pharmacol.* 1991;17:854–859.
31. Kocovic D, Velimirovic D, Djordjivic M, Pavlovic S, Savic D, Stoganov P. Association between stimulated QT interval and ventricular rhythm disturbances: influences of autonomic nervous system. *Pacing Clin Electrophysiol.* 1988;11:1722–1731.
32. Circa J, Moya A, Figueros J, Roma F, Rius J. Circadian variations in the electrical properties of the human heart assessed by sequential bedside electrophysiologic testing. *Am Heart J.* 1986;112:315–321.
33. Huikuri HV, Linnaluoto MK, Seppänen TV, et al. Circadian rhythm of heart rate variability in survivors of cardiac arrest. *Am J Cardiol.* 1992;70:610–615.
34. Lanza GA, Cartellesa MC, Rebuzzi AG, et al. Reproducibility in circadian rhythm of ventricular premature complexes. *Am J Cardiol.* 1990;66:1099–1106.
35. Canada WB, Woodward W, Lee G, et al. Circadian rhythm of hourly ventricular arrhythmia frequency in man. *Angiology.* 1983;34:274–282.

36. Anastasiou-Nana MI, Menloue RC, Nanus JN, Anderson JL. Changes in spontaneous variability of ventricular ectopic activity as a function of time in patients with chronic arrhythmias. *Circulation.* 1988;78: 286:295.
37. Bassingthwaite JB, Liebovitch LS, West BJ. Introduction: fractals really are everywhere. In: *Fractal Physiology.* New York, NY: Oxford University Press; 1994:3–44.
38. Stein KM, Borer JS, Hochreiter C, Kligfield P. Fractal clustering of ventricular ectopy and sudden death in mitral regurgitation. *J Electrocardiol.* 1992;25(suppl):178–181.

Chapter 7

The Primary Prevention of Sudden Cardiac Death:
Prospective Identification of the Problem. Noninvasive and Invasive Techniques for Risk Stratification

Alfred E. Buxton, MD

Prospective Identification of the Problem: Rationale

Sudden cardiac death occurs 1000 times every day in the United States. Although effective treatments are available for survivors of out-of-hospital cardiac arrest, only 2% to 30% of out-of-hospital arrest victims survive to benefit from such treatments.[1-5] Clearly, primary prevention is preferable and necessary, if we are to improve the survival of patients with heart disease. In almost every type of cardiac disease, half of the deaths occur suddenly and unexpectedly.

Effective primary prevention in a resource-limited environment is dependent on several factors. First, the populations at highest risk of sudden death must be identified. Second, the mechanisms responsible for sudden death in each at-risk population must be understood. Third, understanding of these mechanisms should be used to develop tests to identify subpopulations of patients at highest risk. Fourth, based on understanding of these mechanisms, treatments specific for each mechanism must be applied.

At the present time, our understanding of these factors is incomplete. We do know that a majority of sudden death victims have structural heart disease, and in 80%, sudden death is not the

From: Dunbar SB, Ellenbogen KA, Epstein AE, (eds). *Sudden Cardiac Death: Past, Present, and Future.* Armonk, NY: Futura Publishing Company, Inc.; © 1997.

initial manifestation of cardiac disease. We know that in ≈75% of sudden death victims, coronary artery disease is the major anatomic substrate. It is clear that a variety of mechanisms may precipitate sudden death in patients with coronary disease. However, we have a very poor understanding of the mechanisms causing sudden death in persons without coronary artery disease.

The variety of mechanisms capable of precipitating sudden death means that no single test will permit identification of all patients at risk. Each patient must be approached individually, and preliminary simple and cheap screening methods must be applied to identify those patients likely to fall into broad, relatively high-risk categories and likely to benefit from preventive therapy.

Further complicating the appropriate use and interpretation of tests to screen for patients at risk for sudden death is the fact that patients and their diseases are not static. Rather, disease processes evolve over time, resulting in the potential for dynamic changes in mechanisms causing cardiac arrest and sudden death. Take, for example, the case of coronary artery disease. Early in its course, the most common factor precipitating cardiac arrest is acute ischemia, as in the early phase of acute myocardial infarction. Although survivors of acute infarction may remain at risk for ischemically mediated cardiac arrest, the most prominent cause of sudden death after remote myocardial infarction is ventricular tachycardia resulting from intramyocardial reentry. In later stages of the disease, some patients develop the syndrome of congestive heart failure, with its attendant neurohormonal, fluid, electrolyte, and other perturbations. These abnormalities in turn predispose to other mechanisms of ventricular tachyarrhythmias. In addition, drugs used to treat the various symptomatic manifestations of coronary disease may further alter arrhythmia substrates. It should be clear, then, that even in the case of patients with coronary artery disease, mechanisms causing ventricular tachyarrhythmias evolve over time, and thus, no single screening test is likely to be appropriate throughout the course of the disease.

Populations at Risk of Sudden Death

Screening tests all carry expenses and risks, both direct and indirect. Therefore, to apply them intelligently, one must have an idea of the patient populations most likely to benefit from interventions based on the test results. For example, although out-of-hospital cardiac arrests do occur in persons without recognizable heart disease, the incidence of this is so rare that it is not realistic or appropriate to apply any screening test to asymptomatic, apparently healthy individuals. The populations most likely to benefit from screening may be determined from examination of reports of victims of out-of-hospital cardiac arrest. These studies have consistently shown a prevalence of 70% to 80% of coronary artery disease in victims of out-of-hospital arrest.[6-9] Excluded from most of these series are patients in whom the cardiac arrest complicated acute myocardial infarction. If such patients are included, the relative prevalence of coronary artery disease in patients suffering out-of-hospital cardiac arrest obviously increases. However, it should be noted that earlier series found evidence of acute myocardial infarction in far fewer than 50% of out-of-hospital cardiac arrests.[1-3] Cardiomyopathies, both dilated and hypertrophic, constitute the next most common anatomic abnormality. Apparently even less frequent are arrests in patients with hypertension, valvular disease, and miscellaneous conditions such as cardiac sarcoidosis and right ventricular dysplasia. Much less common are primary electrical abnormalities such as the long-QT syndromes, Wolff-Parkinson-White syndrome, and other idiopathic types of ventricular tachycardia and fibrillation.

The remainder of this chapter will review the role of screening tests in the most common cardiac conditions associated with sudden death. We will consider the utility of screening tests to predict both overall cardiac mortality and sudden cardiac deaths. Although some investigators argue about limitations in our ability to accurately classify deaths as sudden and presumably due to arrhythmias, experience with an ongoing multicenter trial has convinced us that this is usually possible. The importance of finding a test that can specifically predict sudden, arrhythmic death lies in its clinical utility. The usefulness of tests that merely indicate patients at increased mortality risk is limited to our being able to advise patients of this fact. Nonspecific tests do not permit physicians to institute specific treatments that may alter the mortality risk. On the other hand, if one knows that a certain positive test predicts tachyarrhythmic death specifically, there is a rationale to institute a specific type of antiarrhythmic therapy, with the hope of altering the course of the disease.

Coronary Artery Disease

As noted above, the dynamic nature of coronary artery disease makes it unlikely that any single screening test will be found to be appropriate and useful in all patients. Furthermore, any test that correctly identifies patients at risk at one stage in their disease may lose its usefulness as the disease evolves in the same patients. Nonetheless, there are several times in the course of coronary artery disease at which patients have been identified as being at especially high risk for sudden death, and a number of screening tests have been evaluated for utility in these settings.

The period of highest risk is the first 24 hours (and especially the first hour) after the onset of acute myocardial infarction. The recognition of this association led to the development of mobile rescue units and the coronary care unit in the 1960s, permitting rapid defibrillation. Continuous electrocardiographic (ECG) monitoring of patients with acute infarction revealed that in the minutes preceding primary ventricular fibrillation, there is often an increase in the frequency and "complexity" of ventricular ectopy and the development of paroxysms of nonsustained ventricular tachycardia. However, it was also observed that about half of the patients who developed primary ventricular fibrillation in the intensive care unit did not display these so-called "warning arrhythmias."[10] In addition, the occurrence of nonsustained ventricular tachycardia during the first 24 hours of acute myocardial infarction does not carry an increased risk for subsequent overall cardiac mortality or sudden death, either in-hospital or long-term.[11]

Although several series have shown that the mortality of patients who do experience primary ventricular fibrillation in the early phase of acute myocardial infarction is increased, it is not clear that this adverse prognosis is due to the arrhythmia itself. The usefulness of any test to screen for risk of cardiac arrest in acute infarction patients, who are already monitored in intensive care units, is likely to be limited. Ventricular tachyarrhythmias in this setting are treated rapidly and effectively, and the morbidity associated with prophylactic antiarrhythmic therapy limits the cost-effectiveness of such therapy.

Survivors of Acute Myocardial Infarction

A far larger group of patients at risk for sudden death comprises survivors of the acute phase of myocardial infarction. Most research has been centered on this group of patients. The risk of sudden death in myocardial infarction survivors is time-dependent: the period of highest risk is the first 6 to 12 months after infarction, although a substantial remainder of cardiac arrests occur years after the index infarction.[12] We have found that the median time from index infarction to event in a group of 86 patients referred after resuscitation from out-of-hospital cardiac arrest was 11 months. (A.E.B., unpublished data).

Clinical Factors

A number of factors obtained from the history and physical examination have been found to be useful in identifying patients at increased mortality risk (although they do not specifically predict sudden death). These include a history of previous infarction and congestive heart failure complicating the infarction.[13] Tests that have been used to further stratify risk of sudden death include those that assess nonarrhythmic factors, such as the presence of residual myocardial ischemia, functional status (exercise testing), and left ventricular function (gated blood pool scans or echocardiograms). Other tests, such as the Holter monitor, have assessed the presence and extent of spontaneous arrhythmias, ie, ventricular ectopy and nonsustained ventricular tachycardia, which have been presumed to act as triggers to initiate sustained ventricular tachycardia or fibrillation. Another group of tests have been aimed at detecting the presence of a substrate for reentrant ventricular tachycardias. This group includes both noninvasive studies, such as the signal-averaged ECG and measurement of QT dispersion, and invasive electrophysiological studies. Finally, a third group of tests has evaluated abnormalities of the autonomic nervous system, which are thought to play a role in modulating the interaction between the presumed triggers (ventricular ectopy) and the reentrant substrate. Included in this group are assessment of heart rate variability and baroreflex sensitivity.

Exercise Testing

Exercise testing is now recognized as a standard prognostic test in all survivors of acute myocardial infarction. The presence of ST-segment changes, inappropriate blood pressure response, and angina at sub-maximal exercise testing before hospital discharge and maximal (symptom-limited) testing 1 month after infarction predicts the occurrence of ischemic events, such as angina pectoris, recurrent infarction, need for coronary artery bypass graft surgery, and overall cardiac mortality, with good sensitivity and specificity.[14,15] Of interest, a patient's inability to perform a predischarge exercise test, when due to a cardiac problem, is also a powerful predictor of mortality. The ability of myocardial ischemia or ventricular arrhythmias (ie, ventricular ectopy or nonsustained ventricular tachycardia) elicited by exercise testing in the postinfarction patient to specifically identify patients prone to subsequent sudden death is controversial. Some investigators have noted a relation between ventricular arrhythmias and sudden death,[16] but most have not found exercise results to predict sudden death specifically.[14,15,17]

Left Ventricular Ejection Fraction

Left ventricular dysfunction has proved to be a key factor in stratifying mortality risk of patients after infarction. Left ventricular function is a continuous variable, with the risk of death increasing progressively as the ejection fraction decreases.[18] To express this information in a manner that can be used to provide practical guidelines, the ejection fraction is usually dichotomized around a value that distinguishes patients at relatively low from those at higher mortality risk. Most often, the best single value of ejection fraction at which to make this discrimination has been 0.40.[19,20] Ejection fraction is an independent predictor of mortality. That is, even in the absence of other factors, such as the presence of spontaneous arrhythmias or abnormalities of the signal-averaged ECG, an ejection fraction ≤0.40 indicates increased mortality risk (by at least threefold to fourfold).[18] When left ventricular dysfunction is accompanied by other abnormalities, such as evidence of arrhythmias, the mortality risk increases further. However, a major limit to the usefulness of ejection fraction is its lack of specificity for predicting sudden death: the presence of an ejection fraction <0.40 indicates similarly increased risks for both sudden and nonsudden cardiac death. It is noteworthy that left ventricular dysfunction remains an independent predictor of mortality in recent studies of patients who have undergone thrombolytic therapy.[18]

Ambulatory ECG Monitoring

Multiple studies have confirmed the prognostic significance of frequent premature ventricular complexes and nonsustained ventricular tachycardia documented anytime from 1 week to 3 months after acute myocardial infarction.[21-24] The occurrence of nonsustained ventricular tachycardia in the late hospital phase of myocardial infarction more than doubles the risk of subsequent sudden death. Nonsustained ventricular tachycardia detected 3 months to 1 year after myocardial infarction is also associated with a significantly higher mortality rate,[25,26] and frequent ventricular ectopy (>10 premature ventricular complexes per hour on a 24-hour monitor) recorded 1 year after acute infarction predicts increased mortality over the subsequent 2 years.[27] The prognostic significance of frequent ventricular ectopy and nonsustained ventricular tachycardia in the first month after acute infarction is preserved in patients who have received thrombolytic therapy.[24] However, just as was noted for left ventricular dysfunction, the specificity of spontaneous ventricular ectopy is limited. In each of the quoted studies, the rates of nonsudden cardiac death are increased in proportion to the increase in rates of sudden death.[24]

It is important to note that, contrary to intuition, mortality is not influenced by the frequency, duration, or rate of nonsustained ventricular tachycardia episodes.[22,23,28] That is, a single three-beat run of nonsustained ventricular tachycardia at 110 bpm on a 24-hour monitor carries the same adverse prognostic significance as 10 episodes of 14 beats of nonsustained ventricular tachycardia at 200 bpm.

Signal-Averaged Electrocardiography

Tests aimed at detecting specific electrophysiological factors predisposing patients to reentrant ventricular tachyarrhythmias include the signal-averaged ECG, dispersion of the QT interval, and electrophysiological studies. A number of studies have examined the prognostic significance of the signal-averaged ECG alone in unselected groups of patients early after acute infarction and in combination with other tests, such as ambulatory ECG monitoring and measurement of ejection fraction.[29–36] A majority of the studies have used time-domain rather than frequency-domain analysis of the signal-averaged ECG. In these studies, the test has been abnormal in 50% to 90% of patients who died suddenly or experienced spontaneous sustained ventricular tachycardia during follow-up periods of 6 to 24 months. Thus, it seems to have moderate to good sensitivity. Its primary benefit in these reports appears to be its ability to identify patients at low risk for developing arrhythmic events, because the reported negative predictive values are ≈95%. The risk of arrhythmic events in patients with an abnormal result (ie, the positive predictive value) has been far lower, averaging 20% in these reports. The true risk of sudden death is often difficult to determine, because many of the reports present outcomes as sudden death or cardiac arrest grouped together with sustained ventricular tachycardia. Furthermore, the quoted reports have not provided the rates of nonsudden cardiac deaths in patients with abnormal signal-averaged ECGs. Thus, we cannot be certain of the ability of the signal-averaged ECG to predict sudden death specifically. One recent report based on patients screened for participation in the Cardiac Arrhythmia Suppression Trial ("CAST") did state that the test did not identify patients experiencing nonsudden death (implying that the test specifically predicted arrhythmic deaths).[33] However, a report from Sydney showed a similar increase in sudden death and nonsudden cardiac death in patients with abnormal signal-averaged ECGs (ratio of "electrical" events to all cardiac deaths, 0.8).[35] On the other hand, a study from Japan reported a ratio of 6:1.[36] Thus, it is not clear at this time whether this test is a specific predictor of sudden death in postinfarction patients, as opposed to all-cause mortality.

Electrophysiological Testing

In the early 1970s, Wellens et al[37] demonstrated that pacing techniques (programmed stimulation) could safely and reproducibly initiate ventricular tachycardia in the majority of patients who had experienced prior episodes of spontaneous sustained ventricular tachycardia. Subsequent studies confirmed his observations and demonstrated reproduction of spontaneous sustained ventricular tachycardia by programmed stimulation in >90% of patients.[38] Subsequently, other clinical and experimental studies of postinfarction arrhythmias demonstrated that most monomorphic sustained tachycardias are due to intramyocardial reentry. This led to the application of programmed stimulation to survivors of out-of-hospital cardiac arrest.[39,40] Survivors of cardiac arrest were found to differ from patients presenting with stable sustained ventricular tachycardia in a number of respects, including the fact that monomorphic sustained ventricular tachycardia was inducible in only 30% to 40% of cases. Nonetheless, investigators then proceeded to apply programmed stimulation as a tool for risk stratification for sudden death in patients recovering from acute infarction. Greene et al[41] were the first to apply electrophysiological studies for this purpose, using as an end point the induction of the repetitive ventricular response. A number of other laboratories followed, using the induction of ventricular tachycardia as the end point for stimulation.[42-50] The results of these studies are difficult to compare because of differences in patient populations (some studied only patients with complicated infarctions; most excluded patients with unstable angina or uncontrolled congestive heart failure), stimulation protocols (numbers of extrastimuli, stimulation sites, stimulating energy), and timing of electrophysiological study (ranging from 5 days to 1.8 months). However, the results may be summarized. Monomorphic sustained ventricular tachycardia is inducible in 6% to 30% of patients. Ventricular fibrillation or polymorphic ventricular tachycardia is induced in a smaller percentage. Stimulation protocols limited to two or fewer ventricular extrastimuli result in significantly lower rates of inducible tachycardias. Patients given thrombolytic therapy are reported to have lower rates of inducible ventricular tachycardia: 0% to 10% in streptokinase-treated patients versus 12% to 74% in untreated patients.[51,52] The early (day-to-day, week-to-week) and long-term (8 months) reproducibility of inducible tachycardia has ranged from 50% to 80% and seems to be significantly greater when the induced tachycardias are slower (cycle length >240 ms).[53-57]

The prognostic significance of ventricular tachyarrhythmias induced early after myocardial infarction has been evaluated by several groups. As might be suspected, the clinical utility has varied, partly because of the variations in stimulation protocols used and patient populations, as noted above. The second factor influencing the interpretation of reports is the use of antiarrhythmic therapy. Very few groups have been able to resist giving antiarrhythmic drugs to patients with inducible tachycardias. Those studies using stimulation protocols limited to two or fewer ventricular extrastimuli or with follow-up <1 year have reported low sensitivity and low positive predictive values for inducible ventricular tachycardia.[48,53] Studies using stimulation protocols with three or more ventricular extrastimuli and follow-up of at least 1 year have found arrhythmic event rates of 25% to 36% in patients with inducible sustained ventricular tachycardia.[50,58] The group in Sydney has the most extensive controlled experience in this area. They have reported results in >1200 patients followed for at least 2 years.[58] They have shown that patients in whom only polymorphic ventricular tachycardia or ventricular fibrillation could be induced have no higher risk of arrhythmic events that patients without any induced arrhythmia.[59] Their work suggests that only induced tachycardias having cycle lengths ≥230 ms have prognostic significance. What seems very consistent in all reports is a negative predictive value of the response to programmed stimulation of ≈98%.

The group in Sydney has also compared the prognostic utility of a number of tests in the same patient group (Table 1).[35] Although the electrophysiological study was not the most sensitive test for identifying patients at risk for sudden death, it did have the highest positive predictive value (30%). Furthermore, it was the only test that specifically identified patients at risk for sudden death: the ratios of electrical events to all cardiac deaths for the sensitivity and positive predictive values of electrophysiological study were more than twice those for any other test. Thus, it appears that early after acute infarction, inducible sustained ventricular tachycardia not only identifies patients at increased risk for any cardiac death (ie, a population of generally "sick" patients) but also predicts how the deaths will occur.

TABLE 1

Comparison of Tests for Mortality Prediction in Myocardial Infarction Survivors

	Sensitivity, %	Specificity, %	Positive Predictive Value, %	Negative Predictive Value, %	References
Prediction of electrical events by test					
EPS	50-82	87-96	5-36	97-99	35,46,48,58
EF≤0.40	50-71	61-74	11-24	94-98	30,31,35
SAECG	48-93	62-90	10-27	93-99	29,31,33,35,36
Holter	44-82	40-73	6-23	91-98	30,31,35
ETT (ischemia)	20-91	83	2-16	98	16,35
Prediction of all cardiac deaths by test					
EPS	25	94	17	96	35
EF≤0.40	75	76	16	98	35
SAECG	71	83	22	98	35
Holter	81	40	8	97	35
ETT (ischemia)	23-89	63-83	6-24	96-98	14,16,35
Ratio of electrical to all cardiac events by test					
EPS	2.32		1.76		35
EF≤0.40	0.95		0.69		35
SAECG	0.8		0.77-6		35,36
Holter	1.01		0.75		35
ETT (ischemia)	0.87		0.33-1.7		16,35

Reported follow-up was 7.5 to 28 months. Electrical events include resuscitated ventricular fibrillation or ventricular tachycardia, or sudden death. EPS indicates electrophysiological study; EF, left ventricular ejection fraction; SAECG, signal-averaged electrocardiogram; and ETT, treadmill exercise test.

Programmed stimulation has been applied to another high-risk subgroup of patients with coronary artery disease: those with spontaneous nonsustained ventricular tachycardia. Five studies reported to date have examined the results of programmed stimulation in at least 35 patients with coronary disease and nonsustained ventricular tachycardia.[60-64] These studies have demonstrated inducible ventricular tachycardia in 21% to 45% of patients. If we limit our examination to protocols including three ventricular extrastimuli, we find rates of inducible sustained ventricular tachycardia of 40% to 45%. These three reports examined patients an average of 3 years after acute infarction. The increase in the numbers of patients having inducible ventricular tachycardia in comparison with those studied early after infarction is of interest, as is the relation of inducible ventricular tachycardia to prognosis in this population. After a mean follow-up ranging from 14 to 30 months in these three studies, arrhythmic events (sudden death, resuscitated cardiac arrest, or sustained ventricular tachycardia) occurred in 12.5% to 23% of patients. These studies again demonstrated the high specificity of programmed stimulation for predicting arrhythmic events: only 4% to 12% of patients without inducible sustained ventricular tachycardia experienced arrhythmic events. Thus, in this population, the negative predictive value of electrophysiological studies ranges from 88% to 96%. Unfortunately, the majority of patients with inducible sustained ventricular tachycardia in these studies received antiarrhythmic therapy guided by serial electrophysiological studies. The rates of arrhythmic events in these patients ranged from 11% to 31%. In contrast, in the smaller number of patients with inducible sustained ventricular tachycardia receiving empirical antiarrhythmic therapy, arrhythmic event rates were 50% to 88%. Almost all of the arrhythmic events occurred in patients with inducible sustained ventricular tachycardia and left ventricular ejection fractions ≤ 0.40. In the study by Wilber et al,[64] all patients with inducible sustained ventricular tachycardia received antiarrhythmic therapy guided by the results of programmed stimulation. However, therapy was able to suppress inducible sustained ventricular tachycardia in only 50% of patients. The rate of arrhythmic events in patients whose inducible sustained ventricular tachycardia was suppressed was 5% (1/20), whereas the arrhythmic event rate in the patients whose inducible sustained ventricular tachycardia could not be suppressed was 35% (7/20).

A major problem facing us today is how to apply the results of the electrophysiological study in the postinfarction population. Such testing cannot practically be applied to all infarction survivors or even to the 20% to 30% who have a left ventricular ejection fraction

≤0.40. There is clearly a need for better noninvasive tests to more precisely identify the one third of patients with inducible ventricular tachycardia reported to suffer a life-threatening arrhythmic event over a 1- to 2-year follow-up period. In interpreting these results, it is also necessary to realize that a subpopulation of patients at risk continues to develop sudden death for many years after the acute infarction.[12] Furthermore, it remains to be proved that current antiarrhythmic therapy can reduce mortality in a cost-effective manner even if an appropriate group of high-risk patients can be identified.

Heart-Rate Variability

The tests discussed above have focused on identifying patients having the substrate to support intramyocardial reentry (the signal-averaged ECG, electrophysiological studies) or the triggers presumed to activate the reentrant substrate (ventricular ectopy and nonsustained ventricular tachycardia on ambulatory ECG monitoring). However, although these tests are fairly sensitive, the positive predictive value is less than desired. In search of the "missing link" to explain why not all patients with substrate present develop spontaneous ventricular tachycardia and to explain factors responsible for activating the reentrant substrate, a number of investigators have studied the potential role of disturbances in autonomic nervous system function in survivors of myocardial infarction. Much evidence in humans and experimental studies suggests that relative decreases in parasympathetic tone are associated with poor prognosis. One reason for this may be the effects of acute ischemia: in the presence of acute ischemia, increased vagal tone protects against ventricular fibrillation. One method of characterizing the balance between the sympathetic and parasympathetic nervous systems has been the assessment of heart-rate or heart-period variability by use of ambulatory ECG monitoring. Beat-to-beat variations around the mean heart rate reflect the balance between the sympathetic and parasympathetic nervous systems. In general, increases in vagal tone cause an increase in heart rate variability. The variability has been characterized by a number of different methods using both time-domain measures (based on measurements of the standard deviation of heart rates) and frequency-domain measures (based on the relative amount of energy contained in the spectra describing the frequency with which the rate variations occur).   ·

A number of studies describing the prognostic significance of abnormally low heart-rate variability in patients with recent myocardial infarction have been reported.[65-70] Kleiger et al[65] first demonstrated the close relation between increased mortality and abnormally low heart-rate variability after acute infarction in 808 patients. They showed that abnormal heart-rate variability correlated with a number of other risk factors, including abnormal ejection fraction, congestive heart failure, and abnormal exercise duration. Of interest was their observation that the heart-rate variation correlated to a much lower degree with spontaneous ventricular ectopy variables, suggesting that these two factors worked independently in their association with mortality. Other large trials confirmed this relation.[66-70] Farrell et al[66] found the sensitivity of heart-rate variability (92%) in the prediction of arrhythmic events (sudden death and spontaneous sustained ventricular tachycardia) to be higher than other risk factors, including exercise testing, ejection fraction, ventricular ectopy, and the signal-averaged ECG. Abnormal heart-rate variability parameters also predict cardiac mortality 1 to 2 years after infarction, not only in the earlier high-risk period 6 to 12 months after the acute infarction.[70] However, as with other tests, over a mean follow-up of 612 days, the positive predictive value was only 17%. The other limitation to the potential clinical utility of heart-rate variability relates to its specificity for predicting sudden death and sustained ventricular tachycardia. In each of the studies reporting both overall cardiac mortality and sudden death or arrhythmic events, the increase in risk associated with abnormal heart-rate variability almost parallels the increase in overall cardiac mortality risk.[66-69] Thus, this test too appears to tell the clinician not how an individual patient will die but only that the patient is at increased overall mortality risk.

At this time, the optimal methodology for measuring heart-rate variability has not yet been standardized. Comparative studies suggest that measures of frequency- and time-domain rate variability give similar results. Likewise, short-term measures of variability acquired over just 2 to 15 minutes have been reported to give results very close to those obtained from longer monitoring periods (24 hours),[69] which increases the ease of acquiring data. However, the optimal sampling time and measurement methodologies have not yet been determined. Further evaluation of heart-rate variability in large-scale, prospective trials is needed before its use in the management of the postinfarction patient can be recommended.

In summary, then, for patients with coronary artery disease and prior myocardial infarction, all the above factors can be used to distinguish patients at low and high risk for both sudden and overall cardiac death. However, the only test that has been shown to identify patients specifically at increased risk for sudden death is the electrophysiological study. Some studies suggest that the signal-averaged ECG and heart-rate variability may be specific predictors of sudden death, but more data are needed to clarify the role of these tests in predicting risk for sudden death. Other tests are being investigated actively, including the dispersion of QT intervals on the standard 12-lead ECG and baroreflex sensitivity, but currently available data are insufficient to determine their utility in patients with coronary artery disease.

If one knew that a specific intervention could significantly reduce the risk of sudden death in high-risk patients with coronary artery disease, what would be a logical algorithm with which to identify the high-risk patient today? I believe the initial step should involve two tests. First, exercise testing should be performed to search for evidence of residual myocardial ischemia after infarction. If ischemia is found, it should be treated either pharmacologically or by an appropriate intervention, especially if the patient has abnormal ventricular function. Second, the left ventricular ejection fraction should be quantified. If the ejection fraction is >0.40, I would not perform further tests. If the ejection fraction is ≤0.40, it might make sense to perform a signal-averaged ECG, given the reported high negative predictive value of this technique. If the signal-averaged ECG is abnormal, I would perform an electrophysiological study. As alluded to earlier, the question then becomes, What should be done with this information? At this time, in the absence of data showing that therapy can effectively reduce the risk of sudden death at acceptable costs in terms of both money and side effects, we are at a loss to recommend specific interventions based on the risk stratification other than encouraging the use of β-adrenergic blocking agents and converting-enzyme inhibitors. Fortunately, a number of multicenter trials nearing completion are evaluating pharmacological and implantable defibrillator therapy in high-risk postinfarction patients. The results of these trials should demonstrate the degree to which currently available therapy can reduce the risk of sudden death in these patients. It may be reasonable to modify the proposed algorithm in patients with a first infarction who have received thrombolytic therapy or in whom coronary angiography has demonstrated effective reperfusion if the reports of very low rates of inducible sustained ventricular tachycardia in such cases are corroborated.

Hypertrophic Cardiomyopathy

Sudden death is a significant cause of mortality in patients with hypertrophic cardiomyopathy (HCM), with the yearly incidence reported to be 2% to 3% in selected, adult referral populations.[71,72] More recent studies in less selected groups of asymptomatic or minimally symptomatic patients report a lower annual risk, ranging from 0.1% to 0.7%.[73,74] The potential mechanisms causing sudden death in this entity are multiple. The frequent occurrence of sudden death in association with exercise (40% of episodes) has raised the question of the contribution of dynamic outflow tract obstruction and subendocardial ischemia, while ventricular fibrillation occurring de novo has also been documented.[75-77] A number of clinical, hemodynamic, and electrical parameters have been investigated for potential links to sudden death. Most sudden deaths in HCM occur in persons <30 years old. Some victims have a family history of sudden death. Sudden death appears to be more common in patients with more extensive hypertrophy and evidence of systolic dysfunction, but these findings are not specific enough to be useful prognostic indexes in individual patients.[78,79] Hemodynamic abnormalities, including the degree of left ventricular outflow tract obstruction, do not correlate well with the risk of sudden death.[75] Likewise, the existence of symptoms and functional class are not useful in predicting sudden death. Even a history of syncope has not appeared to increase the risk for sudden death in some studies, although it has correlated with risk in others.[72,75] In 40% to 50% of cases, sudden death is the first manifestation of cardiac disease.[75]

The association between exertion and sudden death in HCM has led to the evaluation of exercise tests to identify patients at risk. Exercise testing has not been useful to expose ventricular arrhythmias,[80-82] although evidence of ischemia on thallium scans is reported to correlate with prior cardiac arrest and syncope in young persons with HCM.[83] Limited data suggest little utility of exercise testing in the prediction of subsequent sudden death in this disease.[80]

The documentation of ventricular arrhythmias during episodes of cardiac arrest has led to extensive evaluation of the potential utility of ambulatory ECG monitoring in patients with HCM. Holter monitoring in this condition frequently reveals both supraventricular and ventricular arrhythmias. Nonsustained ventricular tachycardia has been documented in 17% to 28% of idiopathic HCM patients without a history of cardiac arrest during 24 to 72 hours of ambulatory ECG monitoring.[80,81,84-86] The occurrence of nonsustained ventricular tachycardia is not influenced by therapy with β-adrenergic blocking agents.[81] Patients with more severe hypertrophy are significantly more likely to exhibit ventricular tachycardia.[87] In contrast to almost every other cardiac disease, the presence of nonsustained ventricular tachycardia seems to indicate an increased risk specifically for sudden death: patients with nonsustained ventricular tachycardia have a yearly sudden death rate reported at 8% to 10% compared with 1% in patients without nonsustained ventricular tachycardia.[84,85] Unfortunately, these reports are derived from two specialized centers and are based on highly selected referral populations. Thus, it may be difficult to extrapolate these data to less selected patient populations. However, a recent report from Italy sheds some light on this issue.[88] In 151 asymptomatic or minimally symptomatic patients followed for an average of 4.8 years, the incidence of sudden death was 1.4% yearly in patients with nonsustained ventricular tachycardia versus 0.6% yearly in patients without ventricular tachycardia.[88] This analysis found a relative risk for sudden death of 2.6 to 3.5 for patients with ventricular tachycardia.

Several groups have evaluated the utility of electrophysiological studies in patients with HCM. Abnormalities of the atrioventricular conduction system and inducible atrial and ventricular arrhythmias are found frequently.[89] Programmed ventricular stimulation incorporating stimulation protocols with one to three extrastimuli has induced sustained ventricular tachycardia in one third to two thirds of patients when a maximum of two or three extrastimuli were delivered, respectively.[89–93] Sustained ventricular tachycardia has been induced in 66% to 100% of patients with a history of cardiac arrest.[89–92] The presence of inducible ventricular tachycardia has not correlated with any clinical or hemodynamic findings.[90] The majority of induced arrhythmias have been polymorphic and required triple extrastimuli for induction, raising the question of the specificity of these findings. However, these arrhythmias have been induced significantly more often in patients with a history of cardiac arrest or syncope.[89–92] Fananapazir et al[92] believe that the presence of inducible, sustained ventricular tachycardia carries prognostic significance. In their study, the presence of inducible ventricular tachycardia carried a significantly higher risk for arrhythmic events (sudden death, cardiac arrest, or syncope in association with discharge of an implantable defibrillator) over a 28-month follow-up period. Even in their patients with a history of cardiac arrest or syncope, those who did not have induction of sustained ventricular tachycardia had a 17% arrhythmia event rate compared with a 60% event rate in patients with inducible ventricular tachycardia. The presence of inducible sustained ventricular tachycardia was also associated with a significantly higher arrhythmia event rate in patients without a history of syncope or cardiac arrest. However, this was a highly selected population of patients, with the majority having survived episodes of cardiac arrest or syncope or having a strong family history of sudden death.

In addition, almost all their patients with inducible or spontaneous symptomatic arrhythmias received various treatments in an uncontrolled fashion. Thus, it is not clear what the prognostic utility of programmed stimulation is in asymptomatic patients with a negative family history of sudden death.

Several groups have observed the occurrence of unusual fractionated local right ventricular electrograms in response to premature stimuli in the electrophysiology laboratory.[90,93,94] These abnormal electrograms seem to be elicited primarily in survivors of cardiac arrest and patients with nonsustained ventricular tachycardia on Holter monitoring.[93,94] Although the published retrospective analyses suggest potential uses for these electrograms, this preliminary work requires prospective analysis in a large patient group to determine its potential prognostic significance.

Other tests, including the signal-averaged ECG, QT-interval dispersion, and heart-rate variability, have been evaluated for potential prognostic utility in HCM patients. One study comparing both spectral and temporal measures of heart-rate variability failed to find a distinction between patients with and without cardiac arrest.[95] Abnormalities of the signal-averaged ECG have been found in 12% to 20% of patients with HCM.[96] Their presence has correlated with nonsustained ventricular tachycardia on Holter monitoring in some but not all studies[96,97] and with inducible sustained ventricular tachycardia in one study.[97] In one prospective evaluation, the signal-averaged ECG did not distinguish patients with cardiac arrest.[97] Finally, a small (26 patients) retrospective analysis has noted marked differences in QT dispersion between patients with cardiac arrest or spontaneous nonsustained ventricular tachycardia and a control group.[98] Further prospective studies are obviously required to assess the potential prognostic significance of this finding.

Just as was the case for coronary artery disease, the utility of any of the described prognostic tests in patients with HCM is limited by our ability to institute effective therapy in high-risk patients. No pharmacological agent has as yet been found to reliably prevent sudden death in this entity. Although the implantable cardioverter-defibrillator is becoming more widely used, its expense prevents widespread, indiscriminate use in asymptomatic patients at this time.

Dilated Cardiomyopathy

The mortality for patients with nonischemic or idiopathic dilated cardiomyopathy (DCM) is very high, ≈10% yearly in referral practices and 5% yearly in population-based studies.[99,100] Just as is the case for patients with coronary artery disease, sudden death accounts for about 50% of the mortality in patients with DCM. A major problem in developing a rational approach to prevention of sudden death in DCM is our poor understanding of the mechanisms responsible for sudden death in this condition. Although many factors have been identified that may contribute to sudden death in patients with DCM, the actual role of these factors is unknown.[100-103] Another problem is the heterogeneity of causes whose end result is DCM. Furthermore, in contrast to patients with coronary artery disease, bradyarrhythmias are the initial arrhythmias recorded at the onset of cardiac arrest in a significant fraction of patients with advanced heart failure due to DCM. These may represent responses to noncardiac phenomena, such as acute pulmonary embolism.[104] Nonetheless, ventricular tachyarrhythmias do seem to account for the majority of sudden unexpected cardiac arrests in patients with DCM when patients with the full spectrum of the disease are considered.

Although the overall mortality is increased in patients with symptomatic and objective evidence of more severe hemodynamic dysfunction, only one clinical factor seems to predict sudden death with a high specificity. A history of syncope predicts an increased risk for both sudden and nonsudden death, but the risk for sudden death seems to be increased out of proportion to the risk for nonsudden death.[105]

Many studies have evaluated the usefulness of tests of factors that may predispose to tachyarrhythmias, such as the ambulatory ECG. Asymptomatic ventricular arrhythmias discovered by continuous ECG recording are ubiquitous in patients with DCM. Surveys using 24-hour recordings reveal episodes of nonsustained ventricular tachycardia in 40% to 50% of patients with DCM.[106-111] Unlike coronary artery disease, the relation of nonsustained ventricular tachycardia to left ventricular dysfunction is not clear. Some of these studies have demonstrated an increased prevalence of nonsustained ventricular tachycardia in patients with more advanced degrees of left ventricular dysfunction, and others have not.

The prognostic significance of spontaneous ventricular arrhythmias, especially nonsustained ventricular tachycardia, detected by ambulatory monitoring has been investigated extensively.[107-114] Although several of these studies have shown the risk of cardiac mortality to be increased in patients with nonsustained ventricular tachycardia, others have not. Of greater clinical relevance, even those studies that have demonstrated a correlation between nonsustained ventricular tachycardia and overall cardiac mortality have not shown a specific predictive value for sudden death. That is, the odds of sudden death in patients with nonsustained ventricular tachycardia are increased to a degree similar to the odds of nonsudden or overall cardiac death.

The signal-averaged ECG in patients with DCM has been investigated by a number of groups. Retrospective analyses have shown an increased frequency of abnormalities in patients with prior episodes of sustained ventricular tachycardia or cardiac arrest.[115,116] In comparison with studies of the signal-averaged ECG in patients with coronary artery disease, far fewer patients with DCM have been studied prospectively (530 patients in seven studies).[36,117–121] These studies have included patients with previous episodes of symptomatic arrhythmias and asymptomatic patients receiving prophylactic antiarrhythmic agents. For the prediction of sudden death, the positive predictive value has ranged from 0% to 45%, the sensitivity from 0% to 100%, and the negative predictive value from 71% to 100%. Some of the studies suggest that the signal-averaged ECG may be useful in predicting risk for sudden death, and others do not. Thus, the true prognostic value of the time-domain signal-averaged ECG in patients with DCM is far from clear.[122] One preliminary study suggested that analysis of the signal-averaged ECG by alternative methods, such as spectral turbulence, may permit more accurate prediction of sudden death, although this was not verified by another report.[121,123]

Electrophysiological studies have also been evaluated for their potential prognostic value in patients with DCM. Rates for the induction of sustained ventricular tachycardia have ranged between 0% and 13% in patients without a history of symptomatic arrhythmias.[121,124–134] Not only are the rates of inducible sustained monomorphic ventricular tachycardia significantly lower than those observed in patients with coronary artery disease, but the presence of inducible ventricular tachycardia appears to lack prognostic significance in DCM.[125–134] The reported studies have failed to demonstrate any correlation between inducibility of sustained ventricular tachycardia and subsequent sudden death or total cardiac mortality. The positive predictive value of inducible ventricular tachycardia is far less than 20%, and sudden death has occurred more frequently in patients without inducible ventricular tachycardia than in those with inducible arrhythmias. Thus, there appears to be no role for programmed electrical stimulation as a tool for the prediction of sudden death in this group of patients. It should be noted that the aforementioned studies have found inducible monomorphic sustained ventricular tachycardia to be predictive of subsequent spontaneous (but nonfatal) monomorphic sustained ventricular tachycardia, even though it has not predicted sudden death.

Thus, at the present time we are at a loss to recommend risk stratification tests for patients with idiopathic DCM. Tests that appear to have potential clinical utility in patients with prior myocardial infarction do not appear to be useful in DCM. It seems likely that this is because of differing mechanisms of sudden death dependent on the anatomic substrate. This conclusion is supported by the results of experimental models of nonischemic cardiomyopathy.[135,136] These studies suggest that nonreentrant mechanisms, such as abnormal automaticity or triggered activity, are most often responsible for arrhythmias in this setting.

Conclusions

It should be clear from the preceding discussion that the mechanisms responsible for sudden death are dependent on the anatomic substrate. These mechanisms within individual patients may evolve over time with progression of disease. Our understanding of these mechanisms is best (but far from complete) in the case of coronary artery disease and is grossly inadequate in patients with cardiomyopathies. The variations in the mechanisms causing arrhythmias translate into a need for different types of prognostic tests in the various disease states. Furthermore, certain tests may be valid for only certain stages in specific diseases.

The methodology for identification of patients at high risk of sudden death is in a state of flux today. Technological advances in areas such as signal processing are becoming more widely available. These new technologies, in turn, are being applied to various groups of patients without adequate understanding of the mechanisms responsible for sudden death. This often leads to expensive trials involving risk to patients without rationale.

One of our greatest challenges in this area today is to develop tests that will have direct utility in the care of individual patients. To satisfy this need, we must have tests that identify patients specifically at risk for sudden death so that specific and appropriate treatments may be initiated on the basis of the test results. For example, in the case of coronary artery disease, many parameters have been identified that are capable of identifying groups of patients at high mortality risk. However, tests are lacking that have enough specificity to allow the practitioner dealing with an individual patient to know that his or her patient is likely to die of a tachyarrhythmia and therefore that initiation of specific antiarrhythmic therapy is likely to prolong the patient's life. Finally, it should be clear that improved methods of risk stratification will prove beneficial only if safe, cost-effective treatments are available to those patients at high risk. The results of several ongoing multicenter trials evaluating the efficacy of pharmacological and implantable device therapy for the primary prevention of sudden death in patients with coronary artery disease will be available in the near future. This information should help to determine how best to apply risk stratification tools in the coronary disease population. However, we have a long way to go in the development of effective strategy for the primary prevention of sudden death in patients with cardiomyopathies.

References

1. Liberthson RR, Nagel EL, Hirschman JC, Nussenfeld SR. Prehospital ventricular defibrillation: prognosis and follow-up course. *N Engl J Med.* 1974;291:3317–3321.
2. Baum RS, Alvarez H, Cobb LA. Survival after resuscitation from out-of-hospital ventricular fibrillation. *Circulation.* 1974;50:1231–1235.
3. Eisenberg MS, Hallstrom A, Bergner L. Long-term survival after out-of-hospital cardiac arrest. *N Engl J Med.* 1982;306:22:1340–1343.
4. Weaver WD, Hill D, Fahrenbruch CE, et al. Use of the automatic external defibrillator in the management of out-of-hospital cardiac arrest. *N Engl J Med.* 1988;319:661–716.
5. Becker LB, Han BH, Meyer PM, et al. CPR Chicago project: racial differences in the incidence of cardiac arrest and subsequent survival. *N Engl J Med.* 1993;329:600–606.
6. Roy D, Waxman HL, Kienzle MG, Buxton AE, Marchlinski FE, Josephson ME. Clinical characteristics and long-term follow-up in 119 survivors of cardiac arrest: relation to inducibility at electrophysiologic testing. *Am J Cardiol.* 1983;52:969–974.
7. Eldar M, Sauve MJ, Scheinman MM. Electrophysiologic testing and follow-up of patients with aborted sudden death. *J Am Coll Cardiol.* 1987;10:291–298.
8. Myerburg RL, Conde CA, Sung RJ, et al. Clinical, electrophysiologic and hemodynamic profile of patients resuscitated from prehospital cardiac arrest. *Am J Med.* 1980;68:568–576.
9. Wilber DJ, Garan H, Finkelstein D, et al. Out-of-hospital cardiac arrest: use of electrophysiologic testing in the prediction of long-term outcome. *N Engl J Med.* 1988;318:19–24.
10. Campbell R, Murray A, Julian DG. Ventricular arrhythmias in the first 12 hours of acute myocardial infarction. *Br Heart J.* 1981;46:351–357.
11. de Soyza N, Bennett FA, Murphy ML, Bissett JK, Kane JJ. The relationship of paroxysmal ventricular tachycardia complicating the acute phase and ventricular arrhythmia during the late hospital phase of myocardial infarction to long-term survival. *Am J Med.* 1978;64:377–381.
12. Daly L, Hickey N, Graham I, Mulcahy R. Predictors of sudden death up to 18 years after a first attack of unstable angina or myocardial infarction. *Br Heart J.* 1987;58:567–571.
13. Beller GA, Gibson RS. Risk stratification after myocardial infarction. *Mod Concepts Cardiovasc Dis.* 1986;55:5–10

14. Fioretti P, Brower RW, Simoons ML, et al. Prediction of mortality during the first year after acute myocardial infarction from clinical variables and stress test at hospital discharge. *Am J Cardiol.* 1985;55:1313–1318.
15. Waters DD, Bosch X, Bouchard A, et al. Comparison of clinical variables and variables derived from a limited predischarge exercise test as predictors of early and late mortality after myocardial infarction. *J Am Coll Cardiol.* 1985;5:1–8.
16. Theroux P, Waters DD, Halphen C, Debaisieux J-C, Mizgala HF. Prognostic value of exercise testing soon after myocardial infarction. *N Engl J Med.* 1979;301:341–345.
17. Starling MR, Crawford MH, Kennedy GT, O'Rourke RA. Exercise testing early after myocardial infarction: predictive value for subsequent unstable angina and death. *Am J Cardiol.* 1980;46:909–913.
18. Volpi A, De Vita C, Franzosi MG, et al, for the ad hoc Working Group of the Gruppo Italiano. Determinants of 6-month mortality in survivors of myocardial infarction after thrombolysis: results of the GISSI-2 data base. *Circulation.* 1993;88:416–429.
19. Bigger JT, Fleiss JL, Kleiger R, Miller JP, Rolnitzky LM, and the Multicenter Post-Infarction Research Group. The relationships among ventricular arrhythmias, left ventricular dysfunction, and mortality in the 2 years after myocardial infarction. *Circulation.* 1984;69:250–258.
20. Schulze RA, Strauss HW, Pitt B. Sudden death in the year following myocardial infarction: relation to ventricular premature contractions in the late hospital phase and left ventricular ejection fraction. *Am J Med.* 1977;62:192–199.
21. Ruberman W, Weinblatt E, Goldberg JD, Frank CW, Shapiro S. Ventricular premature complexes and mortality after myocardial infarction. *N Engl J Med.* 1977;297:750–755.
22. Anderson KP, DeCamilla J, Moss AJ. Clinical significance of ventricular tachycardia (3 beats or longer) detected during ambulatory monitoring after myocardial infarction. *Circulation.* 1978;57:890–897.
23. Bigger JT, Weld FM, Rolnitzky LM. Prevalence, characteristics and significance of ventricular tachycardia (three or more complexes) detected with ambulatory electrocardiographic recording in the late hospital phase of acute myocardial infarction. *Am J Cardiol.* 1981;48: 815–823.
24. Maggioni AP, Zuanetti G, Franzosi MG, et al, on behalf of GISSI-2 Investigators. Prevalence and prognostic significance of ventricular arrhythmias after acute myocardial infarction in the fibrinolytic era: GISSI-2 results. *Circulation.* 1993;87:312–322.
25. Tominaga S, Blackburn H, for the Coronary Drug Project Research Group. Prognostic importance of premature beats following myocardial infarction: experience in the Coronary Drug Project. *JAMA.* 1973;223:1116–1124.
26. Hallstrom AP, Bigger JT, Roden D, et al. Prognostic significance of ventricular premature depolarizations measured 1 year after myocardial infarction in patients with early postinfarction asymptomatic ventricular arrhythmia. *J Am Coll Cardiol.* 1992;20:259–264.
27. Hallstrom AP, Bigger JT, Roden D, et al. Prognostic significance of ventricular premature depolarizations measured 1 year after myocardial infarction in patients with early postinfarction asymptomatic ventricular arrhythmia. *J Am Coll Cardiol.* 1992;20:259–264.
28. Denes P, Gillis AM, Pawitan Y, Kammerling JM, Wilhelmsen L, Salerno DM, and the CAST Investigators. Prevalence, characteristics and significance of ventricular premature complexes and ventricular tachycardia

detected by 24-hour continuous electrocardiographic recording in the Cardiac Arrhythmia Suppression Trial. *Am J Cardiol.* 1991;68:887–896.
29. Breithardt G, Schwarzmaier J, Borggrefe M, Haerten K, Seipel L. Prognostic significance of late ventricular potentials after acute myocardial infarction. *Eur Heart J.* 1983;4:487–495.
30. Gomes JA, Winters SL, Stewart D, Horowitz S, Milner M, Barreca P. A new noninvasive index to predict sustained ventricular tachycardia and sudden death in the first year after myocardial infarction: based on signal-averaged electrocardiogram, radionuclide ejection fraction and Holter monitoring. *J Am Coll Cardiol.* 1987;10:349–357.
31. Steinberg JS, Regan A, Sciacca RR, et al. Predicting arrhythmic events after acute myocardial infarction using the signal-averaged electrocardiogram. *Am J Cardiol.* 1992;69:13–21.
32. Kuchar DL, Thorburn CW, Sammel NL. Prediction of serious arrhythmic events after myocardial infarction: signal-averaged electrocardiogram, Holter monitoring and radionuclide ventriculography. *J Am Coll Cardiol.* 1987;9:531–538.
33. El-Sherif N, Denes P, Katz R, et al. Definition of the best prediction criteria of the time domain signal-averaged electrocardiogram for serious arrhythmic events in the postinfarction period. *J Am Coll Cardiol.* 1995;25:908–914.
34. Cain ME, Anderson JL, Arnsdorf MF, Mason JW, Scheinman MM, Waldo AL. Signal-averaged electrocardiography. *J Am Coll Cardiol.* 1996;27:1:238–249.
35. Richards DAB, Byth K, Ross DL, Uther JB. What is the best predictor of spontaneous ventricular tachycardia and sudden death after myocardial infarction? *Circulation.* 1991;83:756–763.
36. Ohnishi Y, Inoue T, Fukuzaki H. Value of the signal averaged electrocardiogram as predictor of sudden death in myocardial infarction and dilated cardiomyopathy. *Jpn Circ J.* 1990;54:127–136.
37. Wellens HJ, Schuilenburg RM, Durrer D. Electrical stimulation of the heart in patients with ventricular tachycardia. *Circulation.* 1972;56:216–226.
38. Buxton AE, Waxman HL, Marchlinski FE, Untereker WJ, Waspe LE, Josephson ME. Role of triple extrastimuli during electrophysiologic study of patients with documented sustained ventricular tachyarrhythmias. *Circulation.* 1984;69:532–540.
39. Ruskin JN, DiMarco JP, Garan H. Out-of-hospital cardiac arrest: electrophysiologic observations and selection of long-term antiarrhythmic therapy. *N Engl J Med.* 1980;303:607–613.
40. Josephson ME, Horowitz LN, Spielman SR, Greenspan AM. Electrophysiologic and hemodynamic studies in patients resuscitated from cardiac arrest. *Am J Cardiol.* 1980;46:948–955.
41. Greene HL, Reid PR, Schaeffer AH. The repetitive ventricular response in man: a predictor of sudden death. *N Engl J Med.* 1978; 299: 729–734.
42. Hamer A, Vohra J, Hunt D, Sloman G. Prediction of sudden death by electrophysiologic studies in high risk patients surviving acute myocardial infarction. *Am J Cardiol.* 1982;50:223–229.
43. Richards DA, Cody DV, Denniss AR, Russell PA, Young AA, Uther JB. Ventricular electrical instability: a predictor of death after myocardial infarction. *Am J Cardiol.* 1983;51:75–80.
44. Marchlinski FE, Buxton AE, Waxman HL, Josephson ME. Identifying patients at risk of sudden death after myocardial infarction: value of the response to programmed stimulation, degree of ventricular ectopic

activity and severity of left ventricular dysfunction. *Am J Cardiol.* 1983; 52:1190–1196.

45. Kowey PR, Friehling T, Meister SG, Engel TR. Late induction of tachycardia in patients with ventricular fibrillation associated with acute myocardial infarction. *J Am Coll Cardiol.* 1984;30:690–695.

46. Roy D, Marchand E, Theroux P, Waters DD, Pelletier GB, Bourassa MG. Programmed ventricular stimulation in survivors of an acute myocardial infarction. *Circulation.* 1985;72:487–494.

47. Waspe LE, Seinfeld D, Ferrick A, Kim SG, Matos JA, Fisher JD. Prediction of sudden death and spontaneous ventricular tachycardia in survivors of complicated myocardial infarction: value of the response to programmed stimulation using a maximum of three ventricular extrastimuli. *J Am Coll Cardiol.* 1985;5:1292–1301.

48. Bhandari AK, Rose JS, Kotlewski A, Rahimtoola SH, Wu D. Frequency and significance of induced sustained ventricular tachycardia or fibrillation two weeks after acute myocardial infarction. *Am J Cardiol.* 1985;56:737–742.

49. Santarelli P, Bellocci F, Liperfido F, et al. Ventricular arrhythmia induced by programmed ventricular stimulation after acute myocardial infarction. *Am J Cardiol.* 1985;55:391–394.

50. Iesaka Y, Nogami A, Aonuma K, et al. Prognostic significance of sustained monomorphic ventricular tachycardia induced by programmed ventricular stimulation using up to triple extrastimuli in survivors of acute myocardial infarction. *Am J Cardiol.* 1990;65:1057–1063.

51. Kersschot IE, Brugada P, Ramentol M, et al. Effects of early reperfusion in acute myocardial infarction on arrhythmias induced by programmed stimulation: a prospective, randomized study. *J Am Coll Cardiol.* 1986;7:1234–1242.

52. Bourke JP, Young AA, Richards DAB, Uther JB. Reduction in incidence of inducible ventricular tachycardia after myocardial infarction by treatment with streptokinase during infarct evolution. *J Am Coll Cardiol.* 1990;16:1703–1710.

53. Roy D, Marchand E, Theroux P, et al. Long-term reproducibility and significance of provocable ventricular arrhythmias after myocardial infarction. *J Am Coll Cardiol.* 1986;8:32–39.

54. Kuck KH, Costard A, Schluter M, Kunze KP. Significance of timing programmed electrical stimulation after acute myocardial infarction. *J Am Coll Cardiol.* 1986;8:1279–1288.

55. Bhandari AK, Au PK, Rose JS, Kotlewski A, Blue S, Rahimtoola SH. Decline in inducibility of sustained ventricular tachycardia from two to twenty weeks after acute myocardial infarction. *Am J Cardiol.* 1987;59:284–290.

56. Bhandari AK, Hong R, Kulick D, et al. Day to day reproducibility of electrically inducible ventricular arrhythmias in survivors of acute myocardial infarction. *J Am Coll Cardiol.* 1990;15:1075–1081.

57. Nogami A, Aonuma K, Takahashi A, et al. Usefulness of early versus late programmed ventricular stimulation in acute myocardial infarction. *Am J Cardiol.* 1991;68:13–20.

58. Bourke JP, Richards ADB, Ross DL, Wallace EM, McGuire MA, Uther JB. Routine programmed electrical stimulation in survivors of acute myocardial infarction for prediction of spontaneous ventricular tachyarrhythmias during follow-up: results, optimal stimulation protocol and cost-effective screening. *J Am Coll Cardiol.* 1991;18:780–788.

59. Bourke JP, Richards DAB, Ross DL, McGuire MA, Uther JB. Does the

induction of ventricular flutter or fibrillation at electrophysiologic testing after myocardial infarction have any prognostic significance? *Am J Cardiol.* 1995;75:431–435.

60. Gomes JAC, Hariman RI, Kang PS, El-Sherif N, Chowdhry I, Lyons J. Programmed electrical stimulation in patients with high-grade ectopy: electrophysiologic findings and prognosis for survival. *Circulation.* 1984;70:43–51.

61. Buxton AE, Marchlinski FE, Flores BT, Miller JM, Doherty JU, Josephson ME. Nonsustained ventricular tachycardia in patients with coronary artery disease: role of electrophysiologic study. *Circulation.* 1987;75:1178–1185.

62. Klein RC, Machell C. Use of electrophysiologic testing in patients with nonsustained ventricular tachycardia: prognostic and therapeutic implications. *J Am Coll Cardiol.* 1989;14:155–161.

63. Manolis AS, Estes NAM. Value of programmed stimulation in the evaluation and management of patients with nonsustained ventricular tachycardia associated with coronary artery disease. *Am J Cardiol.* 1990;65:201–205.

64. Wilber DJ, Olshansky B, Moran JF, Scanlon P. Electrophysiological testing and nonsustained ventricular tachycardia: use and limitations in patients with coronary artery disease and impaired ventricular function. *Circulation.* 1990;82:350–358.

65. Kleiger RE, Miller P, Bigger JT, Moss AJ. Decreased heart rate variability and its association with increased mortality after acute myocardial infarction. *Am J Cardiol.* 1987;59:256–262.

66. Farrell TG, Bashir Y, Cripps T, et al. Risk stratification for arrhythmic events in postinfarction patients based on heart rate variability, ambulatory electrocardiographic variables and the signal-averaged electrocardiogram. *J Am Coll Cardiol.* 1991;18:687–697.

67. Odemuyiwa O, Malik M, Farrell T, Bashir Y, Poloniecki J, Camm AJ. Comparison of the predictive characteristics of heart rate variability index and left ventricular ejection fraction for all-cause mortality, arrhythmic events and sudden death after acute myocardial infarction. *Am J Cardiol.* 1991;68:434–439.

68. Bigger JT, Fleiss, JL, Steinman RC, Rolnitzky LM, Kleiger RE, Rottman JN: Frequency domain measures of heart period variability and mortality after myocardial infarction. Circulation 1992;85:164–171.

69. Bigger JT, Fleiss JL, Rolnitzky LM, Steinman RC. The ability of several short-term measures of RR variability to predict mortality after myocardial infarction. *Circulation.* 1993;88:927–934.

70. Bigger JT, Fleiss JL, Rolnitzky LM, Steinman RC. Frequency domain measures of heart period variability to assess risk late after myocardial infarction. *J Am Coll Cardiol.* 1993;21:729–736.

71. Maron BJ, Fananapazir L. Sudden cardiac death in hypertrophic cardiomyopathy. *Circulation.* 1992;85(suppl I):I-57–I-63.

72. McKenna WJ, Deanfield J, Faruqui A, England D, Oakley C, Goodwin J. Prognosis in hypertrophic cardiomyopathy: role of age and clinical, electrocardiographic and hemodynamic features. *Am J Cardiol.* 1981;47:532–538.

73. Cannan CR, Reeder GS, Bailey KR, Melton LJ, Gersh BJ. Natural history of hypertrophic cardiomyopathy: a population-based study, 1976 through 1990. *Circulation.* 1995;92:2488–2495.

74. Cecchi F, Olivotto I, Montereggi A, Santoro G, Dolara A, Maron BJ. Hypertrophic cardiomyopathy in Tuscany: clinical course and out-

come in an unselected regional population. *J Am Coll Cardiol.* 1995;26: 1529–1536.

75. Maron BJ, Roberts WC, Epstein SE. Sudden death in hypertrophic cardiomyopathy: a profile of 78 patients. *Circulation.* 1982;65:1388–1394.
76. Nicod P, Polikar R, Peterson KL. Hypertrophic cardiomyopathy and sudden death. *N Engl J Med.* 1988;318:1255–1257.
77. Fananapazir L, Epstein SE. Hemodynamic and electrophysiologic evaluation of patients with hypertrophic cardiomyopathy surviving cardiac arrest. *Am J Cardiol.* 1991;67:280–287.
78. Newman H, Sugrue D, Oakley CM, Goodwin JF, McKenna WJ. Relation of left ventricular function and prognosis in hypertrophic cardiomyopathy: an angiographic study. *J Am Coll Cardiol.* 1985;5: 1064–1074.
79. Spirito P, Maron BJ. Relation between extent of left ventricular hypertrophy and occurrence of sudden death in hypetrophic cardiomyopathy. *J Am Coll Cardiol.* 1990;15:1521–1526.
80. Savage DD, Seides SF, Maron BJ, Myers DJ, Epstein SE. Prevalence of arrhythmias during 24-hour electrocardiographic monitoring and exercise testing in patients with obstructive and nonobstructive cardiomyopathy. *Circulation.* 1979;59:866–875.
81. McKenna WJ, Chetty S, Oakley CM, Goodwin JF. Arrhythmia in hypertrophic cardiomyopathy: exercise and 48 hour ambulatory electrocardiographic assessment with and without beta adrenergic blocking therapy. *Am J Cardiol.* 1980;45:1–5.
82. Jansson K, Dahlstrom U, Karlsson E, Nylander E, Walfridsson H, Sonnhag C. The value of exercise test, Holter monitoring, and programmed electrical stimulation in detection of ventricular arrhythmias in patients with hypertrophic cardiomyopathy. *PACE.* 1990;13:1261–1267.
83. Dilsizian V, Bonow RO, Epstein SE, Fananapazir L. Myocardial ischemia detected by thallium scintigraphy is frequently related to cardiac arrest and syncope in young patients with hypertrophic cardiomyopathy. *J Am Coll Cardiol.* 1993;22:796–804.
84. Maron BJ, Savage DD, Wolfson JK, Epstein SE. Prognostic significance of 24 hour ambulatory electrocardiographic monitoring in patients with hypertrophic cardiomyopathy: a prospective study. *Am J Cardiol.* 1981;48:252–257.
85. McKenna WJ, England D, Doi YL, Deanfield JE, Oakley C, Goodwin JF. Arrhythmia in hypertrophic cardiomyopathy, I: influence on prognosis. *Br Heart J.* 1981;46:168–172.
86. Mulrow JP, Healy MJ, McKenna WJ. Variability of ventricular arrhythmias in hypertrophic cardiomyopathy and implications for treatment. *Am J Cardiol.* 1986;58:615–618.
87. Spirito P, Watson RM, Maron BJ. Relation between extent of left ventricular hypertrophy and occurrence of ventricular tachycardia in hypertrophic cardiomyopathy. *Am J Cardiol.* 1987;60:1137–1142.
88. Spirito P, Rapezzi C, Autore C, et al. Prognosis of asymptomatic patients with hypertrophic cardiomyopathy and nonsustained ventricular tachycardia. *Circulation.* 1994;90:2743–2747.
89. Fananapazir L, Tracy CM, Leon MB, et al. Electrophysiologic abnormalities in patients with hypertrophic cardiomyopathy: a consecutive analysis in 155 patients. *Circulation.* 1989;80:1259–1268.
90. Watson RM, Schwartz JL, Maron BJ, Tucker E, Rosing DR, Josephson ME. Inducible polymorphic ventricular tachycardia and ventricular

fibrillation in a subgroup of patients with hypertrophic cardiomy-opathy at high risk for sudden death. *J Am Coll Cardiol.* 1987;10: 761–764.

91. Geibel A, Brugada P, Zehender M, Stevenson W, Waldecker B, Wellens HJJ. Value of programmed electrical stimulation using a standardized ventricular stimulation protocol in hypertrophic car-diomyopathy. *Am J Cardiol.* 1987;60:738.

92. Fananapazir L, Anthony AC, Epstein SE, McAreavey D. Prognostic determinants in hypertrophic cardiomyopathy: prospective evalua-tion of a therapeutic strategy based on clinical, Holter, hemody-namic, and electrophysiologic findings. *Circulation.* 1992;86: 730–740.

93. Saumarez RC, Slade AKB, Grace AA, Sadoul N, Camm AJ, McKenna WJ: The significance of paced electrogram fractionation in hyper-trophic cardiomyopathy: a prospective study. *Circulation.* 1995;91: 2762–2768.

94. Saumarez RC, Camm AJ, Panagos A, et al. Ventricular fibrillation in hypertrophic cardiomyopathy is associated with increased fractiona-tion of paced right ventricular electrograms. *Circulation.* 1992; 86:467–474.

95. Counihan PJ, Fei L, Bashir Y, Farrell TG, Haywood GA,McKenna WJ. Assessment of heart rate variability in hypertrophic cardiomyopathy: association with clinical and prognostic features. *Circulation.* 1993;88:1682–1690.

96. Cripps TR, Counihan PJ, Frenneaux MP, Ward DE, Camm AJ, McKenna WJ. Signal-averaged electrocardiography in hypertrophic cardiomyopathy. *J Am Coll Cardiol.* 1990;15:956–961.

97. Kulakowski P, Counihan PJ, McKenna WJ. Prognostic implications of alterations in the initial portion of the signal-averaged QRS com-plex in hypertrophic cardiomyopathy. *Circulation.* 1991;84(suppl II):II-417. Abstract.

98. Buja G, Miorelli M, Turrini P, Melacini P, Nava A. Comparison of QT dispersion in hypertrophic cardiomyopathy between patients with and without ventricular arrhythmias and sudden death. *Am J Cardiol.* 1993;72:973–976.

99. Redfield MM, Gersh BJ, Bailey KR, Ballard DJ, Rodeheffer RJ. Nat-ural history of idiopathic dilated cardiomyopathy: effect of referral bias and secular trend. *Am J Coll Cardiol.* 1993;22:1921–1926.

100. Dec GW, Fuster V. Idiopathic dilated cardiomyopathy. *N Engl J Med.* 1994;331:1564–1575.

101. Stevenson WG, Stevenson LW, Middlekauf HR, Saxon LA. Sudden death prevention in patients with advanced ventricular dysfunction. *Circulation.* 1993;88:2953–2961.

102. Tomaselli GF, Beuckelmann DJ, Calkins HG, et al. Sudden death in heart failure: the role of abnormal repolarization. *Circulation.* 1994;90:2534–2539.

103. Dean JW, Lab MJ. Arrhythmia in heart failure: role of mechanically induced changes in electrophysiology. *Lancet.* 1989;1309–1312.

104. Luu M, Stevenson WG, Stevenson LW, Baron K, Walden J. Diverse mechanisms of unexpected cardiac arrest in advanced heart failure. *Circulation.* 1989;80:1675–1680.

105. Middlekauf HR, Stevenson WG, Stevenson LW, Saxon LA. Syncope in advanced heart failure: high risk of sudden death regardless of ori-gin of syncope. *J Am Coll Cardiol.* 1993;21:110–116.

106. Suyama A, Anan T, Araki H, Takeshita A, Nakamura M. Prevalence of ventricular tachycardia in patients with different underlying heart disease: a study by Holter ECG monitoring. *Am Heart J.* 1986;112:44–51.
107. Neri R, Mestroni L, Salvi A, Camerini F. Arrhythmias in dilated cardiomyopathy. *Postgrad Med J.* 1986;62:593–597.
108. Meinertz T, Hofmann T, Kasper W, et al. Significance of ventricular arrhythmias in idiopathic dilated cardiomyopathy. *Am J Cardiol.* 1984;53:902–907.
109. Huang SK, Messer JV, Denes P. Significance of ventricular tachycardia in idiopathic dilated cardiomyopathy: observations in 35 patients. *Am J Cardiol.* 1983;51:507–512.
110. Olshausen KV, Stienen U, Math D, Schwarz F, Kubler W, Meyer J. Long-term prognostic significance of ventricular arrhythmias in idiopathic dilated cardiomyopathy. *Am J Cardiol.* 1988;61:146–151.
111. De Maria R, Gavazzi A, Caroli A, Ometto R, Biagini A, Carmerini F, on behalf of the Italian Multicenter Cardiomyopathy Study (SPIC) Group. Ventricular arrhythmias in dilated cardiomyopathy as an independent prognostic hallmark. *Am J Cardiol.* 1992;69:1451–1457.
112. Gradman A, Deedwania P, Cody R, et al, for the Captopril-Digoxin Study Group. Predictors of total mortality and sudden death in mild to moderate heart failure. *J Am Coll Cardiol.* 1989;14:564–570.
113. Holmes J, Kubo SH, Cody RJ, Kligfield P. Arrhythmias in ischemic and nonischemic dilated cardiomyopathy: prediction of mortality by ambulatory electrocardiography. *Am J Cardiol.* 1985;55:146–151.
114. Unverferth DV, Magorien RD, Moeschberger ML, Baker PB, Fetters JK, Leier CV. Factors influencing the one-year mortality of dilated cardiomyopathy. *Am J Cardiol.* 1984;54:147–152.
115. Poll DS, Marchlinski FE, Falcone RA, Josephson ME, Simson MB. Abnormal signal-averaged electrocardiograms in patients with nonischemic congestive cardiomyopathy: relationship to sustained ventricular tachyarrhythmias. *Circulation.* 1985;72:1308–1313.
116. Lindsay BD, Ambos HD, Schechtman KB, Arthur RM, Cain ME. Noninvasive detection of patients with ischemic and nonischemic heart disease prone to ventricular fibrillation. *J Am Coll Cardiol.* 1990;16:1656–1664.
117. Middlekauf HR, Stevenson WG, Woo MA, Moser DK, Stevenson LW. Comparison of frequency of late potentials in idiopathic dilated cardiomyopathy and ischemic cardiomyopathy with advanced congestive heart failure and their usefulness in predicting sudden death. *Am J Cardiol.* 1990;66:1113–1117.
118. Keeling PJ, Kulakowski P, Yi G, Slade AKB, Bent SE, McKenna WJ. Usefulness of signal-averaged electrocardiogram in idiopathic dilated cardiomyopathy for identifying patients with ventricular arrhythmias. *Am J Cardiol.* 1993;72:78–84.
119. Mancini DM, Wong KL, Simson MB. Prognostic value of an abnormal signal-averaged electrocardiogram in patients with nonischemic congestive cardiomyopathy. *Circulation.* 1993;87:1083–1092.
120. Silverman ME, Pressel MD, Brackett JC, Lauria SS, Gold MR, Gottlieb SS. Prognostic value of the signal-averaged electrocardiogram and a prolonged QRS in ischemic and nonischemic cardiomyopathy. *Am J Cardiol.* 1995;75:460–464.
121. Turitto G, Ahuja RK, Caref EB, El-Sherif N. Risk stratification for arrhythmic events in patients with nonischemic dilated cardiomyopathy and nonsustained ventricular tachycardia: role of programmed

ventricular stimulation and the signal-averaged electrocardiogram. *J Am Coll Cardiol.* 1994;24:1523–1528.
122. Cain ME, Anderson JL, Arnsdorf MF, Mason JW, Scheinman MM, Waldo AL. Signal-averaged electrocardiography. *J Am Coll Cardiol.* 1996;27:238–249.
123. Yi G, Keeling PJ, Goldman JH, Jian H, Poloniecki J, McKenna WJ. Prognostic significance of spectral turbulence analysis of the signal-averaged electrocardiogram in patients with idiopathic dilated cardiomyopathy. *Am J Cardiol.* 1995;75:494–497.
124. Buxton AE, Waxman HL, Marchlinski FE, Josephson ME. Electrophysiologic studies in nonsustained ventricular tachycardia: relation to underlying heart disease. *Am J Cardiol.* 1983;52:985–991.
125. Gomes JA, Hariman RL, Kang PS, El-Sherif N, Chowdhry I, Lyons J. Programmed electrical stimulation in patients with high-grade ventricular ectopy: electrophysiologic findings and prognosis for survival. *Circulation.* 1984;70:43–51.
126. Veltri EP, Platia EV, Griffith L, Reid PR. Programmed electrical stimulation and long-term follow-up in asymptomatic, nonsustained ventricular tachycardia. *Am J Cardiol.* 1985;56:306–314.
127. Meinertz T, Treese N, Kasper W, et al. Determinants of prognosis in idiopathic dilated cardiomyopathy as determined by programmed electrical stimulation. *Am J Cardiol.* 1985;56:337–341.
128. Stamato NJ, O'Connell JB, Murdock DK, Moran JF, Loeb HS, Scanlon PJ. The response of patients with complex ventricular arrhythmias secondary to dilated cardiomyopathy to programmed electrical stimulation. *Am Heart J.* 1986;112:505–508.
129. Das SK, Morady F, DiCarlo L, et al. Prognostic usefulness of programmed ventricular stimulation in idiopathic dilated cardiomyopathy without symptomatic ventricular arrhythmias. *Am J Cardiol.* 1986;58:998–1000.
130. Poll DS, Marchlinski FE, Buxton AE, Josephson ME. Usefulness of programmed stimulation in idiopathic dilated cardiomyopathy. *Am J Cardiol.* 1986;58:992–997.
131. Kharsa MH, Gold RL, Moore H, Yazaki Y, Haffajee CI, Alpert JS. Long-term outcome following programmed electrical stimulation in patients with high-grade ventricular ectopy. *PACE.* 1988;11:603–609.
132. Buxton AE, Marchlinski FE, Waxman HL, Flores BT, Cassidy DM, Josephson ME. Prognostic factors in nonsustained ventricular tachycardia. *Am J Cardiol.* 1984;53:1275–1279.
133. Stevenson WG, Stevenson LW, Weiss J, Tillisch JH. Inducible ventricular arrhythmias and sudden death during vasodilator therapy of severe heart failure. *Am Heart J.* 1988;116:1447–1454.
134. Brembilla-Perrot B, Donetti J, de la Chaise AT, Sadoul N, Aliot E, Juilliere Y. Diagnostic value of ventricular stimulation in patients with idiopathic dilated cardiomyopathy. *Am Heart J.* 1991;121: 1124–1131.
135. Li HG, Jones DL, Yee R, Klein GJ. Electrophysiologic substrate associated with pacing-induced heart failure in dogs: potential value of programmed stimulation in predicting sudden death. *J Am Coll Cardiol.* 1992;19:444–449.
136. Pogwizd SM. Nonreentrant mechanisms underlying spontaneous ventricular arrhythmias in a model of nonischemic heart failure in rabbits. *Circulation.* 1995;92:1034–1048.

Chapter 8

Cardiac Rhythm Monitoring Advances

Barbara J. Drew, RN, PhD

Cardiac rhythm monitoring has become routine ever since the first coronary care units were introduced in the early 1960s. In the early years, single bipolar leads requiring just a positive, a negative, and a ground electrode were used simply to track heart rate and to detect cardiac arrest, ie, asystole or ventricular fibrillation. In the ensuing decades, the goals of cardiac monitoring have become extremely sophisticated. For example, clinicians use the bedside monitor to diagnose right and left bundle-branch block, to determine right versus left ventricular pacing rhythms, to distinguish ventricular tachycardia (VT) from supraventricular tachycardia (SVT) with aberrant conduction, to match recurrent wide-QRS complex tachycardias occurring with telemetry monitoring to specific QRS morphologies induced during invasive cardiac electrophysiological studies, and to detect episodes of myocardial ischemia with continuous ST-segment monitoring. Such sophisticated goals of monitoring require analysis of electrocardiographic (ECG) criteria from specific leads that are comparable to those recorded with a standard 12-lead ECG machine. The challenge is to have a bedside cardiac monitoring system that is both diagnostically accurate and yet simple enough to be practical for patients who are mobilized very early after myocardial infarction and revascularization procedures.

The purpose of this discussion is to raise several clinically relevant questions related to cardiac rhythm monitoring of patients in coronary care and telemetry units. Some of these questions have been the focus of prior research, and others require additional study. The questions include the following. (1) What is the best way

From: Dunbar SB, Ellenbogen KA, Epstein AE, (eds). *Sudden Cardiac Death: Past, Present, and Future.* Armonk, NY: Futura Publishing Company, Inc.; © 1997.

to monitor patients for accurate analysis of wide-QRS-complex tachycardia? (2) Can the MCL_1 monitoring lead be substituted for V_1 in the use of morphological criteria for diagnosing VT? (3) How important is accurate lead placement in distinguishing VT from SVT with aberrant conduction? (4) Are we monitoring the wrong thing?—ie, Is monitoring of ischemia more important than monitoring of arrhythmia for early warning of sudden cardiac death? (5) Is a derived 12-lead ECG advantageous for cardiac monitoring?

Diagnosis of Wide-QRS-Complex Tachycardia in the Immediate Care Setting

The standard 12-lead ECG remains the "gold standard" for distinguishing VT from SVT with aberrancy or bundle-branch block in the immediate care setting, because clinical findings, such as the patient's blood pressure or level of consciousness, may be misleading. In fact, when patients' signs and symptoms are used to make the diagnosis, wide-QRS-complex tachycardias are frequently misdiagnosed and patients suffer disastrous outcomes. For example, in two important reports,[1,2] when patients with hemodynamically stable VT were misdiagnosed as having SVT with aberrant conduction and were treated with intravenous verapamil, outcomes included persistent hypotension requiring vasopressors, acceleration of the tachycardia, degeneration of VT into ventricular fibrillation requiring defibrillation, and asystole after cardioversion.

We recently reported[3] that the 12-lead ECG was valuable in distinguishing between aberrantly conducted SVT and VT, even when limb electrodes were placed on the body torso and highly detailed criteria were modified for practical application in the immediate care setting. We concluded that multiple leads were required for accurate measurement of QRS width, presence of atrioventricular dissociation or ventriculoatrial block, QRS axis, and precordial lead morphological criteria. Using the standard 12-lead ECG and blinded to all clinical information, we were able to correctly identify 90% of wide-QRS-complex tachycardias induced during invasive cardiac electrophysiological study. Our findings were similar to those of Wellens et al[4] and Akhtar et al,[5] both of whom correctly identified 92% of wide-QRS-complex tachycardias with the 12-lead ECG. It is important to point out, however, that in the best of circumstances with experts analyzing the ECG, still about 1 in 10 wide-QRS-complex tachycardias defy differentiation. This is especially true of tachycardias >190 bpm, which deserve the most urgent attention in the immediate care setting.[3]

Although the 12-lead ECG is valuable for diagnosing wide-QRS-complex tachycardia, immediate treatment of a symptomatic patient should not be delayed until a standard ECG machine is located and all the necessary lead wires are attached. In such circumstances, 12-lead documentation of the tachycardia is often missed because the tachycardia is nonsustained. Although 12-lead cardiac monitoring has recently been made available, the cumbersome 10-electrode lead configuration is impractical because the left precordial electrodes are difficult to maintain in female patients with pendulous breasts or in men with hairy chests. Moreover, the multiple electrodes and lead wires interfere with recording echocardiograms, taking portable chest x-rays, and initiating emergency resuscitation, including defibrillation. Continuous 12-lead monitoring also curtails a patient's mobility and creates a noisy signal with body movement because electrodes are placed near moving joints (ie, shoulders and hips).

Although 12-lead monitoring may not be practical, it is possible to select cardiac monitoring leads that are more valuable than the routinely used lead II in the diagnosis of wide-QRS-complex tachycardia (Figure 1).[6] For example, we demonstrated that the combination of leads I, aVF, and V_1 were nearly as accurate as the full 12-lead ECG in distinguishing VT from SVT with aberrant conduction.[7] Leads I and aVF were valuable for identifying the highly abnormal right superior axis quadrant, which strongly suggests VT during a wide-QRS-complex tachycardia, and lead V_1 contained the valuable morphological criteria suggestive of VT or aberrancy. Another advantage of monitoring several leads is that more accurate measurement of QRS width can be made because wide QRS complexes may be partially isoelectric in a given lead, causing one to underestimate the true width of a tachycardia, which, if >0.16 second, is indicative of VT. Monitoring more than one lead also aids in the detection of dissociated P waves, which, if visible, provide strong evidence of VT. We found V_1 to be the most useful lead in observing atrioventricular dissociation; this, combined with its valuable morphological criteria, makes it an essential lead for arrhythmia monitoring.[3] Whereas lead V_1 is considered to contain the most information about disturbances of rhythm and conduction,[8] recent surveys[9,10] indicate that the vast majority of patients are monitored with lead II.

Use of MCL_1 for Cardiac Monitoring

Since its introduction in 1970,[8] monitoring with MCL_1 has become popular, especially for ambulatory telemetry and Holter applications, because of its simple three-electrode lead configuration. The

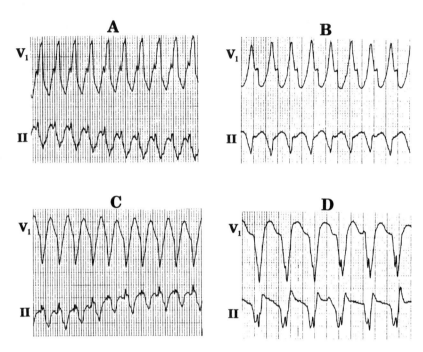

FIGURE 1. *Four patients with wide-QRS complex tachycardia induced during invasive cardiac electrophysiological study illustrate the value of V_1 and inadequacy of lead II for distinguishing SVT with aberrant conduction from VT. Patient A, with Wolff-Parkinson-White syndrome, has atrioventricular reciprocating (supraventricular) tachycardia. While lead II records a nonspecific pattern, V_1 records a triphasic pattern correctly indicative of right bundle-branch block–type aberrancy.[3–5] Patient B has VT, which can be readily identified by the positive waveform in lead V_1, with a taller left peak pattern.[3–5] Patient C has atrioventricular reciprocating (supraventricular) tachycardia with left bundle-branch block–type aberrancy. Lead V_1 records a negative wide complex with a steep, straight S downstroke reaching its nadir in ≤ 60 ms from QRS onset, which is correctly suggestive of aberrancy rather than VT.[6] Patient D has VT, which can be easily detected with V_1 by the notched S downstroke and delayed S nadir >60 ms.[6] An unhelpful pattern is recorded in lead II, which has a similar morphology in all four patients.*

diagnostic advantages of MCL_1 include the ability to identify right and left bundle-branch block patterns and aberrant ventricular conduction during SVT. However, we found that one could not substitute MCL_1 for V_1 in application of the morphological criteria for diagnosing VT.[3] We observed that MCL_1 looked identical to lead V_1

in a majority (90%) of patients during sinus rhythm; however, it often recorded clearly different QRS morphology during VT (Figure 2). In fact, 39 of 98 VTs (40%) exhibited clearly different QRS morphology in MCL_1 compared with V_1.[3] When we considered making a diagnosis based on QRS morphology from a single V_1 lead versus a single MCL_1 lead, 22% of VTs had morphological criteria in MCL_1 that erroneously favored aberrant SVT, whereas V_1 patterns

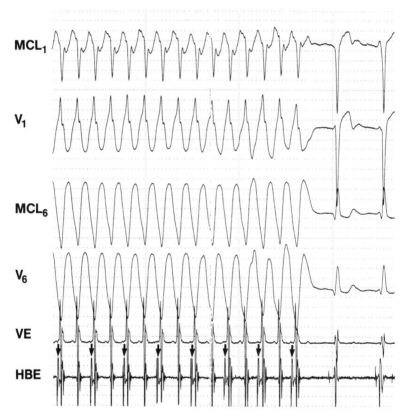

FIGURE 2. *Simultaneous recordings of MCL_1, V_1, MCL_6, V_6, and intracardiac electrograms (VE indicates ventricular electrogram; HBE, His bundle electrogram) in a patient with nonsustained VT. Retrograde conduction to the atria with 2:1 ventriculoatrial block is evident on the HBE recording (arrows). Although MCL_1 and V_1 record identical patterns after the tachycardia, during VT they exhibit clearly different QRS morphology. V_1 records a pattern indicative of VT,[3-5] whereas the negative complex with a steep, straight S downstroke recorded in MCL_1 is erroneously indicative of aberrancy rather than VT.[6]*

correctly suggested VT.[3] Because of these differences in QRS morphology between MCL_1 and V_1 during VT, we advised caution in applying morphological criteria intended for lead V_1 to MCL_1. This means that every attempt should be made to use a five-electrode true unipolar V_1 lead system for continuous cardiac monitoring rather than a three-electrode bipolar MCL_1 lead configuration.

Importance of Accurate Lead Placement

The closer a recording electrode is to the heart, the more exaggerated are QRS waveform changes with slight variations in electrode positioning.[11] Therefore, QRS morphology in the precordial leads, which are in close proximity to the heart, can be altered considerably if an electrode is moved just one intercostal space away from its designated location (Figure 3). Accurate lead placement is not only important for accurate diagnosis; it is also imperative for comparing wide-QRS tachycardias recorded during cardiac monitoring with specific QRS morphologies induced during invasive cardiac electrophysiological studies. For example, it is not uncommon for sudden cardiac death survivors with recurrent monomorphic VT to have ventricular ectopy or nonsustained VT during cardiac monitoring that is unrelated to the tachycardia of concern and that has QRS morphology different from that identified during cardiac electrophysiological study. Such different morphological patterns are not the target of pharmacological treatment. Distinction between such "benign" versus lethal tachycardias can be made only if lead placement for cardiac monitoring is accurate and identical to lead placement during cardiac electrophysiological study.

Importance of Ischemia Monitoring in Patients With Sudden Cardiac Death

Most patients who experience sudden arrhythmic arrest have underlying ischemic heart disease. Transient myocardial ischemia is a common substrate for the development of malignant ventricular arrhythmias. In a recent study examining the relation between sudden death and ischemia,[12] transient ischemic ST changes preceded the terminal event in 52% of patients who died during ambulatory ECG monitoring. Figure 4 illustrates a patient from our institution who developed VT after 30 minutes of progressive ST-segment deviation. It is conceivable that aggressive treatment of transient myocardial ischemia might prevent sudden arrhythmic

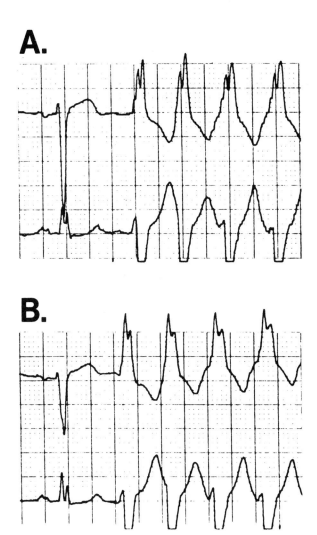

FIGURE 3. *Dual-channel rhythm strips (V_1, top; lead II, bottom) in a patient with recurrent monomorphic VT. In A, lead placement is inaccurate, with the chest electrode for V_1 placed in the fifth rather than the fourth intercostal space. QRS morphology shows a taller right peak pattern that is not indicative of VT.[4] When lead placement is corrected in B, the same monomorphic tachycardia now exhibits the valuable taller left peak pattern in V_1, which correctly indicates VT.[3–5]*

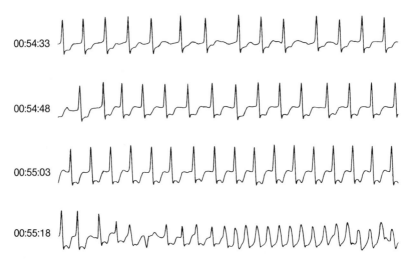

FIGURE 4. *Monitoring of a patient admitted to the coronary care unit with unstable angina and episodes of acute "flash" pulmonary edema. Upon admission, the patient's ST segments were isoelectric in this lead. At 00:54:33 (top strip), several millimeters of J-point depression was evident, with an up-sloping ST segment. Over the next few minutes, ischemic ST-segment abnormalities become more severe, as evidenced by a horizontal (00:54:48) followed by a downsloping (000:55:03) ST segment. With this ischemic substrate present, all that was required to induce VT and sudden cardiac death was a trigger in the form of a ventricular premature beat. In such patients, continuous ischemia monitoring may provide an early warning of sudden cardiac death.*

death in such patients. An important area for future research would be to determine whether "substrate" monitoring (ie, ischemia monitoring) would be more valuable than arrhythmia monitoring in treating patients at risk for sudden cardiac death.

Whereas lead V_1 has been shown to be a valuable lead for arrhythmia monitoring, it is not a valuable lead for ischemia monitoring.[13-18] The ideal laboratory for studying the value of various leads in detecting ischemia due to coronary occlusion is the cardiac catheterization laboratory, because ischemia occurs repeatedly with interruptions of blood flow during angioplasty catheter balloon inflations. We have recorded 12-lead ECG recordings during coronary angioplasty in more than 400 patients to date and have found leads III and aVF to be most sensitive for detecting ischemia related to right coronary artery occlusion and V_3 to be most sensitive for detecting ischemia related to left anterior descending or left circumflex artery occlusions. Others have reported similar findings, with precordial leads V_2 or V_3 often recommended for ischemia monitoring.[13-17] Unfortunately, with the vast majority of current monitoring systems, it is not possible to monitor more than one precordial lead. Therefore, it is impossible to monitor patients with both an ideal arrhythmia lead (V_1) and an ideal ischemia lead (V_2 or V_3).

Potential Advantages of Monitoring a Derived 12-Lead ECG

We recently reported[19] that the "EASI" lead method introduced by Dower et al[20] for deriving 12 ECG leads from three information channels by use of a five-electrode configuration was as valuable as the standard 12-lead ECG for diagnosing wide-QRS complex tachycardia (Figures 5 and 6).[21] Further testing indicated that the derived 12-lead ECG was valuable for diagnosing ischemia during angioplasty balloon inflation.[22] Moreover, ST-segment monitoring of the derived 12-lead ECG was superior to routine monitoring for detecting transient myocardial ischemia in patients admitted to the coronary care unit for unstable angina or acute myocardial infarction.[23] In our study,[23] 55 of 250 patients (22%) had a total of 176 ischemic episodes detected with ST monitoring of the derived 12-lead ECG. Of these 55 patients with ischemia, 75% reported no chest pain, and in 64% no ischemic ST changes were visible with routine monitoring leads.

The potential advantages of monitoring patients with the derived 12-lead ECG are summarized in Table 1. Monitoring the derived ECG provides all 12 leads for arrhythmia and ischemia analysis, with the advantage that transient events can be documented with a full 12-lead ECG. In contrast, routine cardiac monitoring provides a limited number of leads, with typically only one V lead choice. The disadvantage of one V lead choice is that patients cannot be monitored with the best arrhythmia lead (V_1) and the best ischemia lead (V_2 or V_3). As mentioned above, ischemia is an important substrate for the development of life-threatening arrhythmias, so patients should be monitored for both conditions. Routine telemetry monitoring often involves the use of a modified precordial lead (MCL_1), which should not be substituted for V_1 when morphological criteria are applied for diagnosing VT.

Monitoring the derived 12-lead ECG also has advantages over monitoring the standard 12-lead ECG. For example, the standard ECG requires 10 electrodes, which is impractical for bedside moni-

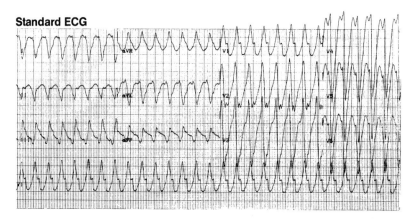

FIGURE 5. *Standard 12-lead ECG recorded in the cardiac electrophysiology laboratory during VT. Numerous ECG criteria are present that are valuable in diagnosing VT, including (1) a QRS axis in the right superior quadrant,[3,4] (2) a positive complex in V$_1$ with a taller left peak pattern,[3–5] (3) a QS complex in V$_6$,[3–5] (4) a QRS width >0.16 second,[3] and (5) a prolonged (>100 ms) RS interval in several precordial leads.[21]*

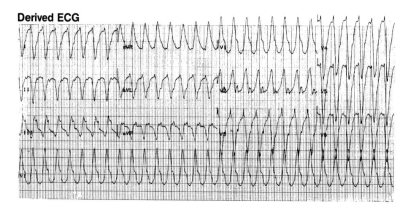

FIGURE 6. *Derived 12-lead ECG recorded simultaneously with Figure 6 exhibits the same valuable criteria for VT as are observed with the standard ECG. Although the standard and derived ECGs record different QRS amplitudes in various leads, these differences do not affect the diagnostic accuracy of the derived ECG for distinguishing SVT with aberrant conduction from VT.[18]*

TABLE 1

Comparisons of Cardiac Rhythm Monitoring Systems

Derived 12-lead	Routine Monitoring
All 12 leads available for: Accurate arrhythmia diagnosis Sensitive ischemia detection Documentation of transient events	Limited number of leads available: Typically, only one V lead choice Best arrhythmia lead is V_1 Best ischemia lead is V_3 MCL leads are unacceptable substitutes for V lead

Derived 12-Lead	Standard 12-Lead
Fewer (3) information channels required Increased capacity for "full disclosure" storage of 12-lead ECGs	More (8) information channels required Reduced storage capacity
Convenient electrode configuration Left precordium free of electrodes	Inconvenient electrode configuration V_2–V_5 in the way of defibrillation, echocar- diography, auscultation, portable chest x-rays Multiple electrodes costly, cause skin irritation
Stable electrode positions Electrodes on upper/lower sternum and under right and left axilla create minimal noise with body movement	Unstable electrode positions near shoulders, hips Noisy signal with body movement Different QRS waveforms with electrodes on torso rather than on extremities

toring, and it also requires eight information channels, which limits the number of ECGs that can be stored with "full disclosure"–type monitoring systems. The eight information channels of the standard 12-lead ECG include the six precordial leads and two standard limb leads, from which the remaining four limb leads are derived. In contrast, the derived ECG requires just three information channels, which increases its storage capacity. Another advantage of the derived ECG is that it has a convenient electrode configuration that leaves the left precordium free for cardiac auscultation, defibrillation, recording of echocardiograms, etc. Finally, the derived electrode positions (Figure 7) are not close to moving joints, and therefore, minimal noise is observed with body movement.

Conclusions

Over the past three decades, enormous improvements have been made in ECG diagnosis of arrhythmias causing sudden cardiac death and in cardiac monitoring techniques. However, many patients are not being monitored with the most valuable leads for ischemia and arrhythmia diagnosis, and inaccurate lead placement is

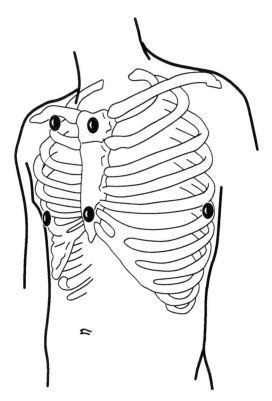

FIGURE 7. *The EASI™ electrode placement for obtaining the derived 12-lead ECG.[20] Electrodes are placed on the upper and lower sternum (level of the fifth intercostal space) and the right and left midaxillary lines at the same level as the lower sternal electrode. The fifth electrode is the ground electrode, which can be placed anywhere (shown here below the right clavicle).*

also a problem in current practice. Future studies need to determine the role of ischemia monitoring in patients with life-threatening arrhythmias and the utility of continuous monitoring with a derived 12-lead ECG.

References

1. Stewart RB, Bardy GH, Greene HL. Wide complex tachycardia: misdiagnosis and outcome after emergent therapy. *Ann Intern Med.* 1986;104:766–771.
2. Buxton AE, Marchlinski FE, Doherty JU, Flores B, Josephson ME. Hazards of intravenous verapamil for sustained ventricular tachycardia. *Am J Cardiol.* 1987;59:1107–1110.
3. Drew BJ, Scheinman MM. ECG criteria to distinguish between aberrantly conducted supraventricular tachycardia and ventricular tachycardia: practical aspects for the immediate care setting. *PACE.* 1995;18:2194–2208.
4. Wellens HJJ, Bär FW, Vanagt EJ, Brugada P, Farre J. The differentiation between ventricular tachycardia and supraventricular tachycardia with aberrrant conduction: the value of the 12-lead electrocardiogram. In: Wellens HJJ, Kulbertus HE, eds. *What's New in Electrocardiography.* The Hague, Netherlands: Martinus Nijhoff; 1981:184–199.
5. Akhtar M, Shenasa M, Jazayeri M, Caceres J, Tchou PJ. Wide QRS complex tachycardia: reappraisal of a common clinical problem. *Ann Intern Med.* 1988;109 905–912.
6. Kindwall KE, Brown J, Josephson ME. Electrocardiographic criteria for ventricular tachycardia in wide complex left bundle branch block morphology tachycardias. *Am J Cardiol.* 1988;61:1279–1283.
7. Drew BJ, Scheinman MM. Value of electrocardiographic leads MCL_1, MCL_6 and other selected leads in the diagnosis of wide QRS complex tachycardia. *J Am Coll Cardiol.* 1991;18:1025–1033.
8. Marriott HJL, Fogg E. Constant monitoring for cardiac dysrhythmias and blocks. *Mod Concepts Cardiovasc Dis.* 1970;39:103–108.
9. Drew BJ, Ide B, Sparacino PSA. Bedside ECG monitoring: a report on current practices of critical care nurses. *Heart Lung.* 1991;20:597–609.
10. Thomason TR, Riegel B, Carlson B, Gocka I. Monitoring electrocardiographic changes: results of a national survey. *J Cardiovasc Nurs.* 1995;9:1–9.
11. Wilson FN. The distribution of the potential differences produced by the heart beat within the body and at its surface. *Am Heart J.* 1929–1930;5:599–616.
12. Pepine CJ, Gottlieb SO, Morganroth J. Ambulatory ischemia and sudden death: an analysis of 35 cases of death during ambulatory ECG monitoring. *J Am Coll Cardiol.* 1991;17:63A. Abstract.
13. Blanke H, Cohen M, Schlueter GU, Karsch KR, Rentrop KP. Electrocardiographic and coronary arteriographic correlations during acute myocardial infarction. *Am J Cardiol.* 1984;54:249–255.
14. Krucoff MW. Identification of high risk patients with silent myocardial ischemia after transluminal coronary angioplasty by multilead monitoring. *Am J Cardiol.* 1988;61:29F–34F.

15. Berry C, Zalewski A, Kovach R, Savage M, Goldberg S. Surface electrocardiogram in the detection of transmural myocardial ischemia during coronary artery occlusion. *Am J Cardiol.* 1989;63:21–26.
16. Mizutani M, Freedman SB, Barns E, Ogasawara S, Bailey BP, Bernstein L. ST monitoring for myocardial ischemia during and after coronary angioplasty. *Am J Cardiol.* 1990;66:389–393.
17. Bush HS, Ferguson JJ, Angelini P, Willerson JT. Twelve-lead electrocardiographic evaluation of ischemia during percutaneous transluminal coronary angioplasty and its correlation with acute reocclusion. *Am Heart J.* 1991;121:1591–1599.
18. Drew BJ, Tisdale LA. ST segment monitoring for coronary artery reocclusion following thrombolytic therapy and coronary angioplasty: identification of optimal bedside monitoring leads. *Am J Crit Care.* 1993;2:280–292.
19. Drew BJ, Scheinman MM, Evans GT. Comparison of a vectorcardiographically derived 12-lead electrocardiogram with the conventional electrocardiogram during wide QRS complex tachycardia, and its potential application for continuous bedside monitoring. *Am J Cardiol.* 1992;69:612–618.
20. Dower GE, Yakush A, Nazzal SB, Jutzy RV, Ruiz CE. Deriving the 12-lead electrocardiogram from four (EASI) electrodes. *J Electrocardiol.* 1988;120–S182–S187.
21. Brugada P, Brugada J, Mont L, Smeets J, Andries EW. A new approach to the differential diagnosis of a regular tachycardia with a wide QRS complex. *Circulation.* 1991;83:1649–1659.
22. Drew BJ, Koops RR, Adams MG, Dower GE. Derived 12-lead ECG: comparison with the standard ECG during myocardial ischemia and its potential application for continuous ST-segment monitoring. *J Electrocardiol.* 1994;27:249–255.
23. Drew BJ, Adams MG, Pelter MM, Wung SF. ST segment monitoring with a derived 12-lead electrocardiogram is superior to routine cardiac care unit monitoring. *Am J Crit Care.* 1996;5:198–206.

Chapter 9

Use of Heart-Rate Variability in Special Populations

Mary A. Woo, DNSc, RN

Introduction

The risk of sudden cardiac death (SCD) is associated with alterations in autonomic nervous system tone in both healthy and ill populations.[1] This association is due primarily to the profound influence of the two branches of the autonomic nervous system, sympathetic and parasympathetic, on cardiac electrophysiological parameters (see Table 1).[2,3] Typically, sympathetic stimulation increases and parasympathetic stimulation decreases the occurrence of ventricular dysrhythmias.[2]

Because of the potent interactions between the autonomic nervous system, ventricular dysrhythmias, and mortality, monitoring and evaluation of sympathetic and parasympathetic activity is an important component in the clinical evaluation and treatment of persons at increased risk for SCD. There are two basic ways to assess autonomic tone: invasive and noninvasive. Invasive methods, such as direct nerve recordings, are expensive, have limited application and repeatability, and require extensive operator training. Because of these problems, many researchers and clinicians have focused on noninvasive methods to assess autonomic tone.

One of the more recent methods developed to evaluate autonomic tone noninvasively is heart-rate variability (HRV). A wide variety of HRV techniques has been used to assess the potential for SCD in several high-risk populations: post–myocardial infarction (MI) patients, heart failure patients, and sudden infant death syndrome (SIDS) survivors. However, before one can fully appreciate

From: Dunbar SB, Ellenbogen KA, Epstein AE, (eds). *Sudden Cardiac Death: Past, Present, and Future.* Armonk, NY: Futura Publishing Company, Inc.; © 1997.

TABLE 1

Effects of the Autonomic Nervous System on the Heart

Parameter	Sympathetic	Parasympathetic
Cardiac automaticity	Increase	Decrease
Conduction velocity	Increase	Decrease
Refractory period	Decrease	Increase
Ventricular dysrhythmias	Increase	Decrease
Heart rate	Increase	Decrease

the application of HRV to SCD risk in these special populations, an initial understanding of HRV is needed.

Heart-Rate Variability

HRV can be defined as the behavior of sinus RR intervals of an electrocardiogram (ECG). HRV reflects a variety of internal and external influences on the autonomic nervous system. These influences are expressed via the two branches of the autonomic nervous system, the sympathetic and parasympathetic, which in turn alter sinoatrial node depolarization and thus HRV (Figure 1). Parasympathetic activity is particularly influential in RR interval behavior, because this part of the autonomic system responds much more rapidly than the sympathetic branch. Because of the rapidity of the parasympathetic response, most investigators consider that measures of HRV primarily reflect the influence of parasympathetic tone.

High HRV is associated with increased parasympathetic activity and relatively low sympathetic tone. High parasympathetic tone is affiliated with a cardioprotective state.[5] Low HRV is associated with decreased parasympathetic activity and relatively high sympathetic tone.[6] High sympathetic tone is associated with decreased ventricular fibrillatory threshold, increased ventricular arrhythmias, and increased mortality risk.[7,8] Thus, high HRV, with its associated increased parasympathetic tone, is considered to be a desirable state.

Advantages and Disadvantages of HRV

There are multiple advantages in the application of measures of HRV to assess a variety of patient populations. A significant advantage is that it can be measured by noninvasive methods with

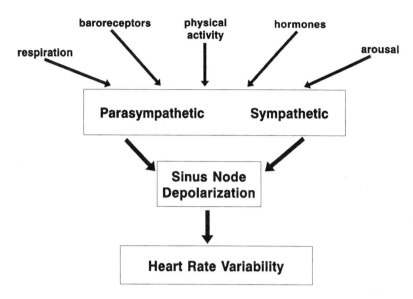

FIGURE 1. *A variety of both internal and external factors affect the autonomic nervous system and are reflected via the parasympathetic and sympathetic branches. These in turn influence sinus node depolarization and thus RR interval behavior (HRV).*

equipment that is currently available in most acute care facilities (Holter scanners), critical care units (monitors), and cardiology laboratories (computerized data acquisition systems, Holter scanners). Another advantage is that many researchers have reported a high degree of association between a variety of HRV measures and other estimates of autonomic nervous system activity. A particularly attractive attribute of HRV is that several investigators have been able to offer convincing evidence that changes in HRV provide an accurate estimate of prognosis in a variety of illnesses. For example, measures of HRV have been used to assess fetal distress and the influence of various maternal drug levels on the fetus,[9] to evaluate prognosis after MI[10] or heart failure,[11] to assess risk of ventricular dysrhythmias and response to antiarrhythmia medications,[12,13] and as a clinical test for autonomic neuropathy in persons with diabetes mellitus.[14] Thus, assessment of HRV can provide clinicians and researchers with valuable information regarding parasympathetic, sympathetic, and overall autonomic nervous system tone.

Unfortunately, there are several drawbacks in the use of HRV. Problems with HRV methodologies include: (1) application only in persons with health conditions in which clinically significant inter-actions between the autonomic nervous system and disease state ex-ist, (2) usefulness only when autonomic tone can be accurately reflected in cardiac RR interval behavior, (3) the indirect nature of the measurement of autonomic activity, and (4) the existence of mul-tiple methods of measuring HRV that are not necessarily equivalent.

Although the autonomic nervous system both influences and reflects internal and external forces in the body, information re-garding autonomic tone may be of minimal assistance in the as-sessment, treatment, or prognosis of patients with certain illnesses. For example, probably autonomic tone information would not sig-nificantly alter the care of persons with appendicitis, fractures, or pneumonia. Additionally, when one considers the rapidly dimin-ishing healthcare funding situation, the allocation of scarce re-sources (money, personnel, and time) to the collection of data with little direct benefit to the patient is a questionable activity for healthcare providers.

An additional problem with HRV exists if prior or current ill-ness conditions diminish direct neurocardiac interaction. This is because reflection of autonomic activity via HRV could be ad-versely affected by such conditions. The sensitivity of HRV to al-terations in neurocardiac communication exists because information regarding autonomic nervous system tone via HRV depends on autonomic influences on sinoatrial node depolariza-tion. Thus, any interference in the transmission or influence of au-tonomic tone on the sinoatrial node could induce error. For example, patients with third-degree heart block, atrial fibrillation or atrial flutter, cardiac pacemakers, or denervated hearts (as after a heart transplantation) may not reflect accurate information re-garding autonomic tone by HRV measures.

HRV is an indirect measure, because it can only infer auto-nomic tone from RR interval behavior. Thus, the precision of mea-sures of HRV depends on both control and consistency of intervening factors that may alter reflection of autonomic tone in RR interval behavior.[15] Examples of intervening factors include changes in environmental temperature, sleep state, and presence of ectopy or recording artifact during RR interval data collection for analysis of HRV.

The existence of multiple measures further confuses potential users of HRV. HRV can be reported with a wide variety of analytic methods, ranging from simple means to nonlinear calculations of fractal behavior. Another complication associated with the pres-ence of numerous methods is the problem that the various mea-sures do not necessarily report the same direction or level of autonomic activity. Examples of this lack of equivalency have been reported in several studies using two or more measures of HRV.[16–18]

Each HRV analysis method has its own strengths and weaknesses that must be considered before it can be applied in a proposed clinical or research situation. These HRV measures can be broadly divided into three groups: linear variance measures, spectral analysis, and nonlinear procedures.

Linear Variance Measures

In general, these methods examine the variability of sequential sinus RR intervals. Although a variety of standard deviation or ratio measures of RR interval behavior have been reported in the literature since the 1960s, it was the research by Kleiger et al[19] in 1987 and his use of a standard deviation measure of HRV in patients after an MI that sparked the interest of cardiologists. They calculated HRV as the standard deviation of the square root of the mean of the squared deviations of each RR interval from the general mean RR interval over a 24-hour recording period (SDNN; Figure 2). Kleiger et al[19] examined 808 post-MI patients and was able to discriminate between individuals at low (SDNN >100 ms), medium (SDNN between 50 and 100 ms), and high (SDNN <50 ms) risk for mortality. He demonstrated that an SDNN of <50 ms had a greater statistical strength of association with mortality than

$$\sqrt{\frac{\sum \left(\text{Mean}_T - \text{R-R}_1\right)^2 + \left(\text{Mean}_T - \text{R-R}_2\right)^2 + \ldots + \left(\text{Mean}_T - \text{R-R}_N\right)^2}{N}}$$

Mean$_T$ = mean of all intervals in the sampling period

N = number of intervals in the sample

FIGURE 2. *HRV formula described by Kleiger et al.[18] It consists of the standard deviation of the square root mean of the squared deviations over a 24-hour period.*

other Holter variables, such as frequency of ventricular ectopy, presence of complex ventricular ectopy, mean RR interval, or mean heart rate. Since the development of the SDNN, a number of alternative variance measures have emerged, including multiple versions of standard deviation tools.[20-22] Popular standard deviation measures include an assessment of the proportion of RR-interval pairs in a recording period with an arbitrary difference of >50 ms (PNN50, Figure 3)[13,22,23] and a sequential difference calculation (RMSSD, Figure 4).[23] However, the SDNN method and Kleiger's risk categories remain the only widely used procedure with standards of normalcy for a post-MI patient population.

Disadvantages of Linear Variance Measures

Linear variance measures of HRV, in common with all linear analytic techniques, make the following assumptions regarding the characteristics and behavior of the variables under examination[24]: (1) measurement or control of all variables that influence the be-

$$RR_n - RR_{n+1} \Big\langle \begin{array}{l} \text{If result is > 50 ms, then add 1 to YES count} \\ \\ \text{If result is < 50 ms, then add 1 to NO count} \end{array}$$

$$\text{Heart Rate Variability} = \left(\frac{\text{YES count}}{\text{YES count + NO count}} \right) * 100$$

- -

$$RR_n = \text{R-R interval}$$

$$RR_{n+1} = \text{following R-R interval}$$

Figure 3. *Formulas for the calculation of the proportion of sinus RR interval pairs with >50 ms difference (PNN50).*

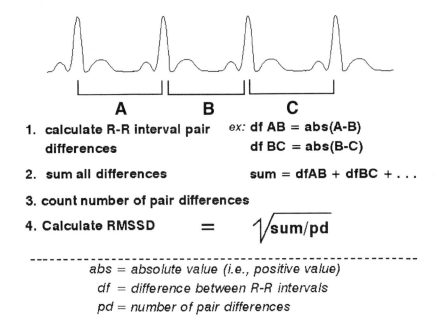

1. **calculate R-R interval pair**   *ex:* **df AB = abs(A-B)**
   differences   **df BC = abs(B-C)**

2. **sum all differences**   **sum = dfAB + dfBC + . . .**

3. **count number of pair differences**

4. **Calculate RMSSD   = $\sqrt{\text{sum/pd}}$**

----

abs = absolute value (i.e., positive value)
df = difference between R-R intervals
pd = number of pair differences

FIGURE 4. *Formulas for the calculation of the root mean square of difference of successive RR intervals (RMSSD).*

havior of interest by the investigator, (2) normal/Gaussian distribution, and (3) stationarity of variable relation. Unfortunately, these conditions are rarely found in biological data and are particularly scarce in the behavior of RR intervals.

As was discussed earlier and briefly illustrated in Figure 1, there are multiple internal and external factors that influence autonomic nervous system activity and are reflected in HRV. Most known factors that influence HRV are either difficult to measure or unethical to control in human subjects. Moreover, there are probably multiple unknown factors that affect HRV.

Normal distribution is a rare occurrence in the behavior of biological phenomena, and it does not often occur in RR intervals (Figure 5). Without normal distribution, interpretation and understanding of standard deviation and other linear analytic measures may be difficult or misleading.

Stationarity refers to the constant and predictive nature of relation between variables of interest. For example, as variable A changes, there would be a predictive and proportional alteration in variable B (Figure 6). Owing in part to the multiple factors that in-

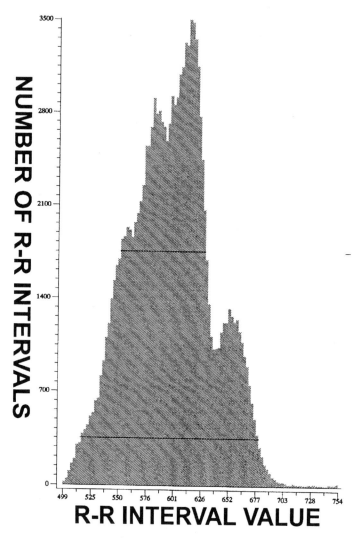

FIGURE 5. *Histogram of RR intervals. Note that the distribution of RR intervals is multimodal and skewed. This non-Gaussian distribution is common in biological data, including RR intervals of the electrocardiogram.*

fluence RR intervals and in part to the inherent nature of RR interval behavior, linear and predictive relation between RR intervals are unlikely. Since RR interval behavior rarely meets the assumptions of linear analysis regarding control, normal distribution, and stationarity, the application and interpretation of these measures must be made with caution.

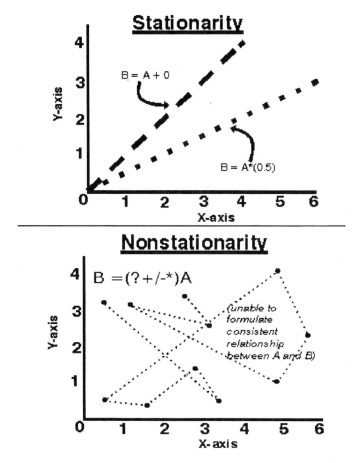

FIGURE 6. *Examples of stationarity and nonstationarity. For these examples, variable A is the x-axis coordinate and variable B is the y-axis coordinate. Stationarity exists when there is a predictive and constant relation between variables (top panel). Nonstationarity exists when there is no predictive and constant relation between the variables (bottom panel).*

Spectral Analysis

Spectral analysis is rapidly becoming one of the most popular measures of HRV. Spectral analysis procedures convert time-domain data into the frequency domain. This conversion into the frequency domain allows the assessment of influential factors that contribute to the behavior of the variable of interest. For example, spectral analysis of HRV would calculate a rate curve from the submitted sinus RR intervals. The frequency components that make up this rate curve then would allow the user to infer physiological mechanisms, such as respiration, baroreceptor reflexes, and physical activity, that influence the behavior of the rate curve. A common way to explain spectral analysis is through the use of the prism analogy (Figure 7). One could think of time-domain data, such as the electrocardiogram, as a beam of white light. To discriminate the various components that make up white light (electrocardiogram), the investigator could pass it through a prism (spectral analysis procedure). The prism (spectral analysis procedure) would break up the white light (RR intervals of the electrocardiogram) into the various colors (physiological variables) that make white light (electrocardiogram) look white (RR interval behavior).

Various researchers have detected at least three distinct components (low, mid, and high) in the frequency domain of spectral analysis of HRV. These components can be described as follows[25,26]: a low-frequency component (0.02 to 0.09 Hz) mediated by sympathetic and parasympathetic nervous systems, thermoregulation, vasomotor tone, and renin-angiotensin systems; a mid-frequency component (0.09 to 0.15 Hz) that primarily reflects

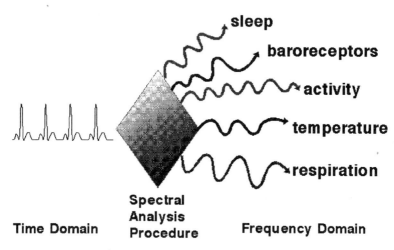

FIGURE 7. *Prism analogy for HRV spectral analysis procedure. For HRV, the electrocardiogram represents white light and the spectral analysis procedure is the prism. As the electrocardiogram (white light) is passed through the spectral analysis procedure (prism), the components (baroreceptor activity, hormones, respiration, etc) that cause the electrocardiogram to behave in its particular manner are converted from the time domain (electrocardiogram) into the frequency domain (usually in Hz).*

baroreflex and blood pressure regulation; and a high-frequency component (0.15 to 0.40 Hz), a respiratory band most closely allied to parasympathetic activity (Figure 8). As can be seen from these frequency components and their ranges, the parasympathetic system can respond over a wide range, whereas the sympathetic nervous system response is limited to relatively low frequencies, often <0.1 Hz. Thus, whereas the low-frequency fluctuations are jointly modulated by both the sympathetic and parasympathetic nervous systems, higher-frequency fluctuations are mediated solely by the parasympathetic nervous system.[27,28]

Spectral analysis has been used with great success in a variety of research and clinical studies.[23,28,29] It has the advantage over other current measures of HRV in its ability to analyze short (<5 minutes) and long (24 hours) data sets and in that it is the only method that can distinguish sympathetic and parasympathetic activity.

However, there are multiple assumptions and disadvantages to this technique that can often be unknown or ignored by its users. Assumptions of spectral analysis include a continuous time series (in both a mathematical and a chronological sense), stationarity of

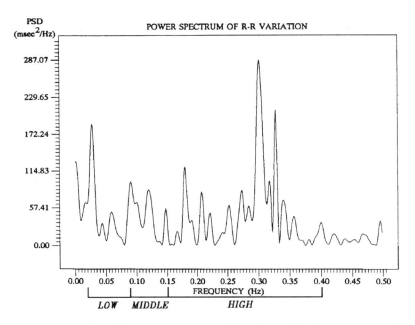

FIGURE 8. *Example of HRV using spectral analysis. The three primary frequency ranges (low, mid, and high) are indicated on the x axis. Note the high-frequency peak in the higher-frequency range (between 0.15 and 0.40 Hz: parasympathetic activity).*

variable relation, whole-number multiple event cycles, and symmetrical distribution of variable behavior around sine-wave peaks of each frequency component.[30,31] Usually such assumptions are not met in biological data, including RR intervals.[30] Violations of these assumptions can lead to erroneous conclusions regarding autonomic nervous system tone as reported by spectral analysis. Another problem is the extreme sensitivity of the spectral analysis procedure to artifact or ectopy.[30,32] Even small perturbations caused by a single artifact or ectopic beat can result in an erroneous or uninterpretable power spectral plot. Another concern is that standards of normalcy have not been established for any spectral analysis procedure of HRV.

Nonlinear Procedures

As has been mentioned previously, most biological variables, including RR intervals, do not behave in the traditional linear manner and often lack normal distribution. Nonlinear analytic techniques are alternative methods of exploring and interpreting the complex actions of data. They do not assume or require linear relation between variables or normal distribution. Thus, some researchers have proposed that nonlinear techniques are more appropriate to examine RR interval characteristics.

A variety of researchers have used nonlinear measures to assess RR interval behavior. Goldberger and Rigney,[33] Guevara and Glass,[34] and Skinner[35] were some of the earliest and most prolific of the adherents of nonlinear analysis for RR interval behavior. They used a variety of nonlinear analysis measures derived from chaos study in physics to provide exciting and alternative views of the dynamic interactions between RR intervals and the autonomic nervous system. However, their applied nonlinear methodologies are mathematically complex and at times may not have completely validated formulas or may be clinically inadequate. Our research has concentrated on the use of a nonlinear measure of HRV called Poincaré plots (also known as Lorenz plots; Figure 9).[36] This method has the advantage of describing both beat-to-beat and overall RR interval behavior, and it is simple both to perform and to interpret. Yet Poincaré plots are inadequate for clinical application in that they lack quantification methods and have not been applied to large numbers or types of patient or healthy populations.

Like the other measures of HRV, nonlinear methods have distinct disadvantages. Nonlinear measures do not allow users to infer causal or directional relation. Of particular concern is the lack

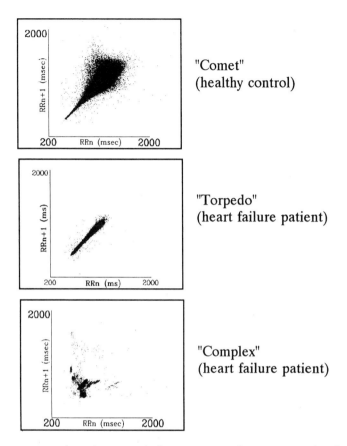

FIGURE 9. *Examples of Poincaré plots. Top panel is an example of a normal Poincaré plot. Normal plots are characterized by increased symmetrical RR interval dispersion at slower heart rates (longer RR intervals). Middle and bottom panels contain examples of abnormal Poincaré plots from heart failure patients (torpedo and complex). Torpedo-shaped plots (middle panel) are characterized by a lack of symmetrical RR interval dispersion at slower heart rates. Complex plots (bottom panel) are characterized by asymmetrical RR interval groups around a small, torpedo-shaped core.*

of standards of normality and the modest assortment of patient populations examined with these techniques.

HRV can be both a promising tool and a source of confusion for clinicians and researchers. Some examples of the use of HRV in the assessment of SCD risk are presented below.

HRV and Sudden Cardiac Death After Myocardial Infarction

SCD is most frequently associated with atherosclerotic heart disease and its induction of lethal dysrhythmias.[37] The increased sympathetic nervous system activity secondary to both acute myocardial ischemia and post-MI decreased ventricular function supports the development and propagation of ventricular dysrhythmias, particularly in the setting of myocardial ischemia.[38-40] Because of the high incidence of MI and SCD, particularly in the industrialized Western countries, the greatest number of HRV investigations have been performed in the post-MI patient population. However, although the predictive value of HRV for overall mortality has been well established by numerous researchers,[10,12,19,20,23] studies of SCD (considered separately from total mortality) have not been as frequent (Table 2, human studies only).[41-46] This lack of differentiation

TABLE 2

Studies on the Association of HRV with Sudden Death in Post-MI Patients

Reference	Clinical Parameter	Number of Subjects	HRV Methods	Associated With SCD?
Bigger JT et al[41]	Short-term measures of HRV	715 Post-MI	Spectral	Yes
Copie X et al[42]	2-Year follow-up	579 Post-acute phase MI	Mean HR SDNN	Yes Yes
Odemuyiwa O et al[43]	LVEF vs HRV	417 Post-MI	SDNN SDANN	Yes Yes
Klingenheben T et al[44]	Circadian variation	14 Hx SCD 14 No Hx SCD	Spectral SDNN PNN50	Yes No No
Hohnloser SH et al[45]	Comparison of SCD survivors vs no SCD	14 Hx SCD 14 No Hx SCD	SDRR PNN50	No No
Odemuyiwa O et al[46]	HRV measured within 6 months after acute MI	433 After first MI	SDNN SDANN	Yes Yes

LVEF indicates left ventricular ejection fraction; Hx, history of; spectral, spectral analysis with fast Fourier transform; HR, heart rate; SDNN, standard deviation of square root of mean of squared deviations of RR intervals; SDANN, standard deviation of 5-minute mean RR intervals; PNN50, proportion of RR intervals >50 ms different; and SDRR, standard deviation of the mean of RR intervals.

between total or all-cause mortality and SCD make the evaluation of HRV for SCD risk in post-MI patients more difficult.

Other problems and differences between studies also create problems for the would-be HRV evaluator or potential operator. Sample sizes can vary widely, with the smaller studies being less likely to discover a link between time-domain/linear-variance measures compared with larger studies. Another hazard is the possible difference in time between the subject's MI and HRV data collection. Both spectral and linear-variance measures of HRV change over a 12-month period after an MI. These HRV measures are low during the early convalescent phase and return to nearly normal by 6 to 12 months after the MI event.[47] Age also can influence HRV results, with a nonlinear decline in HRV with increasing age.[48,49] An additional problem in the comparison of these studies is the small number of spectral analysis HRV investigations with large sample sizes. Although preliminary spectral analysis HRV and SCD studies are impressive,[41,44] further research with spectral analysis HRV and SCD in larger samples would be desirable.

HRV and Sudden Cardiac Death in Heart Failure

Abnormalities in autonomic nervous system tone are common in heart failure patients and are linked to prognosis.[5,50] Multiple investigators have demonstrated both that HRV is decreased in heart failure patients compared with healthy controls[11,17,22] and that there are good associations between a wide variety of HRV methods and 1-year mortality.[11,22] However, SCD is an increasingly important mortality factor in this patient population. Sudden cardiac death now accounts for 30% to 60% of total mortality in persons with the most severe form of heart failure (New York Heart Association functional class III to IV and left ventricular ejection fraction <0.25).[51] Yet despite the autonomic nervous system changes associated with heart failure and the high incidence of SCD, surprisingly few studies have examined the association between HRV and SCD in these patients. (Table 3, human studies only).[52–55]

Examination of Table 3 shows several interesting factors. One factor is the lack of association of spectral-analysis and time-domain (standard deviation) HRV measures with SCD risk in both hypertrophic and dilated heart failure patients. This lack of association between HRV and SCD in heart failure is different from the situation observed in the post-MI population, in whom HRV and SCD appear to be well correlated (Table 2). A significant diffi-

TABLE 3

Studies on the Association of HRV With
Sudden Death in Heart Failure

Reference	Sample Type	Number of Subjects	HRV Methods	Associated With SCD?
Fei L et al[52]	Hypertrophic cardiomyopathy	31 HF 31 Controls	Spectral	No
Counihan PJ et al[53]	Hypertrophic cardiomyopathy	104 HF	Spectral SDRR SDANN PNN50	No No No No
Woo MA et al[54]	NYHA class III-IV, dilated HF	108 HF	SDANN Poincaré	No Yes
Woo MA et al[55]	NYHA class III-IV, LVEF <0.25, dilated HF	113 HF	SDANN Poincaré	Yes Yes

HF indicates heart failure; LVEF, left ventricular ejection fraction; spectral, spectral analysis with fast Fourier transform; SDRR, standard deviation of the mean RR intervals; SDANN, standard deviation of 5-minute mean RR intervals; PNN50, proportion of RR intervals >50 ms different; and Poincaré, Poincaré plots (scattergrams) of RR intervals (nonlinear method).

culty in interpreting the results of HRV data in cardiomyopathy patients is the relatively small sample sizes, particularly in comparison with most of the post-MI studies.

Another interesting trend shown in Table 3 is the apparent difference in SCD risk assessment by the SDANN HRV method in dilated heart failure patients by the same research team.[54,55] There is a difference of only five patients in sample sizes, yet SDANN suddenly became associated with SCD in the larger study. The two studies differed in the inclusion criteria of left ventricular ejection fraction ≤0.25 and the increased use of angiotensin-converting enzyme inhibitors in the larger study. However, the two studies found similar results when evaluating the independent association of SDANN with SCD risk in advanced heart failure patients using a Cox proportional-hazards model. The Poincaré plot HRV measure but not SDANN was an independent predictor of SCD (Table 4).[55]

This now brings up the topic of Poincaré plots. This measure of HRV has been used in only a few patient populations (pediatrics, SIDS, and heart failure), yet it has shown surprisingly good associations with disease progression and SCD risk (Figure 9, control and

TABLE 4

Cox Proportional-Hazards Model of SCD Risk in 113 Advanced Heart Failure Patients

	Sudden Death		
	P (Univariate)	P (Multivariate)	Coefficient±SEM
LVEF	0.66	0.82	. . .
RA	0.16	0.23	. . .
Sodium	0.99	0.54	. . .
SDANN	0.44	0.77	. . .
Plot	0.01	0.0001	7.94±0.19
Walk	0.42	0.14	. . .

LVEF indicates left ventricular ejection fraction; RA, mean right atrial pressure; sodium, serum sodium after pharmacological optimization of heart failure; SDANN, standard deviation of 5-minute mean RR intervals; Plot, Poincaré plot; and Walk, 6-minute walk test.

heart failure). However, there are multiple factors that should inhibit its widespread application. At this time, there is no reliable method to quantify the Poincaré plot patterns, thus leaving the threat of a purely subjective HRV measure. The relatively small sample sizes and limited number of patient types further constrict its usefulness. Also, it shares a similar sensitivity to mislabeled/misidentified artifact and ectopy, which can impair the application of spectral analysis. Of particular concern is the lack of understanding of the physiological regulatory mechanisms that cause alterations in the Poincaré plot patterns. The relative contributions of such varied factors as sinus node dysfunction, respiration, sleep state, ventricular function, and age are poorly understood.

HRV and Sudden Cardiac Death in Sudden Infant Death Syndrome

SIDS is the most common cause of death in children between the ages of 1 month and 1 year in the Western industrialized countries.[56] It has been defined as "the sudden death of any infant or young child which is unexpected by history and in which a thorough post-mortem examination fails to demonstrate an adequate cause of death."[57] Although a number of maternal and prenatal factors, such as inadequate prenatal care, maternal drug or cigarette use, winter season, type B blood type, respiratory anomalies, cardiovascular abnormalities, and immaturity of the autonomic nervous system,[57] have been associated with increased incidence of SIDS, accurate identification techniques for SIDS risk evaluation have yet to be developed. Because of the links of cardiovascular and autonomic nervous system abnormalities with SIDS events, HRV would seem to be a logical and appropriate evaluation method for these patients.

HRV has been applied in a number of studies of infants at increased risk of and infants who later developed SIDS (Table 5).[58-62] Although nonlinear measures (approximate entropy and Poincaré plots) have been successful, there is still some question as to the utility of spectral analysis to assess the risk of SIDS.

The inconclusive spectral HRV results may be a reflection of the very small sample sizes. Although SIDS is a major cause of death in many countries, its incidence is relatively infrequent (1 in every 500 live births in the United States).[56] The relative infrequency of SIDS events coupled with an age group in which Holter or other electrocardiographic studies are unlikely to be performed routinely make data collection for HRV a difficult task.

It is interesting to note that no studies in this group use the more popular time-domain/linear-variance HRV measures frequently used in adult studies. This lack is most likely reflective of the low number of available electrocardiographic studies and the age/heart rate differences in this patient population. In an age group with normally high heart rates (120 to 180 bpm), the sensitivity of standard-variance HRV measures may be diminished and adult standards of normalcy would be inappropriate. Also, because of the relatively small number of both SIDS and control subjects with electrocardiographic data, the establishment of normal criteria is extremely difficult.

TABLE 5

Studies on the Association of HRV With Sids

Reference	Number of Subjects	HRV Methods	Associated With SIDS?
Gordon D et al[58]	10 SIDS, 100 controls	Spectral	No
Kluge KA et al[59]	18 SIDS, 52 controls	Spectral	Yes
Pincus SM et al[60]	14 aborted-SIDS, 45 controls	ApEn	Yes
Schechtman VL et al[61]	13 SIDS, 13 controls	Poincaré	Yes
Antila KJ et al[62]	17 SIDS, 23 controls	Spectral	No

Spectral indicates spectral analysis with fast Fourier transform; ApEn, approximate entropy (nonlinear method); and Poincaré, Poincaré plots (scattergrams) of RR intervals (nonlinear method).

Although the nonlinear HRV methods perform impressively in differentiating between SIDS and healthy control subjects, the small numbers of both subjects and studies that use these methodologies make these techniques as controversial as spectral analysis and the unused time-domain/linear-variance methods.

Summary

HRV is a noninvasive measure of autonomic tone. It has been applied in a variety of clinical situations and patient populations and often is useful in evaluating overall mortality. Yet HRV has a significant problem in the existence of multiple measurement methodologies, which are not necessarily equivalent and do not always report the same level of autonomic tone. Moreover, all of these HRV techniques lack standards of normalcy in most (perhaps in all) adult and pediatric patient populations.

So which is the best HRV method to use? At this time, no HRV technique shows clear superiority. Thus, it seems that the optimal way to apply HRV is to understand both the advantages and disadvantages of the available HRV methodologies and to use the one that a careful consideration of the characteristics of each HRV technique, the patient population, available resources, and clinical/research environment shows to be the most appropriate. In any case, although HRV has demonstrated utility in a variety of patient settings, its clinical application should be done with care and its results interpreted with caution.

References

1. Algra A, Tijssen JG, Roelandt JR, Pool J, Lubsen J. Heart rate variability from 24-hour electrocardiography and the 2-year risk for sudden death. *Circulation.* 1993;88:180–185.
2. Facchini M, De Ferrari GM, Bonazzi O, Weiss T, Schwartz PJ. Effect of reflex vagal activation on frequency of ventricular premature complexes. *Am J Cardiol.* 1991;68:349.
3. Ferguson DW, Berg WJ, Roach PJ, Oren RM, Mark AL, Kempf JS. Effects of heart failure on baroreflex control of sympathetic neural activity. *Am J Cardiol.* 1992;69:523.
4. Ganguly PK. *Catecholamines and Heart Disease.* Boca Raton, Fla: CRC Press; 1991:1.
5. Billmann GE, Schwartz PJ, Stone HL. The effects of daily exercise on susceptibility to sudden cardiac death. *Circulation.* 1984;69:1182–1189.
6. Porter TR, Eckberg DL, Fritsch JM, et al. Autonomic pathophysiology in heart failure patients. *J Clin Invest.* 1990;85:1362–1371.

7. Schwartz PJ, Billman GE, Stone HL. Autonomic mechanisms in ventricular fibrillation induced by myocardial ischemia during exercise in dogs with healed myocardial infarction. *Circulation.* 1984;69:790–800.

8. Billman GE, Schwartz PJ, Stone HL. Baroreceptor reflex control of heart rate: a predictor of sudden cardiac death. *Circulation.* 1982;66: 874–880.

9. Parer WJ, Parer JT, Holbrook RH, Block BSB. Validity of mathematical methods of quantitating fetal heart rate variability. *Am J Obstet Gynecol.* 1985;153:402–409.

10. Malik M, Farrell T, Camm AJ. Circadian rhythm of heart rate variability after acute myocardial infarction and its influence on the prognostic value of heart rate variability. *Am J Cardiol.* 1990;66:1049–1054.

11. Saul JP, Arai Y, Berger RD, Lilly LS, Colucci WS, Cohen RJ. Assessment of autonomic regulation in chronic congestive heart failure by heart rate spectral analysis. *Am J Cardiol.* 1988;61:1292–1299.

12. Odemuyiwa O, Malik M, Farrell T, Bashir Y, Poloniecki J, Camm J. Comparison of the predictive characteristics of heart rate variability index and left ventricular ejection fraction for all-cause mortality, arrhythmic events and sudden death after acute myocardial infarction. *Am J Cardiol.* 1991;68:434–439.

13. Zuanetti G, Latini R, Neilson JMM, Schwartz PJ, Ewing DJ, Antiarrhythmic Drug Evaluation Group. Heart rate variability in patients with ventricular arrhythmias: effect of antiarrhythmic drugs. *J Am Coll Cardiol.* 1991;17:604–612.

14. Bennett T, Fentem PH, Fitton D, Hampton JR, Hosking DJ, Riggott PA. Assessment of vagal control of the heart in diabetes: measuring of RR interval variation under different conditions. *Br Heart J.* 1977;39: 25–28.

15. Dalton KJ, Dawes GS, Patrick JE. The autonomic nervous system and fetal heart rate variability. *Am J Obstet Gynecol.* 1983;146:456–462.

16. Vybiral T, Bryg RJ, Maddens ME, Boden WE. Effect of passive tilt on sympathetic and parasympathetic components of heart rate variability in normal subjects. *Am J Cardiol.* 1989;63:1117–1120.

17. Woo MA, Stevenson WG, Moser DK. Comparison of four methods of assessing heart rate variability in patients with heart failure. *Am J Crit Care.* 1996;5:34–41.

18. Woo MS, Woo MA, Gozal D, Keens T, Harper RM. Heart rate variability in children with congenital central hypoventilation syndrome. *Pediatr Res.* 1992;31:291–296.

19. Kleiger RE, Miller JP, Bigger JT, Moss AJ, Multicenter Post-Infarction Research Group. Decreased heart rate variability and its association with increased mortality after acute myocardial infarction. *Am J Cardiol.* 1987;59:256–262.

20. Martin GJ, Magid NM, Myers G, et al. Heart rate variability and sudden death secondary to coronary artery disease during ambulatory electrocardiographic monitoring. *Am J Cardiol.* 1987;60:86–89.

21. Singer DH, Martin GJ, Magid N, et al. Low heart rate variability and sudden cardiac death. *J Electrocardiol.* 1988;(suppl):S46–S55.

22. Casolo G, Balli E, Taddei T, Amuhasi J, Gori C. Decreased spontaneous heart rate variability in congestive heart failure. *Am J Cardiol.* 1989;64:1162–1167.

23. Bigger JT, Fleiss JL, Steinman RC, Rolnitzky LM, Kleiger RE, Rottman JN. Frequency domain measures of heart period variability and mortality after myocardial infarction. *Circulation.* 1992;85:164–171.

24. Zar JH. *Biostatistical Analysis.* Englewood Cliffs, NJ: Prentice-Hall; 1984.
25. Myers GA, Martin GJ, Magid NM, Barnett PS. Power spectral analysis of heart rate variability in sudden cardiac death: comparison to other methods. *IEEE Trans Biomed Eng.* 1986;33:1149–1156.
26. Mor-Avi V, Abboud S, Akselrod S. Frequency content of the QRS notching in high-fidelity canine ECG. *Comput Biomed Res.* 1989;22: 18–25.
27. Kamath MV, Ghista DN, Fallen EL, Fitchett D. Heart rate variability power spectrogram as a potential noninvasive signature of cardiac regulatory system response, mechanisms, and disorders. *Heart Vessels.* 1987;3:33–41.
28. Kamath MV, Upton ARM, Talalla A, Fallen EL. Effect of vagal nerve electrostimulation on the power spectrum of heart rate variability in man. *PACE.* 1992;15:235–243.
29. Hayano J, Yamada M, Sakakibara Y, et al. Short- and long-term effects of cigarette smoking on heart rate variability. *Am J Cardiol.* 1990;65:84–88.
30. Schechtman VL, Kluge KA, Harper RM. Time-domain system for assessing variation in heart rate. *Med Biol Eng Comp.* 1988;26:367–373.
31. Akselrod S, Gordon D, Shannon DC, Barger AC, Ubel FA. Power spectrum analysis of heart rate fluctuation: a quantitative probe of beat-to-beat cardiovascular control. *Science.* 1981;213:220–222.
32. Xia R, Odemuyiwa O, Gill J, Malik M, Camm AJ. Influence of recognition errors of computerized analysis of 24-hour electrocardiograms on the measurement of spectral components of heart rate variability. *Int J Biomed Comput.* 1993;32:223–235.
33. Goldberger AL, Rigney DR. Sudden death is not chaos. In: Kelso JAS, Mandell AJ, Shlesinger MF, eds. *Dynamic Patterns in Complex Systems.* Teaneck, NJ: World Scientific Publishers; 1988:248–279.
34. Guevara MR, Glass L. Phase-locking, period doubling bifurcations and chaos in a mathematical model of periodically driven oscillators. *J Math Biol.* 1982;14:1–23.
35. Skinner JE. The role of the central nervous system in sudden cardiac death: heartbeat dynamics in conscious pigs during coronary occlusion, psychologic stress and intracerebral propranolol. *Integr Physiol Behav Sci.* 1994;29:355–361.
36. Woo MA, Stevenson WG, Moser DK, Harper RM, Trelease R. Patterns of beat-to-beat heart rate variability in advanced heart failure. *Am Heart J.* 1992;123:704–710.
37. Roberts WC. Sudden cardiac death: a diversity of causes with focus on atherosclerotic coronary artery disease. In: Josephson ME, ed. *Sudden Cardiac Death.* Boston, Mass: Blackwell Scientific Publications; 1993:1–15.
38. Schwartz PJ, Priori SG. Sympathetic nervous system and sudden death. In: Zipes DP, Jalife J, ed. *Cardiac Electrophysiology: From Cell to Bedside.* Philadelphia, Pa: WB Saunders; 1990:330–342.
39. Heathers GP, Yamada KA, Kantor EM, Corr PB. Long-chain acylcarnitine mediates the hypoxia-induced increase in alpha-I adrenergic receptors on adult canine myocytes. *Circ Res.* 1987;61:735–746.
40. Priori SG, Zuanetti G, Schwartz PJ. Ventricular fibrillation induced by the interaction between acute myocardial ischemia and sympathetic hyperactivity: the effect of nifedipine. *Am Heart J.* 1988;116:37–43.

41. Bigger JT, Fleiss JL, Rolnitzky LM. The ability of several short-term measures of RR variability to predict mortality after myocardial infarction. *Circulation.* 1993;88:927–934.
42. Copie X, Hnatkova K, Staunton A, Fei L, Camm AJ, Malik M. Predictive power of increased heart rate vs. depressed left ventricular ejection fraction and heart rate variability for risk stratification after myocardial infarction: results of a 2-year follow-up. *J Am Coll Cardiol.* 1996; 27:270–276.
43. Odemuyiwa O, Malik M, Farrell TG. Multifactorial prediction of arrhythmic events after myocardial infarction: combination of heart rate variability and left ventricular ejection fraction with other variables. *PACE.* 1991;14:1986–1991.
44. Klingenheben T, Rapp U, Hohnloser SH. Circadian variation of heart rate variability in postinfarction patients with and without life-threatening ventricular tachyarrhythmias. *J Cardiovasc Electrophysiol.* 1995; 6:357–364.
45. Hohnloser SH, Klingenheben T, van de Loo A, Hablawetz E, Just H, Schwartz PJ. Reflex versus tonic vagal activity as a prognostic parameter in patients with sustained ventricular tachycardia or ventricular fibrillation. *Circulation.* 1994;89:1068–1073.
46. Odemuyiwa O, Poloniecki J, Malik M, et al. Temporal influences on the prediction of postinfarction mortality by heart rate variability: a comparison with the left ventricular ejection fraction. *Br Heart J.* 1994; 71:521–527.
47. Malliani A, Lombardi F, Pagani M, Cerutti S. Power spectral analysis of cardiovascular variability in patients at risk for sudden cardiac death. *J Cardiovasc Electrophysiol.* 1994;5:274–286.
48. O'Brien IAD, O'Hare P, Corrall RJM. Heart rate variability in healthy subjects: effects of age and the derivation of normal ranges for tests of autonomic function. *Br Heart J.* 1985;55:348–354.
49. Schwartz JB, Gibb WJ, Tran T. Aging effects on heart rate variability. *J Gerontol.* 1991;46:M99–M106.
50. Cohn JN, Levine TB, Olivari MT, et al. Plasma norepinephrine as a guide to prognosis in patients with chronic congestive heart failure. *N Engl J Med.* 1984;311:819–823.
51. American Heart Association. *1995 Heart and Stroke Facts.* Dallas, Tex: American Heart Association; 1995:1.
52. Fei L, Slade AK, Prasad K, Malik M, McKenna WJ, Camm AJ. Is there increased sympathetic activity in patients with hypertrophic cardiomyopathy? *J Am Coll Cardiol.* 1995;26:472–480.
53. Counihan PJ, Fei L, Bashir Y, Farrell TG, Haywood GA, McKenna WJ. Assessment of heart rate variability in hypertrophic cardiomyopathy: association with clinical and prognostic features. *Circulation.* 1993;88:1682–1690.
54. Woo MA, Stevenson WG, Moser DK. Relation of heart rate variability to sudden death in advanced heart failure. *Am J Cardiol.* In press.
55. Woo MA, Moser DK, Stevenson LW, Stevenson WG, Fonarow GC. 6-Minute walk test and heart rate variability: lack of association in heart failure. *Circulation.* 1995;92(suppl I):I-248. Abstract.
56. Goyco PG, Beckerman RC. Sudden infant death syndrome. *Curr Probl Pediatr.* 1990;20:302–346.
57. Bergman AB, Beckwith JB, Ray CG, eds. Epidemiology, sudden infant death syndrome. In: *Proceedings of the Second International Conference*

on *Causes of Sudden Death in Infants.* Seattle, Wash: University of Washington Press; 1970:25–79.

58. Gordon D, Southall DP, Kelly D. Analysis of heart rate and respiratory patterns in sudden infant death syndrome victims and control infants. *Pediatr Res.* 1986;20:680–684.

59. Kluge KA, Harper RM, Schechtman VL. Spectral analysis assessment of respiratory sinus arrhythmia in normal infants who subsequently died of sudden infant death syndrome. *Pediatr Res.* 1988;24:677–682.

60. Pincus SM, Cummins TR, Haddad GG. Heart rate control in normal and aborted-SIDS infants. *Am J Physiol.* 1993;264:R638–R646.

61. Schechtman VL, Raetz SL, Harper RK, et al. Dynamic analysis of cardiac R-R intervals in normal infants and in infants who subsequently succumbed to the sudden infant death syndrome. *Pediatr Res.* 1992;31:606–612.

62. Antila KJ, Valimaki IA, Makela M, Tuominen J, Wilson AJ, Southall DP. Heart rate variability in infants subsequently suffering sudden infant death syndrome (SIDS). *Early Hum Dev.* 1990;22:57–72.

Chapter 10

Overview of Medical and Surgical Treatment Modalities: Pharmacology

D. George Wyse, MD, PhD

This chapter summarizes the current state of knowledge with respect to pharmacological treatment for the prevention of sudden cardiac death (SCD). The future with respect to such treatment is covered in other chapters, particularly those dealing with the emerging interface between molecular biology and sudden cardiac death.

This review of the data supporting our current understanding of the pharmacological treatment of sudden cardiac death will be divided into two sections: primary prevention and secondary prevention. But first, it is important to establish the context within which this review will take place. The first point to be emphasized is that sudden cardiac death is a clinical syndrome and not a precise etiologic diagnosis. In fact, the list of causes that produce the clinical syndrome of sudden cardiac death is extensive. Conventional wisdom states, however, that 80% to 90% of sudden cardiac death is due to hemodynamically unstable ventricular tachycardia or ventricular fibrillation (VT/VF). It is important to recognize that the evidence on which this conventional wisdom is based is not particularly robust. Furthermore, it is not entirely clear in what proportion of patients prevention of terminal VT/VF would produce significant prolongation of life. Given that most such patients have significant underlying structural heart disease, it is probably true that in a substantial proportion of patients, terminal VT/VF may represent a final common pathway leading to the death of a heart that is incapable of extensive further survival and that would soon succumb via another mechanism even if VT/VF were prevented. Nevertheless, it seems clear that VT/VF can occur in hearts

From: Dunbar SB, Ellenbogen KA, Epstein AE, (eds). *Sudden Cardiac Death: Past, Present, and Future.* Armonk, NY: Futura Publishing Company, Inc.; © 1997.

otherwise healthy enough to survive for extensive periods, even though that may not be the situation in 80% to 90% of the cases of sudden cardiac death. Accordingly, the present review will focus specifically on the pharmacological prevention of VT/VF rather than the broader topic of pharmacological prevention of sudden cardiac death. Finally, it must be stated clearly at the outset that there are enormous gaps in our current knowledge concerning the pathophysiology of VT/VF. Consequently, much of the pharmacological approach at this time has been empirical and has sometimes led to surprising and unanticipated results that only highlight our ignorance.

Primary Prevention of Ventricular Tachycardia/Ventricular Fibrillation

The fundamental concept of primary prevention is to identify a high-risk population without prior VT/VF and then to administer a pharmacological therapy that prevents the occurrence of VT/VF. Such an approach has demonstrated limited success when applied in the three settings that have been studied most rigorously: patients presenting with acute myocardial infarction, patients with a recent myocardial infarction (with or without VT/VF risk factors), and patients with reduced ventricular function (regardless of cause) and frequent ventricular premature depolarizations (VPDs).

Acute Myocardial Infarction

The concept underlying treatment of this group of patients is prevention of so-called "primary" VT/VF in otherwise uncomplicated myocardial infarction. It is essentially a prethrombolytic era strategy, and its use has waned considerably. There are some strategic weak points in this prophylactic pharmacological approach. First, the incidence of the target "illness" (VT/VF) is quite low, perhaps <5% overall. Second, the peak incidence of such VT/VF is extremely early (<60 minutes) after the onset of coronary occlusion, a time frame that mitigates against timely intervention. Third, many of the drugs used have important adverse effect profiles. No single study of the class I antiarrhythmics has sufficient power to provide a definitive answer concerning the effectiveness of this strategy using such drugs. A meta-analysis of a few small earlier studies does not suggest any benefit.[1] The class I antiarrhythmic drug most extensively studied is lidocaine, but several meta-analyses (eg, Reference 2) have shown that although the drug may reduce VT/VF incidence in this setting, it actually increases mortality. The only antiarrhythmic drugs shown to have benefit in the prevention of VT/VF without increasing mortality in acute myocardial infarction are the β-adrenergic receptor blocking agents (class II).[3] The calcium channel blockers (class IV) have been used in this setting, but no clear benefit has been demonstrated, and these agents may be harmful when congestive cardiac failure is present.[4] Other drugs, in particular the class III agents, have not been tested in this setting. Furthermore, this particular strategy has not been reevaluated in the postthrombolytic therapy era.

Recent Myocardial Infarction

Clearly, this particular target population has been the most extensively studied. Early studies with class I antiarrhythmic drugs have been summarized by Furberg.[1] The earlier studies of class I antiarrhythmic drugs were badly underpowered and produced no evidence either for or against the prophylactic antiarrhythmic drug strategy in this patient group. Furthermore, these earlier studies were nonselective in that they did not choose patients on the basis of risk factors known to be associated with greater risk of mortality (eg, Reference 5). Once again, however, class II antiarrhythmics (β-adrenergic receptor blocking agents), which have now been studied in tens of thousands of such patients, were conclusively shown to have a beneficial effect,[6] even in unselected groups of patients with a recent myocardial infarction.

The next landmark study that focused on this group of patients was the Cardiac Arrhythmia Suppression Trial (CAST).[7,8] Unlike earlier studies, the CAST attempted to select high-risk patients on the basis of reduced left ventricular function and frequent VPDs. Furthermore, the CAST had a run-in phase that removed from the primary analysis those patients whose VPDs were not suppressed by the CAST antiarrhythmic drugs. The CAST antiarrhythmic drugs were very effective at suppressing VPDs; however, they did not produce the desired effect of preventing sudden cardiac death (the CAST definition included resuscitated VF). In fact, the two class Ic agents used, flecainide and encainide, actually increased sudden cardiac death in comparison with placebo. The third CAST antiarrhythmic drug, moricizine, was a weaker suppressant of VPDs. Moricizine caused a small increase in total mortality during drug titration in the first 2 weeks of use but had no long-term effect in either reducing or increasing sudden cardiac death.

Several small studies that have been examined in a meta-analysis[4] suggested a potential beneficial effect in patients with a recent myocardial infarction for the complex antiarrhythmic agent amiodarone, often over-simplistically characterized as a class III agent. The preliminary results of two recently completed large studies of amiodarone, the Canadian Amiodarone Myocardial Infarction Arrhythmia Trial (CAMIAT) and the European Myocardial Infarct Amiodarone Trial (EMIAT), have been presented at a national meeting. Published reports are not yet available, and the primary result papers are currently under review. Accordingly, the results cannot be published here, although the main data were reviewed orally at the Conference on Sudden Cardiac Death.

The primary end point of CAMIAT was resuscitation from VF or "presumed arrhythmic death," which, as defined in the protocol, is equivalent to sudden cardiac death.[9] Patients with recent myocardial infarction and frequent VPDs or salvos of VT were enrolled within 6 to 45 days of their qualifying myocardial infarction. Ventricular function was not part of the selection criteria. The analysis for the primary end point included both an efficacy analysis and an intention-to-treat analysis.[9] CAMIAT was not powered to provide a definitive result concerning other end points, such as cardiovascular mortality and total mortality. However, there was a favorable trend. The risk reduction for total mortality and cardiovascular mortality was a little over 20% in the efficacy analysis and just under 20% in the intention-to-treat analysis. The treatment effect in CAMIAT with respect to the primary end point of sudden cardiac death was almost 50% reduction in the efficacy analysis and just under 40% reduction in the intention-to-treat analysis; both of these were significant according to the CAMIAT hypothesis.[9] In the efficacy analysis, patients were censored 3 months after permanent discontinuation of the study drug. Such an analysis is important, because the early permanent discontinuation rate for reasons other than an end point was ≈43% in the amiodarone group and 29% in the placebo group 2 years after randomization.

EMIAT differed from CAMIAT primarily in that it selected patients on the basis of reduced left ventricular function, and ventricular arrhythmias were not part of the selection criteria.[10] The entry window was also slightly shorter, being 5 to 21 days after the qualifying myocardial infarction. The primary end point of EMIAT was total mortality, and a two-tailed analysis was planned. Cardiovascular mortality was also assessed, and a secondary end point was resuscitation from VF or presumed arrhythmic death. EMIAT also did both an efficacy analysis and an intention-to-treat analysis. Accordingly, EMIAT and CAMIAT can be compared. With respect to the summary of results given above, EMIAT results agree completely with respect to CAMIAT: amiodarone significantly reduces the combined end point of resuscitated VF or presumed arrhythmic death.

Neither CAMIAT nor EMIAT demonstrated significant reductions in total mortality or cardiovascular mortality, but the two studies again are in full agreement, showing a favorable trend for amiodarone therapy. The trend was obvious and straightforward in the CAMIAT data. In the case of EMIAT, further explanation is necessary, because the trend is not so obvious. In an unadjusted analysis in EMIAT, there is no obvious trend, and the effect of amiodarone appears to be completely neutral with respect to total mortality and cardiovascular mortality. In EMIAT, however, the play of chance resulted in an unfortunate imbalance between the amiodarone-treated and placebo-treated groups. Specifically, there were significant differences between the two treatment groups with respect to three important covariables: proportion of subjects with left ventricular ejection fraction <0.30, history of prior myocardial infarction, and New York Heart Association functional class II/III with respect to symptoms of congestive heart failure. After adjustment for these factors, there was a favorable trend with respect to total mortality and cardiovascular mortality in the amiodarone-treated group in EMIAT.

The earlier small studies showing the potential for the benefit of amiodarone in patients with a recent myocardial infarction encouraged study of other class III antiarrhythmic drugs. A large study of dofetilide in this patient setting is currently in progress, but no results are yet available. A similar study of d-sotalol has just been completed (Survival With Oral d-Sotalol [SWORD]) and the results in SWORD were similar to those in the CAST and were equally disappointing.[11,12] d-Sotalol in this patient setting caused a doubling of the mortality rate in comparison with placebo, from $\approx2\%$ to $\approx4\%$.

Meta-analysis has suggested no benefit of class IV antiarrhythmic drugs (calcium channel blockers) after a recent myocardial infarction, although both harm and benefit have been suggested in subgroup analysis.[4]

In summary, primary prevention of VT/VF in patients with a recent myocardial infarction has met with only mixed success. β-adrenergic receptor blocking agents are clearly beneficial, and amiodarone is also beneficial in selected patients. However, flecainide, encainide, d-sotalol, and probably moricizine are harmful in this patient setting. There are no conclusive data to suggest benefit or harm from all other antiarrhythmic agents. The conflicting results with amiodarone and d-sotalol suggest that a simple classification scheme for antiarrhythmic drugs is not sufficiently robust to allow generalization from one drug to another in the same drug class. Nevertheless, use of any antiarrhythmic drug for this purpose and in this patient setting other than those with proven benefit must be viewed as imprudent.

Reduced Ventricular Function and Frequent Ventricular Premature Depolarizations

The third and final high-risk group that has been studied in some detail with respect to primary prevention of VT/VF comprises patients with reduced left ventricular function and frequent VPDs. There have been three such studies, all investigating amiodarone. Two studies from South America have found the use of amiodarone in this setting to be beneficial.[13,14] The third study was the Veterans Administration's Survival Trial of Antiarrhythmic Therapy in Congestive Heart Failure (CHF-STAT) trial,[15] and it found no benefit from the use of amiodarone in such patients. The reasons for such conflicting results are unclear. A number of potential explanations based on differences in protocols have been proposed, including such factors as drug dosage, patient selection, etc. The most intriguing potential explanation is a different effect of the drug on the basis of the underlying cause of reduced ventricular function. The majority of patients in the two South American studies had reduced ventricular function caused by congestive cardiomyopathy (primarily alcoholic).[13,14] The majority of CHF-STAT patients had reduced ventricular function caused by coronary heart disease.[15] Furthermore, a subgroup analysis of the CHF-STAT data suggests benefit in the subgroup with nonischemic congestive cardiomyopathy but no effect in those with coronary heart disease (Figure 1). However, this particular explanation seems much less tenable given the previously discussed results from CAMIAT and EMIAT, which included only patients with coronary heart disease. A trial of primary prevention in such patients (reduced ventricular function and VPDs) comparing placebo, amiodarone, and the implantable cardioverter-defibrillator (ICD) will soon be under way (Sudden Cardiac Death–Heart Failure Trial [SCD-HEFT], personal communication, G. Bardy).

The Multicenter Unsustained Tachycardia Trial (MUSTT)[16] is investigating the primary prevention strategy using pharmacological therapy directed by programmed stimulation and when two such attempts are unsuccessful, providing an ICD. The MUSTT patients are a high-risk group with coronary heart disease, reduced ventricular function, spontaneous unsustained VT, and inducible sustained VT. The Multicenter Automatic Defibrillator Implantation Trial (MADIT)[17] is a similar primary prevention study that

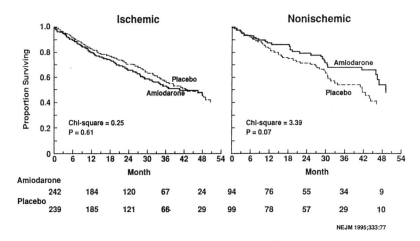

FIGURE 1. *Effect of amiodarone on the CHF-STAT end point of total mortality according to whether the cause of heart failure was ischemic or nonischemic. Reprinted with permission from Reference 15.*

compares ICD therapy with "conventional" therapy. MADIT has recently shown an advantage of the ICD in drug-resistant patients.[17] The overall impact of the MADIT result awaits the context that will be provided by other trials. The Coronary Artery Bypass Graft Patch (CABG-PATCH) Trial is also comparing the ICD with "conventional" therapy as primary prevention of VT/VF in another high-risk population with coronary heart disease. Both MADIT and CABG-PATCH Trial are described elsewhere in this book.

The following primary prevention strategy using antiarrhythmic drugs for VT/VF may be recommended: (1) β-adrenergic receptor blocking agents for patients with acute myocardial infarction; (2) β-adrenergic receptor blocking agents for patients with a recent myocardial infarction; (3) amiodarone for selected patients with a recent myocardial infarction who have reduced left ventricular function and frequent VPDs; and (4) amiodarone for patients with reduced ventricular function due to nonischemic congestive cardiomyopathy and frequent VPDs.

Secondary Prevention of Ventricular Tachycardia/Ventricular Fibrillation

Treatment of survivors of a recent episode of VT/VF without reversible causes to prevent a subsequent episode of VT/VF with pharmacological agents has not been as rigorously studied as primary prevention. In fact, there have been no placebo-controlled studies. The only comparative data available are derived from quasi–natural history studies in patients with implanted ICDs.[18] Such data suggest that the 2-year recurrence rate and the 2-year fatal recurrence rate are ≈50% and ≈25%, respectively.[18] Accordingly, current approaches should be judged against such estimates. Earlier observational studies suggested that therapy directed by the programmed electrical stimulation approach was more effective than therapy directed by the ambulatory ECG approach.[18] Indeed, a small randomized trial confirmed the impression of these earlier nonrandomized reports.[19] A larger randomized trial[20] has raised questions about the conclusions of earlier studies but has been criticized itself for a number of reasons.[18] The Electrophysiologic Study Versus Electrocardiographic Monitoring (ESVEM) Study found little improvement over historical controls with either approach using recurrence of arrhythmia as an end point, although the programmed stimulation approach was superior when total mortality was used as an end point.[20] In a nonrandomized retrospective analysis of the ESVEM data, d,l-sotalol appeared to be superior to the other antiarrhythmic agents tested (Figure 2).[21]

Another recently published trial (Cardiac Arrest in Seattle: Conventional Versus Amiodarone Drug Evaluation, CASCADE[22]) compared "conventional" antiarrhythmic drug therapy, largely guided by programmed stimulation, with therapy with empirical amiodarone. Compared with historical controls, both therapies used in CASCADE were effective, with arrhythmia recurrence at 2 years of 31% for conventional antiarrhythmic drug therapy and 18% for empirical amiodarone (Figure 3). The efficacy of empirical amiodarone was significantly better than the efficacy of conventional antiarrhythmic drug therapy in CASCADE. However, it must be acknowledged that in the conventional-therapy arm of CASCADE, patients were treated with therapies that were predicted to be ineffective. There has been and continues to be interest in the use of β-adrenergic receptor blocking agents as empirical therapy in this patient population, but thus far there are no convincing data that such an approach offers any improvement over results observed in historical controls.[18]

Comparison of secondary prevention of VT/VF by pharmacological versus nonpharmacological therapy is fairly advanced only in the case of the ICD. Three large trials are currently in progress and should be reported in 1998. The Cardiac Arrest Study Hamburg (CASH)[23] is comparing the ICD with empirical amiodarone or empirical metoprolol in a three-arm study. The Canadian Implantable Defibrillator Study (CIDS)[24] is comparing the ICD with

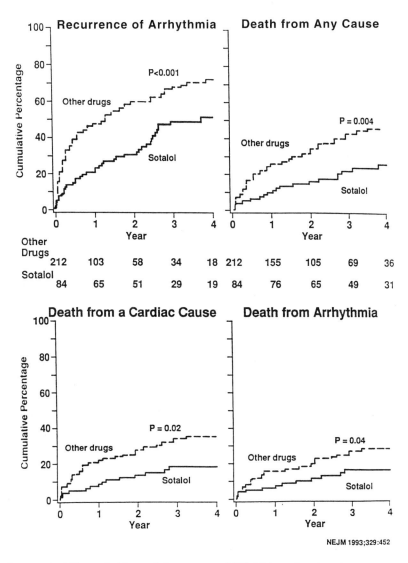

NEJM 1993;329:452

FIGURE 2. *Effect of d,l-sotalol on several ESVEM end points in a nonran-domized analysis. Reprinted with permission from Reference 21.*

empirical amiodarone in a two-arm study. The Antiarrhythmics Versus Implantable Defibrillators (AVID)[25] study is comparing the ICD with empirical amiodarone or guided *d,l*-sotalol in a two-arm study. Although a number of observational studies are reporting on the efficacy of catheter ablation and surgical techniques for sec-ondary prevention of VT/VF, these last two modalities of therapy

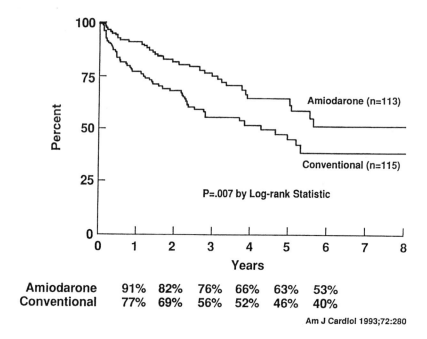

	1	2	3	4	5	6
Amiodarone	91%	82%	76%	66%	63%	53%
Conventional	77%	69%	56%	52%	46%	40%

Am J Cardiol 1993;72:280

FIGURE 3. *Comparison of empirical amiodarone and conventional antiarrhythmic drug therapy in the CASCADE trial for the end point of cardiac survival. Reprinted with permission from Reference 22.*

have not yet advanced sufficiently to be directly compared with pharamacological therapy or the ICD.

Clearly, the secondary prevention treatment strategy has not been studied as rigorously as the primary prevention strategy. From the available data, the strategy of using antiarrhythmic drugs for secondary prevention of VT/VF may be cautiously recommended with the following specifications.

1. When a directed approach is to be used, the programmed stimulation method is preferable (if applicable), but attempts to find effective drug therapy should be limited to three attempts, and preferably fewer. When effective suppressive drug therapy is not found, other modalities of therapy should be used promptly, and the selection of the alternative therapy should be dependent on local experience. Empirical amiodarone and the ICD are the most widely available alternative therapies. However, in the absence of firm data identifying the optimal approach, enrollment in clinical trials designed to define the best treatment strategy is encouraged.

2. *d,l*-Sotalol, if tolerated, may be the best drug to use in the directed approach.

3. Empirical amiodarone therapy is effective and is arguably the best available pharmacological therapy.

4. Other antiarrhythmic drug therapies are unproven in this setting.

Pharamacological Versus Other Forms of Therapy

As has been briefly mentioned, pharmacological versus other forms of therapy for both primary and secondary prevention of VT/VF is the subject of a number of ongoing studies. A detailed discussion of the currently available studies is beyond the scope of the present report. Other forms of therapy are discussed in detail elsewhere in this book. At this time, there are no definitive data and a plethora of opinions. Judging from the trials currently in progress, good comparative data with respect to pharmacological therapy versus device therapy should be available within the next year.

References

1. Furberg CE. Effect of antiarrhythmic drugs on mortality after myocardial infarction. *Am J Cardiol.* 1983;52:32C–36C.
2. MacMahon S, Collins R, Peto R, et al. Effects of prophylactic lidocaine in suspected acute myocardial infarction: an overview of results from randomized, controlled trials. *JAMA.* 1988;260:1910–1916.
3. Ryden L, Ariniego R, Arnman K, et al. A double-blind trial of metoprolol in acute myocardial infarction: effects of ventricular tachyarrhythmias. *N Engl J Med.* 1983;308:614–618.
4. Teo KT, Yusuf S, Furberg CD. Effects of prophylactic antiarrhythmic drug therapy in acute myocardial infarction: an overview of results from randomized controlled trials. *JAMA.* 1993;270:1589–1595.
5. Bigger JT Jr, Fleiss JL, Kleiger R, et al, for the Multicenter Post-Infarction Research Group. The relationships among ventricular arrhythmias, left ventricular dysfunction, and mortality in the 2 years after myocardial infarction. *Circulation.* 1984;69:250–258.
6. Yusuf S, Peto R, Lewis J. Beta blockade during and after myocardial infarction: an overview of the randomized trials. *Prog Cardiovasc Dis.* 1985;27:335–371.
7. Echt DS, Liebson PR, Mitchell LB, et al. Mortality and morbidity in patients receiving encainide, flecainide or placebo: the Cardiac Arrhythmia Supression Trial. *N Engl J Med.* 1991;324:781–788.
8. The Cardiac Arrhythmia Suppression Trial-II Investigators. Effect of the antiarrhythmic agent moricizine on survival after myocardial infarction. *N Engl J Med.* 1992;327:227–233.
9. Cairns JA, Connolly SJ, Roberts R, et al. Canadian Amiodarone Myocardial Infarction Arrhythmia Trial (CAMIAT): rationale and protocol. *Am J Cardiol.* 1993;72:87F–94F.

10. Camm AJ, Julian D, Janse G, et al. The European Myocardial Infarct Amiodarone Trial (EMIAT). *Am J Cardiol.* 1993;72:95F–98F.
11. Waldo AL, Camm AJ, dePuyter H, et al. Effect of *d*-sotalol on mortality in patients with left ventricular dysfunction after recent and remote myocardial infarction. The SWORD Investigators. Survival with Oral *d*-Sotalol. *Lancet.* 1996;348:7–12.
12. Waldo AL, Camm AJ, dePuyter H, et al. Survival with oral *d*-sotalol in patients with left ventricular dysfunction after myocardial infarction: rationale, design, and methods (the SWORD Trial). *Am J Cardiol.* 1995;75:1023–1027.
13. Doval HC, Nul DR, Grancelli HO, et al. Randomized trial of low-dose amiodarone in severe congestive heart failure. *Lancet.* 1994;344:493–498.
14. Garguichevich JJ, Ramos JL, Gambarte A, et al. Effect of amiodarone therapy on mortality in patients with left ventricular dysfunction and asymptomatic complex ventricular arrhythmias: Argentina Pilot Study of Sudden Death and Amiodarone (EPAMSA). *Am Heart J.* 1995;130:494–500.
15. Singh SN, Fletcher RD, Gross-Fisher S, et al. Amiodarone in patients with congestive heart failure and asymptomatic ventricular arrhythmia. *N Engl J Med.* 1995;333:77–82.
16. Buxton AE, Fisher JD, Josephson ME, et al. Prevention of sudden death in patients with coronary artery disease: the Multicenter Unsustained Tachycardia Trial (MUSTT). *Prog Cardiovasc Dis.* 1993;36:215–226.
17. MADIT Executive Committee. Multicenter Automatic Defibrillator Implantation Trial (MADIT): design and clinical protocol. *PACE.* 1991;14:920–927.
18. Wyse DG, Mitchell LB. Selection of antiarrhythmic therapy: ESVEM in focus and in context. *Cardiol Rev.* 1994;2:291–302.
19. Mitchell LB, Duff H, Manyari D, et al. A randomized clinical trial of the noninvasive and invasive approaches to drug therapy of ventricular tachycardia. *N Engl J Med.* 1987;317:1681–1687.
20. Mason JW, and the ESVEM Investigators. A comparison of electrophysiologic testing with Holter monitoring to predict antiarrhythmic-drug efficacy for ventricular tachyarrhythmias. *N Engl J Med.* 1993;329:445–451.
21. Mason JW, and the ESVEM Investigators. A comparison of seven antiarrhythmic drugs in patients with ventricular tachyarrhythmias. *N Engl J Med.* 1993;329:452–458.
22. CASCADE Investigators. The CASCADE Study: randomized antiarrhythmic drug therapy in survivors of cardiac arrest in Seattle. *Am J Cardiol.* 1993;72:280–287.
23. Siebels J, Kuck K-H, and the CASH Investigators. Implantable cardioverter defibrillator compared with antiarrhythmic drug treatment in cardiac arrest survivors (the Cardiac Arrest Study Hamburg). *Am Heart J.* 1994;127:1139–1144.
24. Connolly SJ, Gent M, Roberts RS, et al. Canadian Implantable Defibrillator Study (CIDS): study design and organization. *Am J Cardiol.* 1993;72:103F–108F.
25. AVID Investigators. Antiarrhythmics Versus Implantable Defibrillators (AVID): rationale, design and methods. *Am J Cardiol.* 1995;75:470–475.

Chapter 11

Ablative Therapy for Ventricular Tachycardia in Chronic Coronary Artery Disease

Francis E. Marchlinski, MD, Charles D. Gottlieb, MD, David J. Callans, MD, David Schwartzman, MD, David C. Man, MD, Brian H. Sarter, MD, Dina R. Yazmajian, MD, and Erica S. Zado, PA-C

Ablative therapy for sustained ventricular tachycardia and fibrillation is the only therapeutic option that can "cure" these arrhythmias by permanently altering or removing the electrophysiological substrate. This chapter will begin by describing the developmental history and current status of surgical ablative therapy for patients with ventricular tachycardia occurring in the setting of coronary artery disease. The evolution of catheter ablative techniques using direct-current and radiofrequency energy in these patients is then described. Subsequently, arrhythmia localization techniques, anticipated efficacy rates, and end points for judging efficacy of catheter ablative therapy are reviewed. Recommendations for techniques that can improve the success of catheter ablation in patients with coronary artery disease are suggested. We conclude with a summary of anticipated future developments in catheter-based ablative therapy for ventricular tachycardia occurring in the setting of chronic coronary artery disease. A discussion of information related to catheter ablation for ventricular tachycardia in the absence of structural heart disease and other disease settings is beyond the scope of this review; the reader is referred to a number of excellent reference and review articles on those subjects.[1-10]

From: Dunbar SB, Ellenbogen KA, Epstein AE, (eds). *Sudden Cardiac Death: Past, Present, and Future.* Armonk, NY: Futura Publishing Company, Inc.; © 1997.

Surgical Ablative Therapy

Currently, surgical ablative therapy for ventricular tachycardia is performed infrequently. However, the development of surgical ablative techniques is important from more than just a historical perspective. The information learned about the pathophysiology of ventricular tachycardia from the surgical ablation experience provides a valuable guide for the development of catheter-based ablative techniques. In addition, the success of surgical ablation of ventricular tachycardia provides an important reference for judging the efficacy of catheter-based ablative techniques.

Coronary artery bypass graft surgery, which was developed in the 1960s, was found to be useful in treating polymorphic ischemia–induced ventricular arrhythmias.[11] However, coronary artery bypass graft surgery alone, with or without aneurysmectomy, failed to control recurrent unimorphic sustained ventricular tachycardia.[12-14] These results suggested that in most patients, the anatomic and electrophysiological substrate for unimorphic ventricular tachycardia extended outside the densely infarcted aneurysm. In addition, the results suggested that ischemia was not required for the initiation or maintenance of sustained unimorphic ventricular tachycardia in humans. In the mid-1970s, Josephson and colleagues[15,16] described techniques for endocardial catheter mapping during presumed reentrant tachycardia observed in the setting of chronic coronary artery disease (Figure 1). Using multipolar-electrode catheter recording techniques, these investigators identified regions of myocardium extending from the border zone of the aneurysm that demonstrated mid to early diastolic electrical activity. The diastolic electrical activity maintained a constant relation to the subsequent QRS complex during the tachycardia and after transient stimulation techniques introduced during the tachycardia.[17,18] The investigators reasoned that if reentry was indeed the mechanism of the sustained ventricular tachycardia, then the described recordings represented endocardial activation of a critical part of the reentrant circuit. Working with their surgical colleague Alden Harken, these investigators documented that the subendocardial resection guided by preoperative and intraoperative activation mapping during ventricular tachycardia was a potentially curative ablative procedure.[19-22]

On the basis of extensive surgical experience with map-guided subendocardial resection, it appears that 70% to 80% of ventricular tachycardias in the setting of chronic coronary artery disease have at least a portion of the reentrant circuit within a 2 to 4-mm intramural margin of the scarred endocardium.[23-26] Just as importantly,

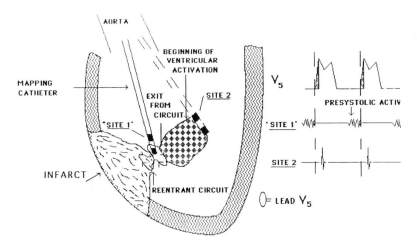

FIGURE 1. *Localization of reentrant ventricular tachycardia associated with chronic coronary artery disease with prior myocardial infarction. The reentrant tachycardia circuit is represented schematically at the border zone of the infarction. Electrical activity continues throughout electrical systole and diastole in the circuit. A catheter-based electrode recording demonstrating presystolic (diastolic) activity (site 1) suggests a recording near or at the reentrant circuit. As the catheter is moved away from the reentrant circuit (site 2), recorded electrical activity is coincident with the repolarization of the rest of the myocardium and the QRS complex generated on the body surface ECG recording. The earliest presystolic activity identifies an appropriate site for catheter ablation.*

the surgical experience suggested that a more completely intramural location or an epicardial location was present in about 20% to 30% of ventricular tachycardias occurring in the setting of chronic coronary artery disease.[22-25] Work from a number of investigators supported the latter conclusion. Krafchek and colleagues[23] documented that ablative therapy directed at the right ventricular septum was necessary in 14% of ventricular tachycardias and that ablative therapy directed outside the area of grossly visible scar was necessary in 21% of ventricular tachycardias. Haines and colleagues[24] documented additional efficacy with sequential map-guided subendocardial resection and cryoablation. The initial endocardial resection was followed by repeat stimulation and additional mapping of any induced ventricular tachycardia. Additional resection and cryoablation was directed at the map-guided site of origin of any additional induced ventricular tachycardia. The supplemental cryoablative procedure allowed for intramural lesion generation after the subendocardial resection. Svenson and colleagues[25] documented that epicardial laser photocoagulation was capable of eliminating reentrant ventricular tachycardia in the setting of coronary artery disease in approximately one third of the patients. Finally, the results of blind subendocardial resection of all visible scar resulted in arrhythmia cure rates of only 70% to 80%.[26] An endocardial location for even part of the reentrant circuit responsible for all ventricular tachycardias associated with chronic coronary artery disease was convincingly refuted by these data.

Several additional lessons may be learned from the surgical experience (Table 1). As will be emphasized later in this chapter, these lessons play an important role in optimizing results with catheter-based ablation. Extensive surgical experience has documented that the endocardial mapped site of origin of most ventricular tachycardias that occur in the setting of chronic coronary artery disease has a septal or paraseptal location.[27] Specifically, all tachycardias with a left bundle-branch block morphology and half of the tachycardias with a right bundle-branch block morphology have a site of origin localized to the intraventricular septum or paraseptal regions (Figure 2). Only those ventricular tachycardias that occur in association with a prior inferior infarction and demonstrate a right bundle-branch block pattern are likely to be localized away from the septal region. The latter tachycardias typically have a basal, mid, or lateral left ventricular location. Information on the most common sites of origin

---

TABLE 1

Major Lessons Learned From the Surgical VT Ablation Experience in the Setting of Chronic Coronary Artery Disease

1. Substrate for sustained VT usually extends beyond the border of dense infarction
2. Initiation and maintenance of VT not critically dependent on presence of ischemia
3. Left ventricular endocardium/subendocardium incorporated in reentrant circuit in 70% to 80% of VTs
4. Left ventricular endocardial septum usually incorporated as critical portion of the reentrant circuit in VT with a left bundle-branch block pattern
5. Mapped site of origin of most VT is located in close proximity to the septum
6. Isthmus between mitral annulus and dense infarction is important for arrhythmogenesis in the setting of inferior infarction
7. Reentrant VT circuit confined to a more intramural, right ventricular septal, or epicardial location in 20% to 30% of VTs

VT indicates ventricular tachycardia.

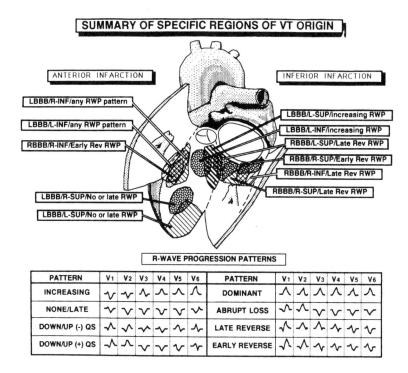

FIGURE 2. *Most common sites of origin of ventricular tachycardia and associated characteristic morphological features found on 12-lead electrocardiogram. Locations were based on analysis of 182 ventricular tachycardias with the site of origin confirmed by catheter and intraoperative mapping techniques. Most ventricular tachycardias originate from septal or paraseptal locations. The bundle-branch block (BBB; L, left; R, right) pattern, frontal plane axis, and precordial R-wave transition (RWP) noted on the 12-lead electrocardiogram obtained during ventricular tachycardia provide helpful clues for regionalizing the origin of ventricular tachycardia. INF indicates inferior; SUP, superior. Reprinted with permission from Reference 14.*

for ventricular tachycardia may play a critical role in optimizing catheter design for achieving adequate mapping and good contact for ablative energy delivery.

The surgical experience has also documented the importance of the isthmus between the mitral annulus and the area of dense inferior infarction for the maintenance of ventricular tachycardia.[28] Although initial results of surgical ablative therapy appear promising for patients with anterior infarctions, the results of surgical ablation for patients with inferior myocardial infarction appear to be only modestly successful. It was initially thought that the poor outcome was secondary to surgical technique and the difficulty in accessing the inferior wall. Importantly, Hargrove and colleagues[28] recognized the importance of the mitral valve isthmus for arrhythmogenesis associated with inferior infarctions. They advocated extending the ventriculotomy/aneurysmectomy from the dense inferior scar to the mitral annulus by use of cryoablative techniques (Figure 3). This modification of the surgical procedure dramatically improved the outcome of surgical ablative therapy for arrhythmia control in patients with ventricular tachycardia associated with inferior infarction. As will be noted below, a similar technique using radiofrequency catheter ablation has been documented to be successful in eliminating ventricular tachycardia associated with prior inferior infarctions.[29]

Surgical techniques evolved throughout the 1980s. The importance of detailed endocardial mapping to maximize elimination of arrhythmia was confirmed. The use of sequential map-guided resection with supplemental cryoablative therapy became the "gold standard" and therefore the preferred surgical technique in most institutions.[14,23,24] Cryoablative therapy was used to achieve deeper intramural lesions, to ablate ventricular tachycardia from the base of the papillary muscle, and to ablate ventricular tachycardia originating from normal-appearing endocardium at the edge of visible endocardial scar. Arrhythmia control after the surgical procedure could be anticipated (Table 2). Despite refinements in the surgical techniques for myocardial preservation and the increasing skill of our surgical colleagues, surgical mortality from even the most experienced centers ranged from 8% to 15%.[14,23,24] Techniques that could mimic the results of surgery in terms of arrhythmia control but eliminate the mortality risk were clearly needed.

Direct-Current Catheter Ablation

In 1982, Scheinman and colleagues[30] and Gallagher and colleagues[31] described a technique for catheter-based direct-current energy delivery for the creation of heart block in patients with uncontrolled atrial fibrillation. Shortly thereafter, the effects of direct-current shock energy delivery on normal ventricular myocardium were described (Table 3).[32] An international registry for assessing efficacy and complications associated with direct-current shock catheter ablation for ventricular tachycardia was established.[33] Although the results of the experience from the registry suggested the

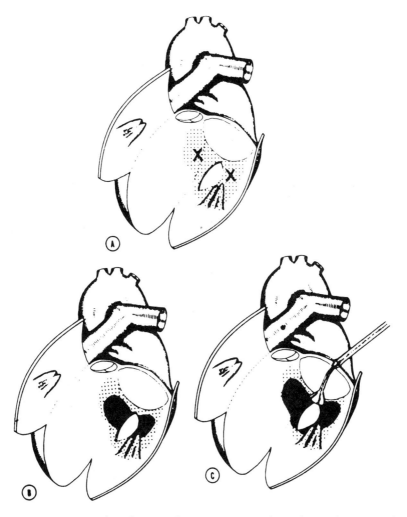

FIGURE 3. *Surgical technique for interrupting the isthmus between the mitral annulus and dense inferior scar described by Hargrove and colleagues.[28] Panel A demonstrates the extent of endocardial scar (stippled area) emanating from dense infarction and the site of the ventriculotomy. The sites of origin of ventricular tachycardia identified during intraoperative mapping are marked by an X on both sides of the ventriculotomy scar. Panel B shows standard subendocardial resection directed at map sites of origin. Panel C shows supplemental cryolesion at mitral annulus that improved outcome of surgical therapy for ventricular tachycardia associated with inferior infarction. A similar technique for successful catheter-based ablation of ventricular tachycardia has been suggested (see Figure 9). Reprinted with permission from Reference 28.*

TABLE 2

Surgical Ablative Therapy for Ventricular Tachycardia in the
Setting of Chronic Coronary Artery Disease

	Penn[14]	Baylor[23]	Virginia[24]
No. of patients	282	39	45
Operative mortality, %	15	10	9
Arrhythmia cure, %	92	89	85

TABLE 3

Comparison of Surgical and Catheter-Based Ablation for
Ventricular Tachycardia

	Subendocardial Resection	Direct-Current Energy	Radiofrequency Energy (4 mm Tip)
Cardiopulmonary bypass allows for mapping of rapid ventricular tachycardia	Yes	No	No
Opportunity to improve coronary blood flow	Yes	No	No
Eliminate aneurysm and improve hemodynamics	Yes	No	No
Serious morbidity/ mortality, %	8-15	8-10	1-3
Endocardial lesion size, cm^2	>16.0	1.0	0.2-0.4
General anesthesia required	Yes	Yes	No
Intramural lesion	Yes, adjunctive cryoablation	Yes, but limited	Very limited
Repeated lesion possible	No	Yes, but limited	Yes
Temperature monitoring to avoid coagulum	Not applicable	No	Yes

potential for arrhythmia cure in up to 70% of patients, the risks of serious complications and/or death still approach 10% (Table 4). The search continued for a technique that could mimic the surgical experience for arrhythmia control but reduce the risk of ablative therapy in patients with life-threatening ventricular arrhythmias.

TABLE 4

Complications of Direct-Current Catheter Ablation for Ventricular Tachycardia (n=164 Patients)[33]

Procedural deaths, m (%)	11 (6.7)
Systemic embolization, m (%)	4 (2.4)
Ventricular perforation, m	1

Radiofrequency Energy Catheter Ablation in Patients With Coronary Artery Disease

In the late 1980s, a number of investigators began to use radiofrequency energy to create a small endocardial lesion and safely eliminate focal sites responsible for the genesis or maintenance of supraventricular tachycardias.[34-37] Importantly, the lesion created was small and had a maximum depth of only 3 to 4 mm. The technique rapidly began to be applied to treatment of focal ventricular tachycardias that occur in the absence of structural heart disease and in the setting of bundle-branch reentrant ventricular tachycardia.[1-10] Despite the small lesion size, three factors made radiofrequency energy delivery the preferred catheter-based energy delivery technique for the treatment of sustained ventricular tachycardia in the setting of chronic coronary artery disease: (1) the ability to apply energy without significant pain or discomfort, thus eliminating the need for general anesthesia; (2) the ability to apply multiple lesions safely; and (3) the ability to monitor impedance and, more recently, temperature to avoid coagulum formation.

Simultaneously with the development of catheter-based ventricular tachycardia ablation techniques, attempts have been made to refine techniques that might facilitate more precise localization of the optimum site for catheter-based energy delivery (Table 5, A and B).[17,38,39] The movement from subendocardial resection to direct-current energy and then to radiofrequency energy limited the size of endocardium destroyed with a single energy application and thus merited a more vigorous attempt to precisely define the optimum site to direct ablation attempts. The role of the 12-lead ECG recorded during ventricular tachycardia to identify the origin of ventricular tachycardia was documented. A detailed retrospective analysis of 182 ventricular tachycardias that were subsequently mapped by catheter and intraoperative recording techniques confirmed the usefulness of certain electrocardiographic patterns for

TABLE 5A

Stimulation Techniques Used to Increase Accuracy of Mapping

Stimulation at distant site (right ventricular apex): good for distinguishing dead
 end versus activity that is part of or near reentrant circuit
Stimulation at site demonstrating presystolic activity ideal response
  Stimulus to QRS during pacing = electrogram to QRS during ventricular
   tachycardia
  Return cycle equal to tachycardia cycle length over a range of pacing cycle
   lengths with or without concealed entrainment on body surface ECG

TABLE 5B

Indications for Stimulation of Ventricular
Tachycardia Mapping Site

1. Extensive area of presystolic activity documented
2. Only limited area of presystolic activity documented after attempt at detailed
   mapping. Presystolic activity within 60 ms of the onset of QRS complex
3. Very early versus late "dead end" activation needs to be determined

regionalizing the origin of ventricular tachycardia.[38] Specifically,
the bundle-branch pattern, frontal plane axis, and R-wave transition all provide helpful clues (Figure 2).

A detailed review and characterization of recording and stimulation techniques and mapping techniques used to assist in identifying the site of origin of ventricular tachycardia is beyond the
scope of this review. However, several key items related to arrhythmia localization are worth reviewing (Table 5, A and B). The site
demonstrating the earliest diastolic activity recorded during tachycardia remains the starting point for ventricular tachycardia localization (Figure 4). However, as documented previously, the extent
of myocardium demonstrating presystolic activity may be large
(Figure 5), and detailed mapping to identify the earliest presystolic
site may be difficult and time-consuming. In addition, sometimes
very few sites demonstrate presystolic activity, and the degree of
presystolic activity is rather limited. Finally, it may be difficult at
times to distinguish sites demonstrating very early presystolic activity from sites that represent late or dead-end activation of areas
of myocardium not critical for arrhythmogenesis. In each of these
latter three situations, stimulation during the tachycardia at sites
demonstrating the earliest presystolic activity may help identify
those sites most appropriate for energy application (Table 5B). It is

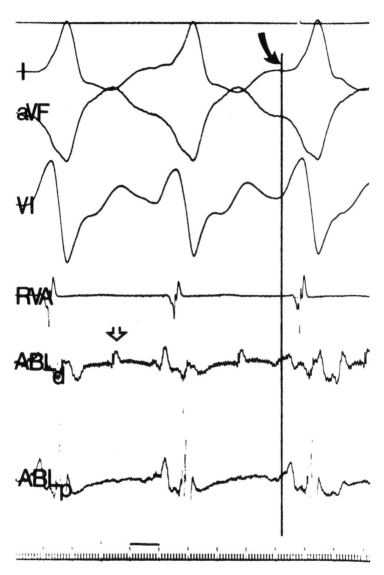

FIGURE 4. *Middiastolic potential (open arrow) recorded at the site of origin of ventricular tachycardia. Onset of QRS complex during VT is indicated (closed arrow). Radiofrequency energy applied to this site terminated ventricular tachycardia. Reprinted with permission from Reference 9.*

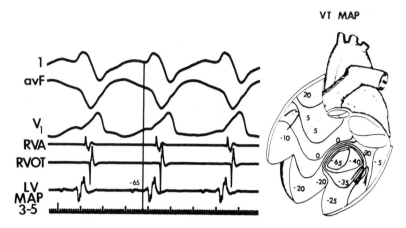

FIGURE 5. *Extensive area of endocardium demonstrating presystolic activity recorded during ventricular tachycardia (VT) mapping. Left panel shows surface ECG recordings, reference recordings from the right ventricle, and recordings from the earliest presystolic site (−65 ms). Right panel shows an isochronic map displayed on a schematic representation of the left ventricular endocardium. Note that presystolic activity was recorded over an extensive area of the inferior and septal endocardium. The earliest presystolic site was recorded 65 ms before the onset of electrical systole. This site was located along the inferior basal septum. Adapted with permission from Reference 17.*

important to recognize that it may not always be advisable to stimulate during ventricular tachycardia to confirm a response that is consistent with a recording at or near the reentrant circuit. The risk of catheter movement from a site that was technically difficult to access and the risk of tachycardia acceleration or change in morphology must be balanced with the additional information gained by performing stimulation techniques before applying energy.

Of note, even a perfect map and perfect response to stimulation at that site may not guarantee successful ablation with energy application. Failure to terminate ventricular tachycardia with energy application despite what appears to be an optimum recording site may occur for two possible reasons: (1) energy application, because of lack of contact, may be inadequate to create sufficient tissue destruction or (2) the critical portion of the reentrant circuit may represent part of a broad activation wave front. A recorded site may demonstrate a middiastolic potential and an appropriate response to stimulation but still not be associated with arrhythmia termination with energy application until the entire band or wave front has been interrupted. This is analogous to what has been observed during mapping and ablation of atrial flutter. A recording from the isthmus of atrial tissue lying between the tricuspid annulus and inferior vena cava may demonstrate pre–P-wave activity and concealed entrainment during pacing, yet focal ablation may not eliminate the flutter circuit. Facilitation of the ablation process will come from further definition of the size and characteristics of the ventricular tachycardia reentrant circuit. There is no reason to believe a priori that the circuit will not vary dramatically from individual to individual; yet, the morphological similarities in ventricular tachycardia from patient to patient suggest that common anatomically determined circuit characteristics may exist.

Outcome Without Radiofrequency Ablation in Ventricular Tachycardia Associated With Coronary Artery Disease

The results of ventricular tachycardia ablation by radiofrequency energy are remarkably consistent from center to center (Table 6). When comparing the results from other centers and our own experience at the Philadelphia Heart Institute in our first 37 patients, we found that the ability to eliminate the targeted ventricular tachycardia approaches 70% to 80% and the ability to eliminate all induced ventricular tachycardia approaches 30% to 40%.[39-42] In assessing long-term outcome and its implications for adjunctive implantable defibrillator therapy after ablation, we took the liberty of combining the results of three centers having the longest duration of reported follow-up in their patients after ventricular tachycardia ablation. The results demonstrated several interesting findings (Figure 6): (1) during an average follow-up of 1 year, ventricular tachycardia is eliminated in >50% of patients who undergo catheter-based ventricular tachycardia ablation with radiofrequency energy; (2) failure to even provide palliative therapy by standard mapping and ablative techniques occurs in ≈20% of patients; and (3) recurrence rates in patients with apparently successful catheter ablation were clearly dependent on the defined end points of the procedure. Patients in whom ablative therapy is aimed at specific targeted tachycardia morphologies have a recurrence rate of ≈40%, whereas patients in whom all uniform ventricular tachycardia morphologies are eliminated at the end of the procedure have documented recurrence rates of ventricular arrhythmias that approach 10% to 20%.

Because of the relatively high rate of life-threatening arrhythmia recurrence, even in patients with apparent successful ablation,

TABLE 6

Catheter-Based Radiofrequency Ablation of VT–Coronary Artery Disease: Overall Success

Institution	No. of Patients	No. (%) of Inducible VTs	No. (%) of Inducible Targeted VTs	Follow-up, Months	Any VT Recurrences, n (%)
Michigan[39]	15	5(33)	11(73)	9	0
UCLA[40]	15	6(40)	10(67)	7	0
Massachusetts General Hospital[41]	21	6(29)	17(81)	13	5(30)
Temple[42]	27	9(33)	22(81)	10	7(32)
Philadelphia Heart Institute	37	12(32)	28(76)	15	10(38)

VT indicates ventricular tachycardia.

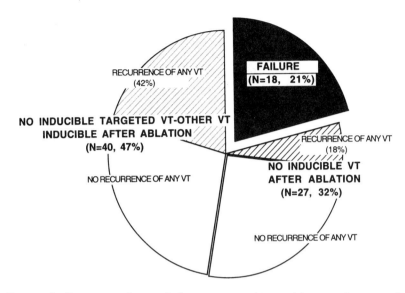

FIGURE 6. *Outcome after radiofrequency catheter ablation of ventricular tachycardia (VT). Because of similar results and length of follow-up, the outcome from reports from the Massachusetts General Hospital,[41] Temple University Hospital,[42] and our own experience at the Philadelphia Heart Institute were combined and are represented in the figure (see also Table 6). The average follow-up was at least 10 months (10 to 15 months). Note that >50% of patients have had no arrhythmia recurrences during follow-up, and in 20% of the patients, targeted ventricular tachycardia could not be eliminated in the electrophysiological laboratory. Outcome appeared to be improved if all inducible ventricular tachycardia could be eliminated.*

we currently advocate the use of hybrid therapy: catheter-based ablation of ventricular tachycardias combined with implantation of an implantable cardioverter-defibrillator. The implanted devices all provide advanced diagnostic information with stored electrograms.[43,44] We use this approach for three reasons: (1) a 10% to 20% recurrence rate, even in patients who have no inducible arrhythmias at the end of the procedure, is too high; (2) the advanced diagnostic information provided in the implantable defibrillator allows for accurate data collection related to the rate and possible morphology of recurrent arrhythmias after ablation; and (3) the improvement in implantable defibrillator system technology with nonthoracotomy lead systems and small devices implanted in the subclavicular area makes this form of adjunctive therapy of minimal risk to the patient.

Suggested Techniques for Improving Results of Catheter Ablation for Ventricular Tachycardia in the Setting of Coronary Artery Disease

Although the early results of catheter ablation for ventricular tachycardia in the setting of coronary artery disease are promising, recurrence rates remain high. In addition, >20% of the patients leave the electrophysiology laboratory without a documented beneficial effect on arrhythmia inducibility. Table 7 lists the various possible recognizable reasons for failure to successfully ablate ventricular tachycardia in the setting of coronary artery disease. The authors of this chapter suggest three basic techniques for improving the results of catheter ablation in this setting. We suggest these techniques from our own personal experience and that of others, but most importantly, because the suggestions are solidly based on surgical experience.

As we have indicated previously, most ventricular tachycardias originate from the septal or paraseptal regions (Figure 2). Access to the septum, especially along the basal septum, can sometimes be difficult by a retrograde aortic approach. For ventricular tachycar-

---

TABLE 7

Failure to Ablate VT–Coronary Artery Disease With Radiofrequency Energy via a Catheter-Based Approach

Left ventricle not accessed with retrograde approach and transseptal approach not attempted

Left ventricle not accessed via retrograde approach and transseptal approach not done

No "marked" presystolic activity identified despite complete mapping

No "marked" presystolic activity identified (technical limitations preventing complete map)

Presystolic activity identified but probably not in VT circuits despite detailed mapping

Presystolic activity identified but probably not in VT circuit (technical difficulties preventing access to suspected appropriate site)

VT termination with radiofrequency but still with inducible VT at appropriate site

Unable to establish good contact as indexed by temperature and impedance changes with radiofrequency and suspect inadequate lesion formation

Cannot initiate clinical VT

VT indicates ventricular tachycardia.

dia with a left bundle-branch block morphology or a right bundle-branch block with a superior axis associated with an anterior infarction, an atrial transseptal approach for introducing the catheter into the left ventricle allows for easy positioning of the catheter (Figure 7). An atrial transseptal technique also allows one to avoid access problems due to the extent of peripheral vascular disease frequently encountered in this patient population.

The second suggested technique to improve the results of catheter-based ablative therapy for ventricular tachycardia occurring in the setting of coronary artery disease is also based on the intraoperative mapping and surgical ablative experience. Krafchek and colleagues[23] documented that >10% of ventricular tachycardias can be localized to the right ventricular septum. In our initial experience with catheter ablation, 2 of our first 20 patients with ventricular tachycardia demonstrating a left bundle-branch block QRS morphology had the earliest presystolic activity localized to the right ventricular endocardial septum (Figure 8). Repeated radiofrequency ablation attempts delivered at the earliest site of activity on the left ventricular endocardium failed to terminate the arrhythmia. Radiofrequency energy application to the right side

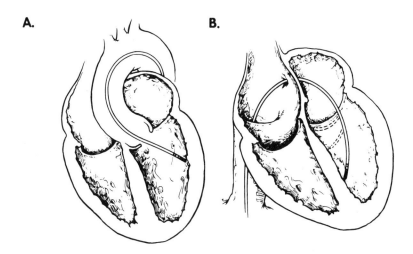

A.   **B.**

FIGURE 7. *Schematic representation of catheter placement in the left ventricle using transaortic (left panel) versus atrial transseptal (right panel) approach. Note that the atrial transseptal approach affords easy access to the septum, especially the basal septum. Since most ventricular tachycardias originate from the septum or paraseptal regions (Figure 2), an atrial transseptal approach may be the preferred technique to ensure adequate mapping and good catheter contact.*

resulted in immediate termination of tachycardia.[45] It is suggested that whenever a ventricular tachycardia with a left bundle-branch block morphology is present, detailed mapping of the right ventricular septem should be strongly considered, particularly when early presystolic activity on the left ventricular septum cannot be identified. Finally, Hargrove and colleagues[28] documented the importance of the isthmus between the mitral annulus and the dense inferior infarction for the genesis and maintenance of sustained ventricular tachycardia (Figure 3). Catheter positioning should begin adjacent to the mitral annulus for initial mapping and subsequent ablation of ventricular tachycardias with a QRS morphology consistent with a very basal location (Figure 9, A and B). Energy

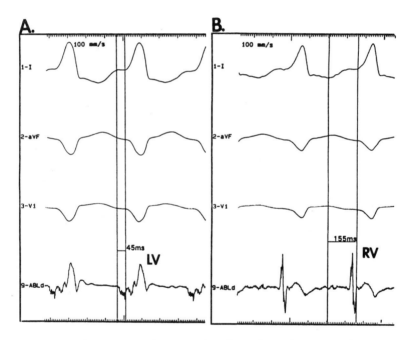

FIGURE 8. *Earliest presystolic recording from the right ventricular (RV) endocardium in patients with chronic coronary artery disease. Panel A shows recording from left ventricular (LV) septum showing earliest presystolic activity recorded 43 ms before the onset of electrical systole. Radiofrequency energy application at this site failed to terminate ventricular tachycardia. Panel B shows a recording from the right ventricular septal endocardium demonstrating electrical earliest activity recorded 155 ms before the onset of electrical systole. Radiofrequency energy application terminated ventricular tachycardia at this site.*

application to the mitral annulus can frequently eliminate both left and right bundle-branch block tachycardia morphologies. Wilber and colleagues[29] have suggested that the periannular tissue may serve as a necessary part of the reentrant circuit for some ventricular tachycardias associated with inferior infarction, somewhat analogously to the way that clockwise and counterclockwise atrial

MITRAL ANNULAR VT ABLATION

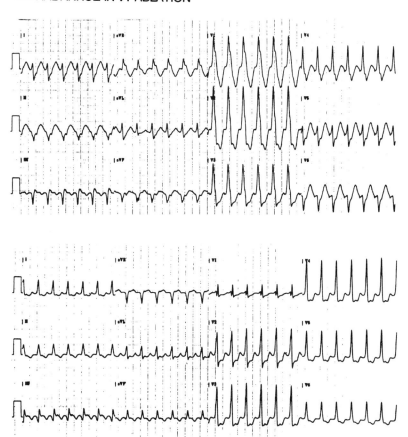

FIGURE 9. *Panel A shows 12-lead electrocardiographic recordings during ventricular tachycardia (VT) induced at the beginning of the electrophysiological study in a patient with an inferior infarction. Radiofrequency energy was applied to the site adjacent (see also Figure 3) to the mitral annulus, and neither ventricular tachycardia could be induced subsequently.*

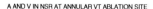

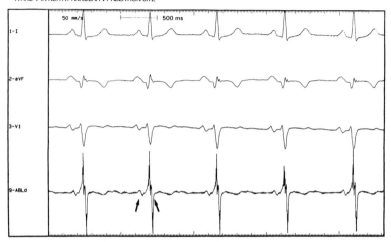

FIGURE 9. (contined) *Panel B shows a recording during normal sinus rhythm (NSR) at the mitral annular site at which radiofrequency energy was applied. Note the recording of atrial activity at this periannular site (arrows).*

flutter uses the isthmus between the tricuspid valve annulus and the inferior vena cava as a critical portion of its reentrant circuit.

Selecting the Appropriate End Point for Catheter Ablation in the Setting of Chronic Coronary Artery Disease

A number of factors need to be taken into consideration when deciding on an end point for ventricular tachycardia ablation in the setting of chronic coronary artery disease. Many patients who present with sustained ventricular tachycardia have multiple spontaneous and induced tachycardia morphologies. The tachycardias may have different rates and produce different hemodynamic effects. The amount of heart disease, although usually extensive, may vary dramatically. Not uncommonly, patients have been given multiple antiarrhythmic drugs before clinical presentation. Antiarrhythmic agents may be continued up to the time of the ablation procedure. Amiodarone, with its complex elimination pharmacokinetics, may have been administered for months or years before the procedure. Frequently, an implantable car-

dioverter-defibrillator is already in place. The frequency of spontaneous arrhythmia occurrence varies considerably from person to
person. A patient with several spontaneous episodes of ventricular
tachycardia, each with a distinct 12-lead QRS morphology, should
be approached differently from the patient with recurrent ventricular tachycardia with each episode demonstrating the same morphology and each episode resulting in an implantable
cardioverter-defibrillator shock. Although the goal of the ablation
procedure should be to eliminate all recognizable spontaneous
and inducible ventricular tachycardias, this approach is not always feasible or practical in the setting of chronic coronary artery
disease. A more practical approach may be necessary. There is no
doubt that the outcome in terms of arrhythmia recurrence is
worse in patients in whom only a specified targeted morphology is
eliminated (Figure 6). There is also no doubt, however, that eliminating the targeted arrhythmia in patients with incessant or frequently recurrent ventricular tachycardia can provide many
months of arrhythmia palliation in most patients.[46] If a patient has
poor left ventricular function and multiple induced tachycardia
morphologies, it is recommended that the electrophysiologist start
the ablation process by trying to target the tachycardia morphology that has been documented to occur spontaneously. A more aggressive approach might be anticipated in patients with preserved
left ventricular function with only a few distinct tachycardia morphologies inducible. A potentially curative ablative procedure
should be attempted by eliminating all spontaneous and induced
ventricular tachycardia morphologies.

These suggestions are meant to serve only as guidelines. It is
obvious that many modifiers exist that can alter the approach to
these patients. The desire to maintain or eliminate antiarrhythmic
drug therapy, the presence or planned use of an implantable defibrillator, difficulty with access, and finally the patient's comfort
and desire and ability to undergo repeated ablation procedures
may all influence the end-point selection. Clearly, the end points for
arrhythmia termination with energy application are not satisfactory. An attempt to reinitiate ventricular tachycardia with programmed stimulation should be performed before the procedure is
declared to be successful.

Future Developments

Further improvements in outcome and extended indications
for catheter-based ventricular tachyarrhythmia ablation in the set-

ting of chronic coronary artery disease should be anticipated. Progress will come with four major developments. The first development will permit more extensive endocardial and deeper intramural tissue destruction by catheter-based energy delivery techniques. Cool-tipped radiofrequency energy delivery, microwave ablation techniques, and others, coupled with altered electrode configuration and design, will permit more extensive endocardial and deeper intramural tissue destruction by catheter-based energy delivery techniques. These developments should more closely mimic successful surgical ablation techniques in terms of the endocardial and intramural extent of tissue ablation. The second development will come from a more complete understanding of the ventricular tachycardia circuit in the setting of coronary artery disease. Animal models that more closely mimic humans have recently been described.[41,47] Detailed mapping and stimulation during ventricular tachycardia will permit a more complete characterization of the size, anatomic boundaries, and physiological response of the arrhythmia circuit. It is expected that the results of this investigation will have direct relevance to arrhythmogenesis in humans and assist in defining techniques to target optimum sites for catheter ablation. The third development will permit more detailed, rapid, and reproducible mapping and processing of recorded data during ventricular tachycardia. Multipolar recording catheter technology coupled with computer software developments will allow for rapid acquisition of multiple recording sites and rapid and accurate processing of recorded data. This should facilitate localization of even rapid ventricular tachycardias that are not amenable to detailed point-by-point catheter mapping. Finally, the relation of anatomy and physiology as it relates to the genesis of ventricular tachycardia and possibly ventricular fibrillation will be defined. Analogous to atrial flutter, one might anticipate that a critical anatomically determined isthmus may be definable for most sustained ventricular tachycardias having a uniform morphology. In addition, the border zone of infarction, which appears to play a significant role in the genesis of most ventricular tachycardias and ventricular fibrillation in the setting of chronic coronary artery disease, may be identifiable by multiple imaging and/or electrical recording techniques.[48] It would not be farfetched to assume that such techniques would be applied to assist in catheter-based ablation. The border zone of infarction might be targeted for ablation in patients defined as having an increased risk of sustained ventricular arrhythmias after myocardial infarctions after a number of well-defined risk-stratifying techniques have been used.

With these four developments, one should anticipate that catheter ablation of ventricular tachycardia will assume a primary role in the management of ventricular arrhythmias by the beginning of the next millennium.

Acknowledgments

The authors would like to thank Susan Shuster for her assistance in the preparation of this manuscript.

References

1. Kottkamp H, Hindricks G, Chen X, et al. Radiofrequency catheter ablation of sustained ventricular tachycardia in idiopathic dilated cardiomyopathy. *Circulation.* 1995;92:1159–1168.
2. Mehdirad A, Keim S, Rist K, et al. Long-term clinical outcome of right bundle branch radiofrequency catheter ablation for treatment of bundle branch reentrant ventricular tachycardia. *PACE.* 1995;18:2135–2143.
3. Kottkamp H, Chen X, Hindricks G, et al. Idiopathic left ventricular tachycardia: new insights into electrophysiological characteristics and radiofrequency catheter ablation. *PACE.* 1995; 18:1285–1297.
4. Zardini T, Thakur R, Klein G, et al. Catheter ablation of idiopathic left ventricular tachycardia. *PACE.* 1995;18:1255– 1265.
5. Wen M, Yeh S, Wang C, et al. Radiofrequency ablation therapy in idiopathic left ventricular tachycardia with no obvious structural heart disease. *Circulation.* 1994;89:1690–1696.
6. Nakagawa H, Beckman J, McClelland J, et al. Radiofrequency catheter ablation of idiopathic left ventricular tachycardia guided by a Purkinje potential. *Circulation.* 1993;88:2607–2617.
7. Jadonath RL, Schwartzman D, Preminger MW, et al. The utility of the 12-lead electrocardiogram in localizing the site of origin of right ventricular outflow tract tachycardia. *Am Heart J.* 1995;130:1107–1113.
8. Duthinh V, Callans DJ, Marchlinski FE. Catheter ablation as therapy for ventricular tachycardia. *Primary Cardiol.* 1995;2:18–22.
9. Callans DJ, Schwartzman D, Gottlieb CD, et al. Insights into the electrophysiology of ventricular tachycardia gained by the catheter ablation experience: "learning while burning." *J Cardiovasc Electrophysiol.* 1994;5:877–894.
10. Movsowitz C, Schwartzman D, Callans DJ, et al. Idiopathic right ventricular outflow tract tachycardia: narrowing the anatomical location for successful ablation. *Am Heart J.* 1996;93:131.
11. Graham AF, Miller DC, Strinson EB, et al. Surgical treatment of refractory life-threatening ventricular tachycardia. *Am J Cardiol.* 1973;32:909.
12. Kim YH, Sosa-Suarez G, Trouton TG, et al. Treatment of ventricular tachycardia by transcatheter radiofrequency ablation in patients with ischemic heart disease. *Circulation.* 1994;89:1094–1102.
13. Harken AH, Horowitz LN, Josephson ME. Comparison of standard aneurysmectomy and aneurysmectomy with directed endocardial

resection for treatment of recurrent sustained ventricular tachycardia. *J Thorac Cardiovasc Surg.* 1980;80:527.

14. Miller JM, Marchlinski FE. Non-pharmacologic therapy of ventricular arrhythmias. In: Brest AN, ed. *Contemporary Management of Ventricular Arrhythmias.* Philadelphia, Pa: FA Davis; 1992:117–146.
15. Josephson ME, Horowitz LN, Farshidi A. Recurrent sustained ventricular tachycardia, II: endocardial mapping. *Circulation.* 1978;57: 440–447.
16. Josephson ME, Horowitz LN, Farshidi A, et al. Sustained ventricular tachycardia: evidence for protected localized reentry. *Am J Cardiol.* 1978;42:416.
17. Marchlinski FE, Almendral JM, Cassidy DM, et al. Localization of endocardial site for catheter ablation of ventricular tachycardia. In: Fontaine G, Sheinman M, eds. *Ablation in Cardiac Arrhythmias.* Mt Kisco, NY: Futura Publishing Co; 1987:289–309.
18. Josephson ME, Horowitz LN, Spielman SR, et al. The role of catheter mapping in the pre-operative evaluation of ventricular tachycardia. *Am J Cardiol.* 1982;49:207.
19. Stevenson WG, Nademanee K, Weiss JN, et al. Programmed electrical stimulation at potential ventricular reentry circuit sites. *Circulation.* 1989;80:793–806.
20. Josephson ME, Harken AH, Horowitz LN. Endocardial excision: a new surgical technique for the treatment of recurrent ventricular tachycardia. *Circulation.* 1979;60:1430.
21. Josephson ME, Waxman HL, Cain ME, et al. Ventricular activation during endocardial pacing, II: role of pace-mapping to localize origin of ventricular tachycardia. *Am J Cardiol.* 1982;50:11–20.
22. Horowitz LN, Harken AH, Kastor JA, et al. Ventricular resection guided by epicardial and endocardial mapping for treatment of recurrent ventricular tachycardia. *N Engl J Med.* 1980;302:589.
23. Krafchek J, Lawrie GM, Roberts R, et al. Surgical ablation of ventricular tachycardias: improved results with map-directed regional approach. *Circulation.* 1986;73:1239.
24. Haines DE, Lerman BB, Kron H, et al. Surgical ablation of ventricular tachycardia with sequential map-guided subendocardial resection: electrophysiologic assessment and long-term follow-up. *Circulation.* 1988;77:131.
25. Svenson RH, Littmann L, Colavita PG, et al. Laser photoablation of ventricular tachycardia: correlation of disastolic activation times and photoablation effects on cycle length and termination-observations supporting a macroreentrant mechanism. *J Am Coll Cardiol.* 1992;19:607–613.
26 Moran JM, Kehoe RH, Loeb JM, et al. Extended endocardial resection for the treatment of ventricular tachycardia and ventricular fibrillation. *Ann Thorac Surg.* 1982;34:538.
27. Miller JM, Kienzle MG, Harken AH, et al. Subendocardial resection for ventricular tachycardia: predictors of surgical success. *Circulation.* 1984;70:624.
28. Hargrove WC, Miller JM, Vassallo JA, et al. Improved results in the operative management of ventricular tachycardia related to inferior wall myocardial infarction: importance of the annular isthmus. *J Thorac Cardiovasc Surg.* 1986;92:726–732.
29. Wilber DJ, Kopp DE, Glascock DN, et al. Catheter ablation of the mi-

tral isthmus for ventricular tachycardia associated with inferior infarction. *Circulation.* 1995;92:3481–3489.

30. Scheinman MM, Morady F, Hess DS, et al. Catheter-induced ablation of the atrioventricular junction to control refractory supraventricular arrhythmias. *JAMA.* 1982;248:851–855.

31. Gallagher JJ, Svenson RH, Kasell JH, et al. Catheter technique for closed-chest ablation of the atrioventricular conduction system. *N Engl J Med.* 1982;306:194–200.

32. Kempf FC, Falcone RA, Iozzo RV, et al. Anatomic and hemodynamic effects of catheter-delivered ablation energies in the ventricle. *Am J Cardiol.* 1985;56:373–377.

33. Evans GT, Scheinmann MM, Zipes DP, et al. The Percutaneous Cardiac Mapping and Ablation Registry: final summary of results. *PACE.* 1988;11:1621–1626.

34. Jackman WM, Wang X, Friday KJ, et al. Catheter ablation of accessory atrioventricular pathways (Wolff-Parkinson-White syndrome) by radiofrequency current. *N Engl J Med.* 1991;324:1605–1611.

35. Calkins H, Sousa J, El-Atassi R, et al. Diagnosis and cure of the Wolff-Parkinson-White syndrome of paroxysmal supraventricular tachycardias during a single electrophysiologic test. *N Engl J Med.* 1991; 324:1612–1618.

36. Jackman WM, Beckman KJ, McClelland JH, et al. Treatment of supraventricular tachycardia due to atrioventricular nodal reentry by radiofrequency catheter ablation of slow-pathway conduction. *N Engl J Med.* 1992;327:313.

37. Morady F, Frank R, Kou WH, et al. Identification and catheter ablation of a zone of slow conduction in the reentrant circuit of ventricular tachycardia in humans. *J Am Coll Cardiol.* 1988;11:775–782.

38. Miller JM, Marchlinski FE, Buxton AE, et al. Relationship between the 12-lead electrocardiogram site of origin in patients with coronary artery disease. *Circulation.* 1988;77:759.

39. Morady F, Harvey M, Kalbfleisch SJ, et al. Radiofrequency catheter ablation of ventricular tachycardia in patients with coronary artery disease. *Circulation.* 1993;87:363–372.

40. Stevenson WG, Khan H, Sager P, et al. Identification of reentry circuit sites during catheter mapping and radiofrequency ablation of ventricular tachycardia late after myocardial infarction. *Circulation.* 1993;88:1647–1670.

41. Chang I, Michele JJ, Dillon SM, et al. Left ventricular endocardial electrical impedance measurement in chronic infarction using a multipolar ("basket") catheter. *PACE.* 1994;19:713.

42. Rothman SA, Hsia HH, Cossu SF, et al. Post infarct ventricular tachycardia: success rate of catheter ablation. *J Am Coll Cardiol.* 1995;25: 705–706:42A. Abstract.

43. Marchlinski FE, Callans DJ, Gottlieb CD, et al. Benefits and lessons learned from stored electrogram information in implantable defibrillators. *J Cardiovasc Electrophysiol.* 1995;6:832–851.

44. Marchlinski FE, Gottlieb CD, Sarter B, et al. ICD data storage: value in arrhythmia management. *PACE.* 1993;16:527–534.

45. Menz V, Duthinh V, Schwartzman D, et al. Radiofrequency current ablation of ventricular tachycardia after myocardial infarction from the right ventricular septum. *PACE.* In press.

46. Schwartzman D, Jadonath RL, Callans DJ, et al. Radiofrequency catheter ablation for control of frequent ventricular tachycardia after myocardial infarction. *Am J Cardiol.* 1995;75:297–299.
47. Kreiner G, Gottlieb CD, Yeh I, et al. Ventricular tachycardia in an ovine model of left ventricular aneurysm. *Surg Forum.* 1989;40: 219–220.
48. Schwartman D, Chang I, Mirotznik MS, et al. Left ventricular catheter mapping during sinus rhythm in chronic myocardial infarction: correlation of electrograms with electrical impedance. *J Am Coll Cardiol.* 1994; Feb;202A.

Chapter 12

Device Therapy and Evolution

Debra S. Echt, MD

Device Evolution

Implantable cardioverter-defibrillator (ICD) device therapy has undergone tremendous technological advancement. The idea was first conceived by Dr Michael Mirowski in 1967. The first breadboard model for the device was designed in 1969.[1] Animal testing began in 1972, and the first animal implantation was performed in 1976.[2] Interestingly, the original lead system tested was a single transvenous lead with two defibrillating electrodes, but it was ineffective. The first human implant in 1980 used a transvenous spring electrode in the superior vena cava and an epicardial cone (not patch) sutured to the left ventricular apex. This device detected only ventricular fibrillation. Rate-sensing leads and circuitry were added in 1982, allowing the detection and treatment of ventricular tachycardia. The epicardial cone shape was changed to a flat patch in 1981, and in 1982 the combination of two patches, one over each ventricle, could be used instead of the spring-patch combination. In 1985, the first ICD device attained FDA approval.[3] It was large (292 g and 162 cm^3) and not programmable: each device had to be custom ordered as to the rate-detection cutoff. These devices were activated and deactivated by a magnet; battery depletion was estimated from prolongation of the time required to charge the capacitors; and the only diagnostic information available was the number of shocks delivered.

Now, 11 years later, devices use one or two transvenous leads, and the pulse generators are implanted pectorally, similar to permanent bradycardia pacemakers. The success of the most significant advancement, the avoidance of thoracotomy with transvenous lead systems, is attributed in large part to the incorporation of biphasic defibrillating waveforms[4,5] (Figure 1). In retrospect, the

From: Dunbar SB, Ellenbogen KA, Epstein AE, (eds). *Sudden Cardiac Death: Past, Present, and Future.* Armonk, NY: Futura Publishing Company, Inc.; © 1997.

BIPHASIC WAVEFORM

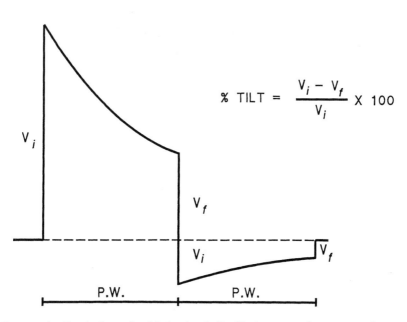

$$\% \text{ TILT} = \frac{V_i - V_f}{V_i} \times 100$$

FIGURE 1. *Depiction of a biphasic defibrillating waveform. V_i indicates initial (peak) voltage; V_f, final voltage; and P.W., pulse width. Formula for the calculation of the percent tilt is shown.*

inefficacy of the original transvenous lead system tested in dogs was because the defibrillating waveform was monophasic. At present, there are a number of electrode configurations that can be used without resorting to a thoracotomy procedure. One or two transvenous leads contain two defibrillating electrodes and a pacing and rate-sensing pair (Figure 2).[6] The pulse generator itself can serve as one defibrillating electrode when implanted in the pectoral region.[7] If two transvenous defibrillating electrodes are ineffective, a third defibrillating electrode, either a patch or an array, can be added in the precordial area subcutaneously.[8]

Another major advance has been the availability of stored electrograms of detected events in retrievable memory[9] (Figure 3). Previously, the interpretation of device therapy was based solely on the patient's history. Unfortunately, the presence or absence of symptoms before device therapy is not specific for ventricular tachycardia or fibrillation. The availability of stored electrograms has resulted in substantial improvements in avoiding inappropriate therapy and op-

TRANSVENOUS LEAD SYSTEMS

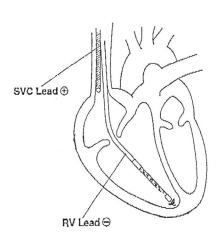

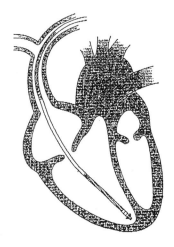

SVC Lead ⊕

RV Lead ⊖

FIGURE 2. *Drawing of two transvenous lead systems. Electrode configuration on the left uses two leads, allowing positioning of each defibrillating electrode. Electrode configuration on the right incorporates both defibrillating electrodes in a single lead.*

timizing individualized parameter settings. Moreover, it often obviates the need to hospitalize patients receiving multiple shocks.

Another major advance has been the improvement in battery longevity. The first device available had a median battery life of 18 months. Some currently available devices last 4 to 6 years. Projected battery longevity information provided by manufacturers is based on prediction and can be inaccurate. Data regarding the longevity of specific devices are limited. Battery drain from ICD power consumption is a function of sensing, pacing, and capacitor discharges. Antibradycardia pacing substantially reduces battery longevity. Continuous pacing at a nominal setting reduces overall ICD device longevity by ≈ 2 years. Each high-energy shock shortens ICD longevity by 1 to 2 weeks.

Other advances include the ability to individually program virtually all parameter settings (Figure 4). Detailed diagnostic data can be obtained noninvasively through interrogation with the programmer. Specific information regarding the arrhythmia episodes detected and therapies delivered is available (Figure 5). Capacitors now re-form automatically, and the most recent capacitor charging

Stored EGM Report

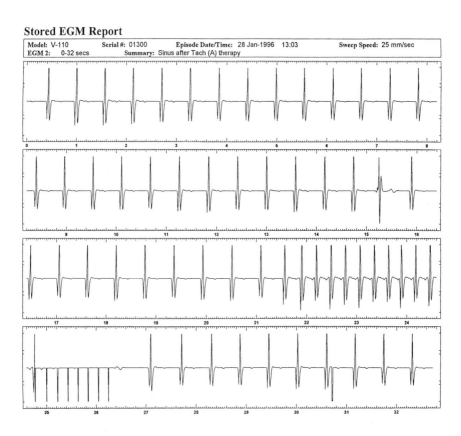

| Model: V-110 | Serial #: 01300 | Episode Date/Time: 28 Jan-1996   13:03 | Sweep Speed: 25 mm/sec |
| EGM 2:   0-32 secs | | Summary: Sinus after Tach (A) therapy | |

FIGURE 3. *Stored electrogram recording of a spontaneous episode of ventricular tachycardia. The recording is continuous: the rhythm in top panel is sinus from a right ventricular recording site; the second panel includes a premature ventricular complex; ventricular tachycardia occurs on the third panel; and the bottom panel reveals antitachycardia burst pacing artifacts with restoration of sinus rhythm.*

Programmed Parameter Summary Report

Model:	V-110 D	Serial #:	01300
Print Report Date/Time:	01-Feb-1996 / 10:42		

Device Configuration
Defibrillator with Single Tach Discrimination

Detection Criteria		Tachyarrhythmia Therapies	
Fib Detection:	270 ms (222 bpm)	Fib/EHR Therapy:	[1] 750 V
			[2] 750 V
EHR Detection:	Same as Tach		[3] 750 V x 4
	for 40 sec		
Tach Detection:	375 ms (160 bpm)	Tach Therapy:	[1] ATP
	for 8 intervals		[2] CVRT 750 V
	Sudden Onset Off		[3] CVRT 750 V
			[4] CVRT 750 V
		Waveform:	Biphasic
			+10.0 ms, -10.0 ms
Bradycardia Pacing		**Anti-Tachycardia Pacing**	
Pacing: VVI 40 ppm		Auto-Dec: On	Output: 10.0 V, 1.0 ms
Brady Output: 5.0 V, 0.5 ms		BCL: 85 %	Min. BCL: 200 ms
Refractory Period: 400 ms		No. Bursts: 4	Stimuli: 8 w/10 ms steps
Post-therapy Pause: 2 events		Scanning: Off	

Capacitor Maintenance	
Maintenance Interval: 6 months	Maintenance Voltage: 750 V

Electrogram Storage Parameters	
Number (Duration) of stored events: 3 Events (32 sec)	Event Trigger: Sinus
Duration of Pre-Trigger: 30 sec	
Events Stored: Fib, EHR, Tach	

Real-Time Measurements	
Unloaded Battery Voltage: >6.3 V	Auto Gain Setting: 0
Pacing Lead Impedance: 1225 ohms	R-Wave Amplitude: >9 mV

FIGURE 4. *Example of a report of the programmed parameters of a third-generation tiered-therapy ICD device.*

time is available. However, the battery voltage is also given, which is used to determine battery depletion directly. Pacing lead integrity can be evaluated with impedance calculation, R-wave amplitude measurement, and real-time electrogram recordings. Antitachycardia pacing modalities allow the termination of slower-rate ventricular tachycardia by low-output pacing stimuli, which avoids the discomfort of high-output capacitor discharges (see example, Figure 3). Newer devices also offer tiered therapy, such that ventricular tachyarrhythmias of different rates can receive different therapies, and for each ventricular tachycardia type, a protocol of increasingly more aggressive therapies can be programmed. Noninvasive programmed stimulation can be performed via the programmer without the need for intravenous catheters. An example of the noninvasive induction of ventricular fibrillation is shown

Initial Diagnostics Report

Model:	V-110 D	Serial #:	01300
Print Report Date/Time:	01-Feb-1996 / 10:43		

Diagnostics Summary

Detections Resulting in Therapy:
Fib: 0
EHR: 0
Tach: 12   Min/Max Cycle Length: 285 ms / 365 ms

Total Number Aborted Shocks: 0
Date/Time Diagnostics Last Cleared: 02 Nov-1995   11:21

Capacitor Maintenance

Maintenance Interval: 6 months   Last Charge Time: 12.9 sec
Last Capacitor Charge Voltage: 750 V
Last Cap. Maintenance Charge: 13 Dec-1995   01:58

Device Charging History

50 - 200 V :   1
250 - 400 V :   2
450 - 600 V :   1
650 - 750 V :   5

Diagnostic Therapy Sequencing

Episode 11 of 11(Most Recent)
                                          Therapy Duration: < 10 sec
Initial Detection: Tach
Therapy: ATP   Result: Below Rate Detection

Last Successful BCL: 265 ms

Episode 10 of 11
                                          Therapy Duration: < 10 sec
Initial Detection: Tach
Therapy: ATP   Result: Below Rate Detection

Episode 9 of 11
                                          Therapy Duration: < 10 sec
Initial Detection: Tach
Therapy: ATP   Result: Below Rate Detection

Episode 8 of 11
                                          Therapy Duration: < 10 sec
Initial Detection: Tach
Therapy: ATP   Result: Below Rate Detection

FIGURE 5. *Example of a report of diagnostic information of tachyarrhythmias detected and therapies delivered.*

in Figure 6. As mentioned previously, currently available ICD devices also have antibradycardia pacing capability in the VVI mode. An example of ventricular demand pacing after shock is also seen in Figure 7.

Indications and Selection

There are two major indications for treating patients with ICD device systems, as originally approved for labeling by the FDA in

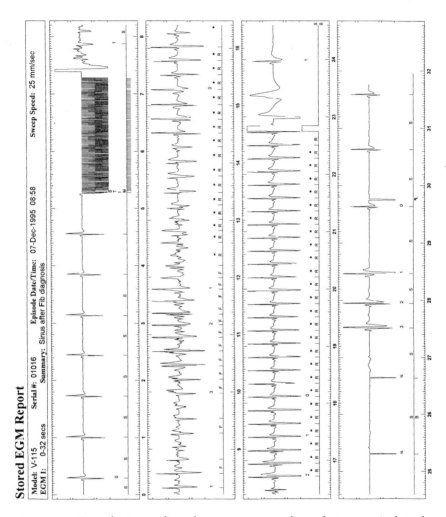

FIGURE 6. *Stored intracardiac electrogram recording of an event induced with noninvasive programmed stimulation. Top panel, ultra-rapid burst pacing via the device converts sinus rhythm into ventricular fibrillation. Second panel, ventricular fibrillation organizes to ventricular flutter and is terminated by a high-voltage discharge. Bottom panel shows two antibradycardia paced beats followed by three beats of ventricular tachycardia and then sinus rhythm.*

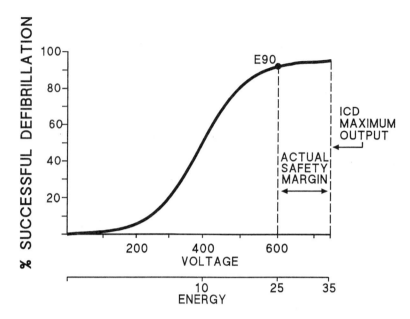

FIGURE 7. *Relation between the energy or peak voltage delivered and the percentage of successful ventricular defibrillation attempts, described as a sigmoid curve. The "safety margin" is defined as the difference between the 90% to 95% effective defibrillation energy or voltage (E90) and maximum output of the ICD device. This illustration depicts a 10-J, 150-V safety margin, which has been shown to be adequate for ICD devices with maximum outputs of ≥32 J.*

1985. They are (1) patients who survive a cardiac arrest presumed to be due to ventricular tachycardia or ventricular fibrillation and not an acute myocardial infarction and (2) patients with sustained ventricular tachycardia or ventricular fibrillation in whom conventional antiarrhythmic drugs are limited by inefficacy, intolerance, or noncompliance. This means that (1) for patients who survive a cardiac arrest, it is not necessary to have ECG documentation of ventricular tachycardia or fibrillation, nor is electrophysiological testing or inducibility required, and (2) for patients with sustained ventricular tachycardia or ventricular fibrillation, the number of conventional drugs evaluated is not specified. Several large organizations have considered additional indications. The North American Society of Pacing and Electrophysiology reported the conclusions of a policy conference,[10] and the American Heart Association and American College of Cardiology published guidelines from a combined task force.[11] There were only minor differences in their recommendations. It is generally agreed that ICD therapy may be indicated for patients with recurrent, unexplained syncope in whom ventricular tachycardia or ventricular fibrillation is inducible and drug therapy is limited by inefficacy, intolerance, or noncompliance. Also, ICD therapy may be indicated for patients with hemodynamically significant ventricular tachycardia or ventricular fibrillation when drug efficacy testing is possible. In fact, these two categories, in which it was concluded in publications 5 years ago that ICD therapy might be indicated, are now accepted as the standard of care. It is generally accepted that ICD therapy is indicated in patients with (1) recurrent, unexplained syncope without inducible ventricular tachycardia or ventricular fibrillation, (2) incessant ventricular tachycardia or ventricular fibrillation, (3) correctable or reversible ventricular tachycardia or ventricular fibrillation, or (4) ventricular fibrillation secondary to Wolff-Parkinson-White syndrome.

A number of clinical studies of ICD systems have been published, reporting either large experiences at one center[12-14] or a multicenter experience with a specific ICD device system.[15,16] Overall, the characteristics of the patients receiving ICD systems are similar among published series, except that the average age is now older, presumably because preventive measures and therapeutic advances for coronary artery disease have resulted in ischemic cardiomyopathy developing in older patients. The average age at ICD implant in earlier studies was about 55 years, but it is now about 65 years. Most (80% to 85%) of the patients are male, consistent with the prevalence of coronary artery disease in men of this age group. The underlying heart disease is coronary artery disease in 70% to 75% of patients. Idiopathic (nonischemic) cardiomyopathy is present in 10% to 15% of patients. Other cardiac disorders, such as the long-QT syndrome, valvular heart disease, congenital heart disease, left ventricular hypertrophy, or hypertrophic cardiomyopathy, are thought to be causative in 10% of patients, and no underlying cardiac disease is apparent in 5% of patients. The majority of patients have significant left ventricular dysfunction, with the average ejection fraction being in the 32% to 35% range.

Patient Management

The ICD implantation procedure is now more commonly performed in the electrophysiology laboratory by a clinical electrophysiologist, rather than in an operating room by a cardiac surgeon. The complication rate and outcome in patients receiving implants by nonsurgeons and outside of the operating room have been found to be equivalent to the implantation of ICD systems with transvenous lead systems in the traditional setting.[17] The choice of anesthesia is based on physician preference.[18] Anesthesia may be achieved with conscious sedation and a brief period of deep sedation for defibrillation threshold testing, or with the more traditional general anesthesia.

It appears that pulse generators <100 cm^3 in volume and 140 g in weight may be implanted safely in the pectoral region. Because pectoral device implantation reduces the surgical procedure to one that is more like a bradycardia pacemaker, it is favored by clinical electrophysiologists. The pulse generator may be implanted either subcutaneously or beneath the pectoral muscle. The subpectoral position is less likely to result in erosion or migration but makes generator replacement a more extensive procedure. It is desirable, if possible, to insert the transvenous leads more laterally in the left cephalic vein rather than in the left subclavian vein to reduce the likelihood of a lead crush injury because of the narrow space between the clavicle and first rib.

The selection of leads and electrode configurations is primarily a matter of physician preference and philosophy. There are two strategies to consider: simplicity and versatility. The strategy to use the simplest lead arrangement begins with the testing of a "unipolar" defibrillating system consisting of a transvenous right ventricular coil and the pulse generator can itself. However, should this be ineffective, a second lead must be inserted transvenously and advanced to an innominate, subclavian, or right atrial position. Another single-lead system is composed of both distal (right ventricular) and proximal (right atrial) defibrillating coils. However, this system does not offer the versatility of variability of the position of the proximal coil electrode. Also, the caliber of the lead causes stiffness, which restricts the ability to vary the position of the lead tip within the right ventricle. The initial testing of a two-lead system has the disadvantage of requiring two venous insertions, but it then provides the flexibility to adjust the position of each defibrillating coil. In all "bipolar" systems using two defibrillating leads, reversing polarity can be tried to improve defibrillation efficacy. Also, a third electrode, either a subcutaneous patch or an array, can be added to attempt to improve efficacy. With a biphasic defibrillating waveform, nonthoracotomy lead systems are effective in ≈ 98% of patients. Therefore, the need for thoracotomy to implant epicardial patch electrodes is now quite rare.

Clinical Results

The most striking benefit of ICD device therapy is the subsequent low incidence of sudden cardiac death and death attributed to ventricular tachycardia or fibrillation. The 1-year actuarial incidence of sudden death is ≤2% in most series[12] and 2% per year thereafter. Nonarrhythmic cardiac death is the major cause of death, with an actuarial incidence of total mortality being ≈ 8% per year. Results of retrospective studies in which therapy was not randomized suggest that patients who receive ICD device systems have improved survival.[19] The most important determinant of outcome for patients who receive ICD systems is left ventricular function, with severe left ventricular dysfunction associated with earlier mortality.[20] Another important determinant of patient outcome is frequent or multiple defibrillator discharges, which are also associated with earlier mortality.[21]

The major complications of ICD therapy are perioperative mortality, infection, and lead problems requiring revision. The incidence of perioperative mortality for patients who receive epicardial patches and require a thoracotomy procedure was ≈ 3% to 5%.[12-16] The incidence has been substantially reduced with the introduction of transvenous lead systems, ranging from 0.5% to 1.0%.[6] However, the avoidance of major surgery has not resulted in an improvement in the long-term incidence of infection, which remains at 2% to 3%. The occurrence of systemic infection is devastating, in that it almost always requires removal of the ICD device and leads. The incidence of problems, including dislodgement, conductor fracture, or insulation discontinuities requiring surgical revision, ranges from 5% to 10% in long-term (3- to 5-year) follow-up. The prevalence has not diminished with the use of transvenous lead systems, even though only 1 to 3 leads are used for transvenous systems, compared with 3 or 4 for epicardial systems. This is probably because transvenous leads are more likely to dislodge and because lead injury may occur at the site of subclavian insertion. Lead continuity should be assessed regularly in all patients, and the incidence of very late complications has not yet been well characterized.

Future of ICD Therapy

In the near future, technological advances for ICD devices will have the primary goal of reducing pulse generator size. The components that compose the bulk of the volume are the capacitors and batteries. Lowering capacitance would result in smaller capacitor size, and it appears that the standard of 120 to 150 μF can be decreased to 85 to 95 μF without adversely affecting defibrillation efficacy. The battery size can be reduced by improving the efficiency of components and thereby lowering power consumption. However, one must be aware that battery size will probably be reduced substantially only through shortening of battery life or reduction in the maximum output of the device. Technological improvements allowing a change in the shape of the capacitors or batteries could also lead to more efficient space utilization within the pulse generator can. New features likely to become available in the future include the incorporation of DDD pacing and perhaps atrial defibrillation.

References

1. Mirowski M, Mower MM, Staewen WS, et al. Standby automatic defibrillator: an approach to prevention of sudden coronary death. *Arch Intern Med.* 1970;126:158–161.
2. Mirowski M, Mower MM, Langer A, et al. A chronically implanted system for automatic defibrillation in active conscious dogs. *Circulation.* 1978;58:90–94.
3. Mirowski M. The automatic implantable cardioverter-defibrillator: an overview. *J Am Coll Cardiol.* 1985;6:461–466.
4. Fain ES, Sweeney MB, Franz MR. Improved internal defibrillation efficacy with a biphasic waveform. *Am Heart J.* 1989;117:358–364.
5. Winkle RA, Mead RH, Ruder MA, et al. Improved low energy defibrillation efficacy in man with the use of a biphasic truncated exponential waveform. *Am Heart J.* 1989;117:122–127.
6. Brooks R, Garan H, Torchiana D, et al. Determinants of successful nonthoracotomy cardioverter-defibrillator implantation: experience in 101 patients using two different lead systems. *J Am Coll Cardiol.* 1993; 22:1835–1842.
7. Bardy GH, Dolack GL, Kudenchuk PJ, et al. Prospective, randomized comparison in humans of a unipolar defibrillation system with that using an additional superior vena cava electrode. *Circulation.* 1994;89: 1090–1093.
8. Saksena S, DeGroot P, Krol RB, et al. Low-energy endocardial defibrillation using an axillary or a pectoral thoracic electrode location. *Circulation.* 1993;88:2655–2660.
9. Marchlinski FE, Callans DJ, Gottlieb CD, et al. Benefits and lessons learned from stored electrogram information in implantable defibrillators. *J Cardiovasc Electrophysiol.* 1995;6:832–851.
10. Lehmann MH, Saksena S. Implantable cardioverter defibrillators in cardiovascular practice: report of the policy conference of the North American Society of Pacing and Electrophysiology. *PACE.* 1991;14:969–979.
11. Dreifus LS, Fisch C, Griffin JC, et al. Guidelines for implantation of cardiac pacemakers and antiarrhythmia devices. *J Am Coll Cardiol.* 1991;18:1–13.
12. Winkle RA, Mead RH, Ruder MA, et al. Long-term outcome with the automatic implantable cardioverter defibrillator. *J Am Coll Cardiol.* 1989;13:1353–1361.
13. Kelly PA, Cannom DS, Garan H, et al. The automatic implantable cardioverter defibrillator: efficacy, complications and survival in patients with malignant ventricular arrhythmias. *J Am Coll Cardiol.* 1988; 11:1278–1286.
14. Grimm W, Flores BT, Marchlinski FE. Shock occurrence and survival in 241 patients with implantable cardioverter-defibrillator therapy. *Circulation.* 1993;87:1880–1888.

15. Fromer M, Brachmann J, Block M, et al. Efficacy of automatic multi-modal device therapy for ventricular tachyarrhythmias as delivered by a new implantable pacing cardioverter-defibrillator. *Circulation.* 1992;86:363–374.

16. Neuzner J. Clinical experience with a new cardioverter defibrillator capable of biphasic waveform pulse and enhanced data storage: results of a prospective multicenter study. *PACE.* 1994;17: 1243–1255.

17. Strickberger SA, Hummel JD, Daoud E, et al. Implantation by electrophysiologists of 100 consecutive cardioverter defibrillators with nonthoracotomy lead systems. *Circulation.* 1994;90:868–872.

18. Tung RT, Bajaj AK. Safety of implantation of a cardioverter-defibrillator without general anesthesia in an electrophysiology laboratory. *Am J Cardiol.* 1995;75:908–912.

19. Newman D, Sauve MJ, Herre J, et al. Survival after implantation of the cardioverter defibrillator. *Am J Cardiol.* 1992;69:899–903.

20. Kim SG, Fischer JD, Choue CW, et al. Influence of left ventricular function on outcome of patients treated with implantable defibrillators. *Circulation.* 1992;85:1304–1310.

21. Villacastin J, Almendral J, Arenal A, et al. Incidence and clinical significance of multiple consecutive, appropriate, high-energy discharges in patients with implanted cardioverter-defibrillators. *Circulation.* 1996;93:753–762.

Chapter 13

Prospects for Gene Therapy of Sudden Cardiac Death:
The Inherited Long-QT Syndrome as a Model

G. Michael Vincent, MD

Introduction

Sudden death due to cardiac disease remains a major health-care issue in the United States, with more than 400 000 deaths occurring each year. The majority of these deaths are due to ventricular tachyarrhythmias, including ventricular fibrillation, tachycardia, and torsade de pointes. This discussion will explore the possibility that the exciting new concepts of gene therapy can be applied to causes of sudden cardiac death.

Gene therapy might be a therapeutic option for some of the conditions associated with sudden death through one of two mechanisms. The first would be by prevention or amelioration of an underlying disease, such as coronary artery disease or hypertrophic cardiomyopathy, whose consequences lead to sudden death. For example, in coronary artery disease, a clinical trial of gene therapy of familial hypercholesteremia is under way, with the expectation that this intervention will reduce the development of atherosclerotic deposits; another approach might use gene therapy to alter the vascular endothelial or smooth muscle cell responses to atherogenic or traumatic stimuli, decreasing atherosclerosis and restenosis.[1] The second mechanism would be through a direct effect on cardiac electrophysiology, altering the basic pathophysiology responsible for the arrhythmia and the sudden death. The inherited long-QT syndrome is the leading model in which to consider this approach. Once the de-

From: Dunbar SB, Ellenbogen KA, Epstein AE, (eds). *Sudden Cardiac Death: Past, Present, and Future.* Armonk, NY: Futura Publishing Company, Inc.; © 1997.

tails of genetic modification of electrophysiology are worked out in this model, the principles might be applied not only to the long-QT syndrome but also to other conditions associated with abnormal electrophysiology and vulnerability to sudden death. Before we discuss the possibilities of gene therapy, a brief introduction to the long-QT syndrome will be useful to understand its clinical manifestations, pathophysiology, and current treatment options; then the discussion of the potential benefits of gene therapy will be more meaningful.

Background and Epidemiology

Historically, the long-QT syndrome has been recognized to have two variants, based on genetic transmission of the disorder. An autosomal recessive form was described in 1957 in a Norwegian family.[2] Four of six children had recurrent "fainting attacks," with sudden death occurring in three of the affected children. They had marked QT prolongation of the electrocardiogram (ECG), unusual T waves, and congenital deafness. Figure 1 shows a representative

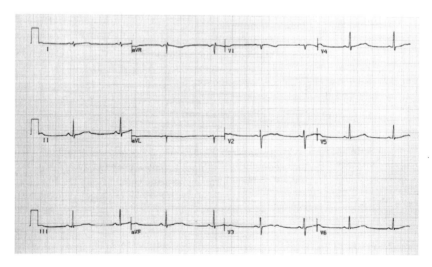

FIGURE 1. *Electrocardiogram from a 22-year-old woman with chromosome 7–linked long-QT syndrome and a history of emotion- and exercise-induced syncope. She was on β-blocker medication at the time the ECG was taken. Note bifid T waves, particularly evident in inferior and lateral precordial leads. Note, too, that the two components look more like a T-U complex in V_2 and V_3, emphasizing the importance of examining all leads before deciding whether a wave is a bifid T or a T-U complex. QT=0.54 seconds, and QT_c=0.49 seconds.*

ECG. Subsequent reports confirmed the condition and the autosomal recessive transmission of the gene.[3-7] This form of the syndrome is rare, and little is known about the molecular genetics. No disease gene has been identified, nor has linkage of the syndrome to any chromosome been found. An autosomal dominant form was described by Romano et al[8] in Italy in 1963 and Ward[9] in Ireland in 1964. Those affected with this form have normal hearing, but otherwise the two forms have appeared to be generally similar. A number of additional reports[10-17] and several reviews of the syndrome[18-20] followed not long after the original reports and can be consulted for additional details. In contrast to the recessive form, which appears to be quite rare, current estimates are that the dominant form may have a frequency of 1 in 5000 to 10 000 persons in the United States. It is being identified with increasing frequency as a cause of unexpected sudden death in children and young adults and may cause as many as 3000 to 4000 sudden deaths in children per year. Because little is known about the molecular genetics and specific pathophysiology of the recessive form, this discussion will focus on the autosomal dominant variant, but as the gene(s) for the recessive form are identified, the concepts presented for gene therapy will probably be applicable to this variant as well.

Symptoms

The principal symptom is episodic syncope due to torsade de pointes ventricular tachyarrhythmia (Figure 2). Syncope usually first appears in adolescence, although symptoms may occur from the first days of life up to 30 to 40 years of age. The syncopal episodes often terminate in sudden death, and in $\approx$40% of patients who die, death occurs with the first or second syncopal spell.[21] In many patients, the torsade de pointes arrhythmia spontaneously reverts to sinus rhythm, and the patients regain consciousness, often without sequelae. Some patients have many, even hundreds, of syncopal spells; others, only a few. In general, the syncope decreases in frequency with increasing age. Curiously, about one third of affected persons never have syncope and lead a normal life with usual longevity.[21] With our current knowledge, it is not possible to distinguish with any confidence which course a given patient will take. Thus, affected children and young persons should be treated once diagnosis is made even if they are asymptomatic, and this concept has considerable importance for gene therapy, with which a cure may be possible.

Most often, the syncope is precipitated by physical and emotional stress. Running, swimming, competitive sports, sudden loud noises, anger, and fright are commonly reported precipitating

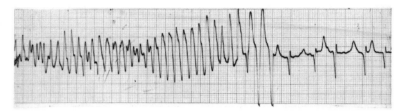

FIGURE 2. *A lead II strip during onset of torsade de pointes.*

events. In some patients, sudden death occurs during sleep, but syncope or sudden death while awake and at rest is uncommon. There is phenotypic heterogeneity among families,[22,23] and recent genotype-phenotype correlation studies have demonstrated differences in the duration of the QT interval, T-wave morphology, the types of precipitating factors, and the frequency of syncope and sudden death among the several genotypes.[23–25]

Diagnosis

The diagnosis may be simple in a patient with a clearly prolonged QT_c interval, for example, ≥0.50 second, as in Figure 1 and exercise-induced syncope or documented torsade de pointes. Unfortunately, even under these circumstances the diagnosis is often missed, resulting in a tragic death of a young person. In many other patients, the diagnosis is more difficult. Approximately 10% of patients have a normal QT_c interval on the presenting ECG (Figure 3). Further, ≈40% of patients have normal to mildly prolonged QT_c intervals that overlap those of normal subjects and are thus difficult to interpret and often overlooked.[21] To aid in the proper identification of patients in this category, a diagnostic scoring system has been developed that includes patient and family history plus several ECG abnormalities in addition to the QT interval.[26] In the future, as additional genes and mutations are identified, genetic testing will become the gold standard for diagnosis and will allow rapid and more precise diagnosis of patients, including those with a normal QT interval and other variations that currently often escape detection.

Pathophysiology

The pathophysiology is not yet completely defined. It has been presumed that cardiac action potential duration is increased, but the

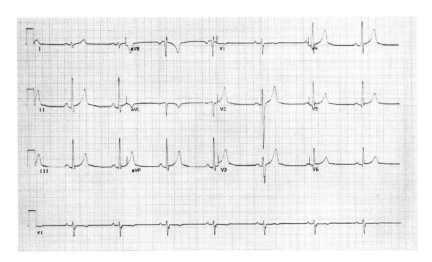

FIGURE 3. *Electrocardiogram from a 17-year-old boy with chromosome 11–linked long-QT syndrome. In this example, the QT interval is normal and the T waveform is normal. QT=0.42 seconds, and QT$_c$=0.41 seconds. ST elevation in leads V$_1$ through V$_4$ is early repolarization, a normal variant, and is not associated with the long-QT syndrome.*

few intracardiac monophasic action potential (MAP) recordings made have demonstrated only modest prolongation of MAP durations, certainly not as prolonged as the QT interval on the surface ECG.[27-29] Although this could be due to a sampling error, the results suggest that other events contribute to the QT lengthening. The surface ECG often shows bifid T waves consistent with two repolarization events, although markedly disparate action potential durations might cause the same surface T-wave pattern. If two separate events are responsible, a proposal is that the first component is due to the action potentials and the second component is due to early afterdepolarizations. Exercise studies support this concept in that the second component of the T wave usually increases considerably during exercise, whereas the first component remains smaller, consistent with the idea that these two components are due to different physiological events. Further, MAP recordings from a few patients show events consistent with early afterdepolarizations,[27-29] and these deflections increase in amplitude during adrenergic stimulation similar to the terminal T-wave increase seen during exercise. The mechanism of the torsade de pointes is thought to be due to early afterdepolarizations[30,31] but will be further defined as the molecular genetics and molecular pathophysiology of the syndrome are further unraveled.

Molecular Genetics of the Syndrome

It appears that mutations of at least five genes can cause the inherited long-QT syndrome. Keating and colleagues[32] provided the breakthrough in the molecular genetics of the syndrome in 1991 by finding linkage of the autosomal dominant long-QT phenotype with the Harvey-*ras*-1 gene locus on chromosome 11p15.5 in a large Utah family of Danish origin.[19,33] Later that year, Keating's group identified H-*ras*-1 linkage in additional families.[34] Although it was therefore initially thought that H-*ras* was the long-QT syndrome gene, Towbin in 1992[35] reported families that did not link to H-*ras*-1, showing genetic heterogeneity, and subsequently other families without H-*ras*-1 linkage were reported.[36–40] In 1994, Jiang et al[41] reported additional linkage results, to chromosome 7q35-36 (*LQT2*) in nine families and to chromosome 3p21-24 (*LQT3*) in three families, all of Northern European origin, and in 1995 Schott et al[42] presented evidence of linkage at chromosome 4q25-27 (*LQT4*) in a French family. Four gene loci have thus been identified: *LQT1* on chromosome 11, *LQT2* on chromosome 7, *LQT3* on chromosome 3, and *LQT4* on chromosome 4, numbered in the order of discovery of the chromosome locus. Along the way, the H-*ras*-1 gene was excluded as the chromosome 11 disease gene.[41,43,44] Further, Jiang et al[41] discovered three families with no linkage to the four known loci, indicating that at least one other gene locus must exist.

Keating's laboratory has now identified three of the disease genes and a number of mutations in each gene (Table 1). Thus, the molecular genetics discoveries are occurring at a furious pace. Brief descriptions of the known disease genes are provided to further our understanding of the molecular pathophysiology.

LQT1 is KVLQT1

KVLQT1, described in January 1996,[45] is a novel potassium channel gene. It appears to be the most common of the *LQT* genes, present in >50% of the patients genotyped thus far.[45] Because it was so recently discovered, studies on the molecular physiology of the potassium ion channel it encodes have not been reported. However, on the basis of its suspected topology, it is thought to be a voltage-gated potassium channel involved in cardiac repolarization, with the mutations resulting in altered channel function and reduced rectifying properties.

TABLE 1

The Inherited Long-QT Syndrome:
Summary of Currently Known Mutations

Coding effect	Nucleotide Δ	Mutation
KVLQT1		
Deletion	ΔTCG	A49P
Missense	GCG to CCC	G60R
Missense	GGG to AGG	R61Q
Missense	GTG to ATG	V125M
Missense	CTC to TTC	L144F
Missense	GGG to AGG	G177R
Missense	ACC to ATC	T183I
Missense	GCG to GAG	A212E
Missense	GCG to GTG	A212V
Missense	GGG to GAG	G216E
HERG		
Deletion	Δ1261	Δ1261
Deletion	Δ27 base pair*	Δ1500-F508
Missense	GCG to GTG	A561V
Missense	AAC to GAC	N470D
Missense	GGC to AGC	G628S
SCN5A		
Deletion	ΔAGAAGCCCC	ΔK1505-Q1507
Missense	CGC to CAC	R1644H
Missense	AAT to AGT	N1325S

*The 27-base-pair deletion=ΔCATCGACATGGTGGCCGCCCATCCCCTT.

LQT2 is HERG

HERG (human ether-à-go-go–related gene) encodes a major subunit of the rapidly activating cardiac delayed rectifier I_{Kr} current, a voltage-gated potassium channel.[46] The physiology of I_{Kr} has been extensively studied.[47–49] A number of drugs that cause acquired long-QT syndrome do so by block of this current.[50] Unlike most other potassium currents, I_{Kr} current increases when intracellular potassium is increased,[51,52] suggesting that elevation of the extracellular potassium in *LQT2* patients may be a therapeutic option. Conversely, lowered extracellular potassium probably potentiates the I_{Kr} abnormality in these patients, similar to the enhancement of drug block of I_{Kr} by hypokalemia.[53] The recognition that I_{Kr} is encoded by a long-QT syndrome disease gene and is also responsible for many cases of acquired long-QT syndrome raises the possibility that patients with acquired long-QT syndrome might have mutations of *HERG* and mild, subclinical impairment of I_{Kr} function that predisposes them to the adverse effects of pharmacological block of this channel. Preliminary genotyping of patients with acquired long-QT syndrome has not demonstrated any of the known genotypes, however.[54] This does not exclude an underlying genetic predisposition in acquired long-QT syndrome patients. They may have a different gene, particularly one that produces a lesser degree of channel impairment than those causing classic inherited long-QT syndrome and that becomes evident only upon further block of the channel when exposed to drugs.

LQT3 is SCN5A

The *SCN5A* gene encodes for the α-subunit of the cardiac sodium channel.[45,55–57] The mutations in *SCN5A* are in a region thought to be important for channel inactivation; thus, it is proposed that the *SCN5A* mutations cause long-QT syndrome through delay in the sodium channel inactivation, resulting in prolonged inward current and, therefore, a prolonged action potential duration, with resultant electrophysiological disturbances such as early afterdepolarization.

A recent extensive review of the known and proposed molecular physiology of the syndrome is recommended to the reader who desires more detailed information.[58]

Genetic Heterogeneity and Treatment Strategies

The discovery of different genotypes has potential implications for treatment strategies. β-Blocker therapy has been quite effective in the majority of long-QT syndrome patients, but the identification of the *SCN5A* sodium channel gene as a cause of the syndrome in some families raised the possibility that a sodium channel blocking drug might be effective therapy. In a pilot study, the effect of mexilitine was compared in patients with the sodium channel *SCN5A* gene (*LQT3*) and in those with the potassium channel *HERG* gene (*LQT2*).[25] The *SCN5A* patients showed a significant shortening of the QT interval, whereas no change was observed in the *HERG* patients, suggesting that the sodium channel blocker drugs may be effective in treating patients with the *SCN5A* genotype. The identification of the two potassium channel genes *HERG* and *KVLQT1* suggests that potassium channel opener drugs might be effective in these genotypes. A report on a single patient of unknown genotype treated with the potassium channel opener drug nicorandil showed shortening of the QT interval, decreased early afterdepolarizations on monophasic action potential recordings, and disappearance of syncope. In addition, the observation that the *HERG* protein function is improved by increased concentration of extracellular potassium[51] suggests that interventions that increase serum potassium in *HERG* gene carriers might be of therapeutic value. Further studies will be necessary to demonstrate the therapeutic efficacy of these pharmacological approaches and to determine whether sodium channel blockers and potassium channel openers are more efficacious than β-blocker therapy or whether these drugs in combination with β-blockers are superior to single-agent treatment.

Prospects for Gene Therapy

Gene therapy is an exciting technology, still in its infancy, and is largely hypothetical as a treatment modality. Many questions remain regarding the mechanics, safety, and efficacy of this approach. This discussion is presented from the perspective of a clinical cardiologist, and the reader is referred to additional sources for more in-depth information and the technical details of gene therapy.[59-62] Although applications of gene therapy are quite new, more than 140 gene therapy protocols are already under way worldwide. It is too early for any long-term successful results to have been reported, but some failures have been identified,[63,64] not particularly surprising or discouraging given the very rudimentary approaches that currently exist. Thus, although there is ample reason for optimism regarding the enormous prospects for this therapy, a careful and cautious approach is warranted.[65]

As currently proposed for the clinical setting, gene therapy is the introduction of new genetic material (DNA) into somatic cells of a host to cause synthesis of missing or defective proteins, the gene products. The goal is to produce a stable, long-term expression of the gene product with little or no toxicity. The new genetic material can modify the host's existing gene structure in three general ways: augmentation, replacement, and correction. Augmentation is the method currently used; it consists of inserting new genetic material into the host in addition to the existing host genome, such that the new material works independently to produce new proteins, thereby augmenting the existing host function. Gene replacement and correction refer to the process of removing abnormal sequences of the defective gene and replacing those sequences with a normal sequence, thus restoring normal function to the existing gene. Gene replacement and correction are technically challenging concepts for the future, as is the possibility of incorporating new genetic material into germ cells, which would allow transmission to offspring.

The complex process of gene therapy may be broken down into six steps (Table 2). The first step is to define the physiological abnormality to be corrected. The second step is to identify the abnormal protein involved, and the third, to identify and characterize the gene that encodes this protein. These are major steps and are incomplete in most genetic disorders. With respect to sudden cardiac death, the model of the long-QT syndrome best fulfills the criteria at the present time. In the long-QT syndrome, the physiological derangements are the abnormalities of cardiac repolarization, including prolonged action potential duration, disparity of ventricular recovery, propensity to develop early afterdepolarizations, and vulnerability to torsade de pointes ventricular tachyarrhythmia and ventricular fibrillation; the abnormal proteins, the ion channel proteins, are known and are being characterized; and the genes involved, the *KVLQT1, HERG,* and *SCN5A* genes, have been identified. Thus, major progress has been made on the first three steps toward gene therapy, and at least for patients with the three known genes, the long-QT syndrome becomes a possible candidate disease for gene therapy.

Once these first steps have been accomplished, the process of genetic manipulation, step 4, can begin, which prepares the gene of interest for use. The sequence of events in this process is shown in a simple schematic in Figure 4. The DNA containing the gene of interest is removed from the cell by cell lysis and digestion in prepa-

---

TABLE 2

Steps in Gene Therapy

1. Recognize the physiological abnormality
2. Identify the missing or defective protein
3. Identify the gene that encodes for the missing or defective protein
4. Insert the desired gene into a vector, producing a recombinant DNA
5. Transfer the new recombinant DNA, via the vector, into the host
6. Monitor the effect of the therapy

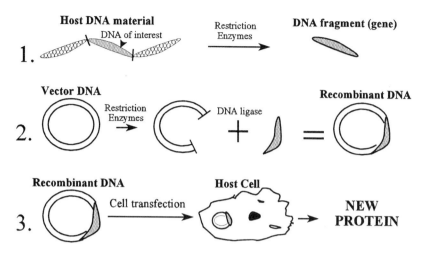

FIGURE 4. *Steps in genetic manipulation. Step 1 involves isolation of the gene of interest, step 2 the incorporation of the gene into a vector, and step 3 the introduction of the recombinant DNA into the host. See text for details.*

ration for the gene of interest to be isolated from the extracted DNA. The isolation is performed with restriction endonucleases, enzymes that cleave the DNA material into fragments by cutting the DNA at specific base-pair sequence sites. Gel electrophoresis is then used to separate the fragments on the basis of the fragment size, and the DNA fragment of interest, the gene of interest, can be isolated and recovered (Figure 4, top). The isolated gene must then be prepared to be inserted into the host. For human in vivo use, this usually involves inserting the DNA fragment into a vector, which is DNA containing a replication initiating sequence, or replicon (Figure 4, middle). To do this, the vector DNA is opened with a restriction enzyme, and the gene of interest is inserted into the open area by use of DNA ligase, producing a recombinant DNA molecule, and this recombinant DNA can replicate in the host cell. The next step is to incorporate or transfer the recombinant DNA into the host cells by some technique. Several methods exist, including chemical methods using calcium phosphate, DEAE-dextran, and liposome delivery systems, as well as physical incorporation by electroporation, but these tools are not necessarily applicable to in vivo transfer, cell access may be quite limited, or they are not cell selective.[59,62] In the current human trials, viruses and plasmids are the most frequently used vectors, with retroviruses being the most common, followed by adenoviruses. There are several concerns regarding the use of recombinant viral vectors. During preparation of the recombinant DNA, the viral DNA sequence responsible for viral replication must be removed, producing a replication-deficient virus; otherwise, the active virus would be transferred into the host, producing the viral disease. Even though this step is taken, there may be some possibility of an active virus emerging. Another concern is the possibility of mutagenesis and development of oncogenes due to the random insertion into the genome of new genetic material. Also, the adenovirus vectors may elicit powerful cytotoxic effects that limit the duration of expression of the gene product and humoral immune responses that preclude the repeated administration of these recombinant vectors.[62,63]

A number of questions remain to be answered before gene therapy can be applied to long-QT syndrome patients. The first question might be which vector to use. The retrovirus vector acts by incorporating its DNA into the host cell genome, and thus the gene of interest is propagated during cell division, allowing for gene expression over an extended period of time. However, target cell replication is necessary for the initial incorporation of viral DNA into the target cell genome. This may pose a significant problem for transfecting the cardiac myocyte, since it is generally thought that the cardiac myocyte does not replicate. In contrast to the retrovirus, the adenovirus does not require host cell replication for gene expression, because the adenovirus efficiently infects nondividing cells and can express large amounts of the gene product. Because the adenovirus DNA is not incorporated into the host cell genome, the recombinant DNA is lost during cell division and the duration of gene expression is short when the target host cells are rapidly dividing. This is not a problem in cardiac cells, of course, because they do not divide. The problem, then, with adenoviral vectors is how to efficiently infect a large number of cardiac myocytes to produce adequate levels of the gene product (the ion channel proteins) and how to limit or prevent the cytotoxic and immune responses mentioned above. Plasmid vectors do not require host cell replication, either, and do not induce the cytotoxic and immune responses of the adenovirus; thus, they may be useful for cardiac myocyte gene transfer. Once the appropriate vector is chosen, the recombinant DNA must be introduced into the host.

There are two strategies for introducing recombinant DNA into the somatic host cells. First, target cells can be removed from the host and cultured, and the new gene can be introduced into the cells in vitro. The genetically modified cells are then returned to the host. As already noted, in the long-QT syndrome the target host cell is the cardiac myocyte. Myocytes probably could be acquired by endocardial biopsy, although the tools for acquiring and culturing healthy myocytes by this technique are at present somewhat limited. The second strategy for delivery involves direct in vivo transfer of the recombinant DNA to the host cells. In either case, the route of administration of the recombinant DNA to transfect the cardiac myocyte is uncertain. Nonselective routes of administration, such as intravenous, subcutaneous, and intranasal sites, are unlikely to lead to selective transfection of cardiac myocytes unless the introduced vector can be designed to have high specificity for the myocyte, perhaps by some form of immunological targeting. However, some cardiac transfer, even though not specific, might be achieved by these means. In a mouse model, intravenous injection of recombinant adenoviral *Escherichia coli* β-galactosidase produced widespread transfer in both cardiac and skeletal muscle and expression of the enzyme over a 12-month period.[66] In another approach, animal studies of direct mechanical injection of recombinant DNA into cardiac or skeletal muscle have shown some expression of the gene.[67-70] Although this probably could be accomplished by catheter techniques in vivo, the ability to transfer the DNA to a large enough number of cardiac myocytes to correct the defect is questionable. Further, as is often the case, the animal model studies may not predict success in humans. Several clinical trials of direct injection of myoblasts into the skeletal muscle of patients with Duchenne dystrophy have been performed in an attempt to cause production of dystrophin, the protein that is deficient in Duchenne dystrophy.[71-73] These trials all failed to show improvement in muscle strength and showed only occasional and low-level expression of dystrophin. Technical advances may improve the results of the direct injection technique, but it may be of limited value for treatment of cardiac disease.

Since we do not know with certainty whether transfer into the cardiac myoctye is necessary for gene therapy of the syndrome, an interesting possibility is that the gene product might be expressed in some other tissue, such as the coronary artery, yet still have a beneficial effect on myocyte ion channel function, particularly if high levels of the expressed protein could be achieved. A number of animal studies have demonstrated the ability to transfer recombinant DNA into vascular endothelial or smooth muscle cells in vivo, including coronary and peripheral vessels, and at least transient expression of the gene product has been observed.[74-78] Whether transfer of recombinant ion channel gene DNA into endothelial cells of the coronary arteries, for example, would correct the physiological abnormalities of the long-QT syndrome is an interesting question. There is no real animal model of inherited long-QT syndrome in which to test these treatment strategies, although an animal model using pharmacological blockade of the channel of interest may provide some insight into the efficacy of myocyte or endothelial cell gene transfer. The transgenic animal model is a very expensive and complex model, but it could also be used for these studies.

Gene therapy is in the early stages of development and has enormous possible consequences for a wide variety of diseases, particularly single-gene disorders. Its application to cardiac diseases, including those associated with sudden death, is hypothetical at present, but long-QT syndrome may be an appropriate model for studies of gene therapy of the physiological disturbances associated with sudden cardiac death. We can expect an exciting, vigorous, and probably bumpy journey over the next few years as gene therapy trials are expanded and we move into this remarkable new phase of treatment for cardiac diseases.

References

1. Rowland RT, Cleveland JC, Meng X, Harken AH, Brown JM. Potential gene therapy strategies in the treatment of cardiovascular disease. *Ann Thorac Surg.* 1995;60:721–728.
2. Jervell A, Lange-Nielsen F. Congenital deaf mutism, functional heart disease with prolongation of the Q-T interval and sudden death. *Am Heart J.* 1957;54:59.
3. Levine S, Woodworth C. Congenital deaf mutism, prolonged Q-T interval, syncopal attacks and sudden death. *N Engl J Med.* 1958;259:412.
4. Fraser GR, Froggatt P, Murphy T. Genetical aspects of the cardio-auditory syndrome of Jervell and Lange-Nielsen (congential deafness and electrocardiographic abnormalities). *Ann Hum Genet.* 1964;28:133–150.
5. Frazer GR, Froggatt P, James TN. Congenital deafness associated with electrocardiographic abnormalities, fainting spells and sudden death: a recessive syndrome. *Q J Med.* 1964;33:361–385.
6. Barlow J, Bosman C, Cochrane J. Congenital cardiac arrhythmia. *Lancet.* 1964;2:531.
7. Jervell A, Thingstad R, Endsjot TO. The Surdo-cardiac syndrome. *Am Heart J.* 1966;72:582–593.
8. Romano C, Genrme G, Pongiglione R. Aritmie cardiache rare dell'eta pediatrica, II: assessi sincopali per fibrillozione ventricolare parossistics. (Presentazione del primo case della letteratura pediatrica italiana.) *Clin Pediatr.* 1963;45–656.
9. Ward O. A new familial cardiac syndrome in children. *J Ir Med Assoc.* 1964;54:103.
10. Gamstorp I, Nilsen R, Westling H. Congenital cardiac arrhythmia. *Lancet.* 1964;2:965.
11. Ward O. The electrocardiographic abnormality in familial cardiac arrhythmia. *Ir J Med Sci.* 1966;6:553.

12. Garza L, McNamara D, Nora J, et al. Familial repolarization myocardiopathy. *Am J Cardiol.* 1969;23:112.
13. Garza LA, Vick RL, Nora JJ, et al. Heritable Q-T prolongation without deafness. *Circulation.* 1970;41:39.
14. Gale GE, Bosman CK, Tucker RBK, et al. Hereditary prolongation of the Q-T interval (study of 2 families). *Br Heart J.* 1970;32:505.
15. Phillips J, Ichinose H. Clinical and pathologic studies in the hereditary syndrome of a long Q-T interval, syncopal spells and sudden death. *Chest.* 1970;58:236.
16. Lipp H, Pitt A, Anderson ST, et al. Recurrent ventricular tachyarrhythmias in a patient with a prolonged Q-T interval. *Med J Aust.* 1970; 1:1296.
17. Karhunen P, Luomanmaki K, Heikkila J, et al. Syncope and Q-T prolongation without deafness: the Romano-Ward syndrome. *Am Heart J.* 1970;80:820.
18. Jervell A, Sivertssen E. Surdo-cardiac syndrome. *Nord Med.* 1967;78: 1433–1450.
19. Vincent GM, Abildskov JA, Burgess MJ. QT interval syndromes. *Prog Cardiovasc Dis.* 1974;16:523–530.
20. Schwartz PJ, Periti M, Malliani A. The long QT syndrome. *Am Heart J.* 1975;89:378–390.
21. Vincent GM, Timothy K, Leppert M, Keating M. The spectrum of symptoms and QT interval in carriers of the gene for the long-QT syndrome. *N Engl J Med.* 1992;327:846–852.
22. Dean JC, Cross S, Jennings K. Evidence of genetic and phenotypic heterogeneity in the Romano-Ward syndrome. *J Med Genet.* 1993;30: 947–950.
23. Vincent GM. Heterogeneity in the inherited long QT syndrome: a review of genetic and clinical observations. *J Cardiovasc Electrophysiol.* 1995;6:137–146.
24. Moss AJ, Zareba W, Benhorin J, et al. Electrocardiographic T-wave patterns in genetically distinct forms of the hereditary long QT syndrome. *Circulation.* 1995;92:2929–2934.
25. Schwartz PJ, Priori SG, Locati EH, et al. Long QT syndrome patients with mutations of the *SCN5A* and *HERG* genes have differential responses to Na+ channel blockade and to increases in heart rate: implications for gene-specific therapy. *Circulation.* 1995;92:3381–3386.
26. Schwartz P, Moss AJ, Vincent GM, Crampton RS. Diagnostic criteria for the long QT syndrome: an update. *Circulation.* 1993;88:782–784.
27. Bonatti V, Rolli A, Botti G. Monophasic action potential studies in human subjects with prolonged ventricular repolarization and long QT syndromes. *Eur Heart J.* 1985;6:131–143.
28. Zhou JT, Zheng LR, Liu WY. Role of early afterdepolarization in familial long QTU syndrome and torsade de pointes. *PACE.* 1992;15:2164–2168.
29. Shimizu W, Ohe T, Kurita T, et al. Early afterdepolarization induced by isoproterenol in patients with congenital long QT syndrome. *Circulation.* 1991;84:1915–1923.
30. El-Sherif N. Early afterdepolarizations and arrhythmogenesis: experimental and clinical aspects. *Arch Mal Coeur Vaiss.* 1991;84:227–234.
31. Roden DM. Early afterdepolarizations and torsade de pointes: implications for the control of cardiac arrhythmias by prolonging repolarization. *Eur Heart J.* 1993;14:56–61.

32. Keating M, Atkinson D, Dunn C, Timothy K, Vincent GM, Leppert M. Linkage of a cardiac arrhythmia, the long QT syndrome, and the Harvey ras-1 gene. *Science.* 1991;252:704–706.
33. Vincent GM. Long-term follow-up of a family with Romano-Ward prolonged QT interval syndrome. In: Butrous GS, Schwartz PJ, eds. *Clinical Aspects of Ventricular Repolarization.* London, UK: Farrand Press; 1989:411–413.
34. Keating AM, Atkinson D, Dunn C, Timothy K, Vincent GM, Leppart M. Consistent linkage of the long QT syndrome to the Harvey ras-1 locus on chromosome 11. *Am J Hum Genet.* 1991;49:1335–1339.
35. Towbin JA, Pagotto L, Siu B, et al. Romano-Ward long QT syndrome (RWLQTS): evidence of genetic heterogeneity. *Pediatr Res.* 1992;31: 23A. Abstract.
36. Curran M, Atkinson D, Timothy K, et al. Locus heterogeneity of autosomal dominant long QT syndrome. *J Clin Invest.* 1993;92:799–803.
37. Benhorin J, Kalman YM, Medina A, et al. Evidence of genetic heterogeneity in the long QT syndrome. *Science.* 1993;260:1960–1962.
38. Akimoto K, Matsuoka R, Kasanuki H, Takao A, Hayakawa K, Hosoda S. Linkage analysis in a Japanese long QT syndrome family. *Kokyu To Junkan.* 1993;41:463–465.
39. Ko YL, Chen SA, Tang K, et al. No evidence for linkage of long QT syndrome and chromosome 11p15.5 markers in a Chinese family: evidence for genetic heterogeneity. *Hum Genet.* 1994;94:364–366.
40. Tanaka T, Nakahara K-i, Kato N, et al. Genetic linkage analyses of Romano-Ward syndrome (RWS) in 13 Japanese families. *Hum Genet.* 1994;94:380–384.
41. Jiang C, Atkinson D, Towbin JA, et al. Two long QT syndrome loci map to chromosome 3 and 7 and evidence for further heterogeneity. *Nat Genet.* 1994;8:141–147.
42. Schott JJ, Charpentier F, Peltier S, et al. Mapping of a gene for long QT syndrome to chromosome 4q25-27. *Am J Hum Genet.* 1995;57: 1114–1122.
43. Russell MW, Brody LC, Munroe D, Dick M II, Collins FS. Characterization of a recombination event excluding the Harvey-ras-1 (H-ras-1) locus in a Romano-Ward long QT syndrome family linked to chromosome 11p15 and isolation of a polymorphic repeat telomeric to H-ras-1. *Am J Hum Genet.* 1994;55:A353. Abstract.
44. Roy N, Kahlem P, Dausse E, et al. Exclusion of HRAS from long QT locus. *Nat Genet.* 1994;8:113–114.
45. Wang Q, Shen J, Splawski I, et al. SCN5a mutations associated with an inherited cardiac arrhythmia, long QT syndrome. *Cell.* 1995;80: 805–811.
46. Curran ME, Splawski I, Timothy KW, Vincent GM, Green ED, Keating MT. A molecular basis for cardiac arrhythmia: HERG mutations cause long QT syndrome. *Cell.* 1995;80:795–803.
47. Balser JR, Bennett PB, Roden DM. Time-dependent outward current in guinea pig ventricular myocytes: gating kinetics of the delayed rectifier. *J Gen Physiol.* 1990;96:835–863.
48. Sanguinetti MC, Jurkiewicz NK. Two components of cardiac delayed rectifier K^+ current: differential sensitivity to block by class III antiarrhythmic agents. *J Gen Physiol.* 1990;96:195–215.
49. Sanguinetti MC, Jurkiewicz NK. I_K is comprised of two components in guinea pig atrial cells. *Am J Physiol.* 1991;260:H393–H399.

50. Sanquinetti MC. Modulation of potassium channels by antiarrhythmic and antihypertensive drugs. *Hypertension.* 1992;19:228–236.
51. Sanquinetti MC, Jiang C, Curran ME, Keating MT. A mechanistic link between an inherited and an acquired cardiac arrhythmia: HERG encodes the I_{Kr} potassium channel. *Cell.* 1995;81:299–307.
52. Trudeau MC, Warmke JW, Ganetsky B, Robertson GA. HERG, a human inward rectifier in the voltage-gated potassium channel family. *Science.* 1995;269:92–95.
53. Yang T, Roden DM. Extracellular potassium modulation of drug block of I_{Kr}: Implications for torsades de pointes and reverse use-dependence. *Circulation.* In press.
54. Wei J, Wathen M, Murray K, Daw R, Roden D, George AL Jr. Absence of HERG and SCN5A mutations in acquired long QT syndrome. *Circulation.* 1995;92(suppl I):I-275. Abstract.
55. Wand Q, Shen J, Li Z, et al. Cardiac sodium channel mutations in patients with long QT syndrome, an inherited cardiac arrhythmia. *Hum Mol Genet.* 1995;9:1603–1607.
56. George AL Jr, Varkony TA, Drabkin HAK, et al. Assignment of the human heart tetrodotoxin-resistant voltage-gated Na^+ channel alpha-subunit gene (SCN5A) to band 3p21. *Cytogenet Cell Genet.* 1995;68:67–70.
57. Bennett PB, Yazawa K, Makita N, George AL Jr. Molecular mechanism for an inherited cardiac arrhythmia. *Nature.* 1995;376:683–685.
58. The SADS Foundation Task Force on LQTS. Multiple mechanisms in the long QT syndrome: current knowledge, gaps, and future directions. *Circulation.* In press.
59. Watt PC, Sawicki MP, Passaro E Jr. A review of gene transfer techniques. *Am J Surg.* 1993;165:350–354.
60. French BA. Gene transfer and cardiovascular disorders. *Herz.* 1993;18:222–229.
61. French BA, Swain JL. Gene transfer in the cardiovascular system. In: Roberts R, ed. *Molecular Basis of Cardiology.* Boston, Mass: Blackwell Scientific Publications; 1993:171–191.
62. Rowland RT, Cleveland JC Jr, Meng X, Harken A, Brown JM. Potential gene therapy strategies in the treatment of cardiovascular disease. *Ann Thorac Surg.* 1995;60:721–728.
63. Knowles MR, Hohneker K, Zhou Z, et al. A controlled study of adenoviral-vector-mediated gene-transfer in the nasal epithelium of patients with cystic fibrosis. *N Engl J Med.* 1995;333:823–831.
64. Mendell JR, Kissell JT, Amato AA, et al. Myoblast transfer in the treatment of Duchenne's muscular dystrophy. *N Engl J Med.* 1995;333:832–838.
65. Leiden JM. Gene therapy: promise, pitfalls, and prognosis. *N Engl J Med.* 1995;333:871–873.
66. Kitsis RN, Buttrick PM, McNally EM, Kaplan ML, Leinwand LA. Hormonal modulation of a gene injected into rat heart in vivo. *Proc Natl Acad Sci U S A.* 1991;88:4138–4142.
67. Stratford-Perricaudet LD, Makeh I, Perricaudet M, Briand P. Widespread long-term gene transfer to mouse skeletal muscles and heart. *J Clin Invest.* 1992;90:626–630.
68. Kirshenbaum LA, MacLellan WR, Mazur W, French BA, Schneider MD. Highly efficient gene transfer into adult ventricular myocytes by recombinant adenovirus. *J Clin Invest.* 1993;92:381–387.

69. Lin H, Parmacek MS, Morle G, Bolling S, Leiden JM. Expression of recombinant genes in myocardium in vivo after direct injection of DNA. *Circulation.* 1990;82:2217–2221.
70. Harsdorf R, Schott RJ, Shen YT, Vatner SF, Mahdavi V, Nadal-Ginard B. Gene injection into canine myocardium as a useful model for studying gene expression in the heart of large mammals. *Circ Res.* 1993;72: 688–695.
71. Law PK, Goodwin TG, Wang MG.Normal myoblast injections provide genetic treatment for murine dystrophy. *Muscle Nerve.* 1988;11: 525–533.
72. Partridge TA, Morgan JE, Coulton GR, Hoffmann EP, Kunkel LM. Conversion of mdx myofibers from dystrophin-negative to -positive by injection of normal myoblasts. *Nature.* 1989;337:176–179.
73. Karpati G, Pouliot Y, Zubrzycka-Gaarn E, et al. Dystrophin is expressed in mdx skeletal muscle fibers after normal myoblast implantation. *Am J Pathol.* 1989;135:27–32.
74. Wilson JM, Birinyi LK, Salomon RN, Libby P, Callow AD, Mulligan RC. Implantation of vascular grafts lined with genetically modified endothelial cells. *Science.* 1989;244:1344–1346.
75. Plautz G, Nabel EG, Nabel GJ. Introduction of vascular smooth muscle cells expressing recombinant genes in vivo. *Circulation.* 1991;83: 578–583.
76. Lemarchand P, Jones M, Yamada I, Crystal RG. In vivo gene transfer and expression in normal uninjured blood vessels using replication-deficient recombinant adenovirus vectors. *Circ Res.* 1993;72:1132–1138.
77. Lim CS, Chapman GD, Gammon RS, et al. Direct in vivo gene transfer into the coronary and peripheral vasculatures of the intact dog. *Circulation.* 1991;83:2007–2011.
78. Chapman GD, Lim CS, Gammon RS, et al. Gene transfer into coronary arteries of intact animals with a percutaneous balloon catheter. *Circ Res.* 1992;71:27–33.

Chapter 14

CPR Training for Families of Patients at High Risk for Sudden Death

Kathleen Dracup, RN, DNSc

Sudden cardiac death is a major public health problem. It is the most frequent cause of death in Western countries, with more than 500 000 deaths each year in the United States alone.[1] The American Heart Association, along with other organizations, has addressed this problem by developing programs to teach cardiopulmonary resuscitation (CPR) methods to individuals in the community and supporting the development of a quick emergency medical response system. As many as 50 million Americans have been trained to perform CPR, making mass CPR training one of the most successful recent public health initiatives.[2]

The hypothesis underlying the American Heart Association effort is that if every individual in the United States is trained to respond to a cardiac emergency appropriately and to initiate CPR, the time between an individual's collapse and the establishment of effective cardiopulmonary circulation will be significantly decreased. Shortening the time before CPR is begun after a cardiopulmonary arrest has been shown to be a critical determinant of survival, with prompt initiation of CPR resulting in significant increases in survival, improved cardiac function, and decreased neurological complications.[3-8]

Researchers have consistently documented the important role of bystanders in the early initiation of CPR. For example, in one retrospective study of 384 cardiac arrests, the investigators found that (1) arrest victims who received bystander CPR had a fourfold increase in ultimate survival compared with those who did not, (2) survival was independent of the adequacy of CPR as judged by the

From: Dunbar SB, Ellenbogen KA, Epstein AE, (eds). *Sudden Cardiac Death: Past, Present, and Future.* Armonk, NY: Futura Publishing Company, Inc.; © 1997.

paramedics who arrived on the scene, (3) bystander CPR was initiated in only 30% of the events, and (4) bystander CPR was least likely to have been initiated if the cardiac arrest occurred in the victim's home.[8] Rapid bystander CPR, combined with appropriate defibrillation· and pharamcological treatment by the emergency medical system, is a rational and effective approach to reducing mortality from sudden cardiac arrest.

However, clinicians and researchers have begun to question the wisdom of community-wide CPR instruction.[9] Hundreds of thousands of individuals are trained to perform CPR but will never be called upon to use it. Scarce resources might be better utilized if subgroups most likely to witness a sudden cardiac arrest were targeted for CPR training. Since three out of four sudden cardiac arrest events occur in the home in the presence of family members,[10] family members of patients at risk for sudden death may yield the greatest benefit from CPR instruction.

Although family members of patients with documented cardiac disease may be the most appropriate target for CPR training, researchers have shown that they are the least likely to attend a community CPR class.[10] Most participants are young, <20 years old, and become CPR certified as part of school or job requirements. For example, in one study of community CPR classes, only 5.6% of students were enrolled because they had a relative with cardiac disease.[11] In a second study, family members of 168 patients with documented coronary heart disease were compared with family members of 159 patients from a general medical clinic and 174 healthy control subjects. The lowest proportion of individuals who had taken a CPR course was in the cardiac family group.[12]

Despite the compelling logic of targeting family members for CPR training, most physicians do not refer the relatives of their patients to CPR classes. For example, in one study, 79% of physicians surveyed stated that CPR training for cardiac family members was important, but only 6% recommended it to the families in their practice.[13] Clinicians worry that family members may not be able to learn CPR, may use it inappropriately during an emergency, or may feel inappropriately burdened by the responsibility it entails.[14] These concerns could explain why health providers believe families should learn CPR but do not actually recommend it to the families in their practice. We have undertaken a series of studies to address the potential concerns of clinicians and policy makers that in the past have served as impediments to teaching CPR to family members of patients at high risk for sudden death.

CPR Learning Capabilities of Cardiac Family Members

We studied learning capabilities in 83 family members of patients at high risk for sudden death who received CPR training.[15] The CPR class was designed to address the special needs of family members by focusing on one-person CPR and keeping class size small (three to six per class) to allow for ample practice time. One-person CPR was taught because most family members lived alone with a cardiac patient as a marital dyad. The steps of CPR (assessment, ventilation, and compression) were divided into discrete segments to allow for return demonstration after each step, with a final demonstration at the end of the training session of the entire procedure.

Eighty-one percent (n=67) successfully learned CPR, as measured by the return demonstration at the end of the training class. Of the demographic and clinical characteristics studied, only sex ($P=0.03$), age ($P=0.004$), and depression (canonical discriminant function coefficient=0.98) were significant in explaining differences in family members' ability to learn CPR. The elderly, the depressed, and men were the most likely to be unsuccessful. These results suggest that most family members of adult cardiac patients can learn to perform CPR successfully in a classroom setting and that concerns about the ability of family members to learn CPR are unfounded.

In a second study of 31 patients,[16] we tested family member's retention of CPR knowledge and skills at 7 and 12 months after initial CPR training. Although knowledge levels remained relatively high even up to 1 year after training, skill retention tested in the home on a mannequin was disappointing. Like other students trained in CPR, the skills of family members degraded quickly and were improved only when family members used a practice packet mailed to the home to review the components of CPR between the time they had learned CPR and retesting.

Psychological Consequences of CPR Training for Families of High-Risk Cardiac Patients

One impediment to targeting family members for CPR training is a concern about the psychological effects of such training on both cardiac patients and their families. To identify these consequences, we conducted two prospective clinical trials.

Research on psychological control was used as the basis for designing the CPR training intervention for families of cardiac patients in both trials. According to this perspective, psychological control is defined as the belief that one has at one's disposal a response that can influence the aversiveness of an event.[17] The types of control relevant to this clinical population are behavioral, cognitive, and informational.[18] Behavioral control is the ability to undertake a specific, behavioral response that can reduce the aversiveness of a noxious event. Cognitive control involves having a cognitive strategy (such as focusing on the benefits of the noxious event or distracting oneself during the event) that can reduce the aversiveness of the noxious event. Informational control refers to a communication delivered to an individual who is a potential recipient of an aversive event concerning the onset, timing, or nature of that event. All three types of psychological control have been found to be effective in reducing the emotional and physiological distress that often accompanies noxious events.[19] We reasoned that providing family members of high-risk cardiac patients with information about the illness and a specific measure (ie, CPR) that could be undertaken in the event of a potential sudden death event constituted examples of informational and behavioral control.

Preliminary Study

Sixty-five patients considered to be at high risk for sudden cardiac death and 69 family members were enrolled. They have been characterized elsewhere.[20] Subjects were randomly assigned to one of two intervention groups or a control group. In the first intervention, which was designed to increase behavioral control, we taught family members CPR using the standard American Heart Association format for basic cardiac life support. The class was taught by a paramedic with Advanced Cardiac Life Support certification and emphasized one-person CPR. In the second intervention, which was designed to increase informational control, we reviewed key cardiac risk factors, taught family members how to recognize important symptoms of cardiac disease, and instructed them how to proceed in the event of a cardiac emergency. This class was taught by clinical nurse specialists and did not cover any information on CPR techniques. Patients were excluded from all intervention classes.

The dependent variables for this study were patient and family member anxiety, depression, and hostility (measured with the Multiple Affect Adjective Checklist[21,22]) and patient psychosocial adjustment to illness (measured by the Psychosocial Adjustment to Illness Scale[23]). The latter measures seven domains: health care orientation, vocational environment, domestic environment, sexual relations, extended family relationships, social environment, and psychological distress. Higher scores indicate higher levels of anxiety, depression, and hostility and poorer adjustment across all domains. The potential intervening effects of marital satisfaction and locus of control were tested with the Spanier Dyadic Adjustment Scale[24] and the Internal/External Locus of Control Scale.[25] Data were collected at baseline, 3 months, and 6 months. The intervention occurred within 24 hours of baseline data collection.

A comparison of the mean family scores at 3- and 6-month follow-up revealed no significant difference among the three groups. In the patient groups, significant differences were noted at 3 and 6 months (Table 1). At 3 months, patients whose family members learned CPR were significantly more anxious ($P<0.01$) than control group patients. Psychosocial adjustment to illness scores were significantly different at both 3 and 6 months. The control group reported increasingly improved adjustment over time, whereas the patients in both intervention groups remained at the same level of psychosocial distress as at study entry. The results were particularly striking given that patients were not present at the experimental sessions but were nonetheless strongly affected. Clearly, a family-mediated effect occurred to increase the anxiety and depression experienced by those patients whose family members learned CPR. Analyses of marital satisfaction and locus of control scores were not enlightening; no significant main effects or interactions were found for either family members or patients.

These findings were the opposite of what had been hypothesized. According to research on control, we expected that family members would experience a decrease in negative emotions and patients would feel reassured that someone in their home would know what to do in case of an emergency. On reflection, it seems that both CPR training and the risk factor education class provided information and specific skills about how to handle a cardiac emergency, but neither provided strategies to increase cognitive control (ie, cognitive mechanisms, such as distraction, to increase an individual's sense of control) or informational control about when the cardiac arrest could be predicted. Nor were the nursing interventions designed to address the emotional response of families to the rehearsal components of CPR training. Family members experienced increased anxiety and depression, feelings that were not resolved in the setting of the intervention and were communicated to the patients. CPR training seems to disrupt denial-based feelings of invulnerability in both the patient and the family member. It may also create interpersonal strain because of the heightened dependency the patient feels toward CPR-trained family members.

TABLE 1

Comparison of Anxiety, Depression, and Psychosocial Adjustment to Illness in Patient Groups by Analysis of Variance

	Control Group		CPR		Education		P
	n	Mean±SD	n	Mean±SD	n	Mean±SD	
Anxiety							
Baseline	24	6.5±4.9	22	6.7±4.2	19	5.4±4.5	0.65
3 mo	16	4.6±4.0	17	8.8±4.9*	14	6.4±5.2	0.05
6 mo	17	5.5±4.2	17	8.0±5.2	16	6.1±4.8	0.29
Depression							
Baseline	24	13.5±7.0	22	13.4±7.1	19	10.2±7.7	0.32
3 mo	16	9.9±6.0	17	15.6±8.3	14	10.0±8.0	0.05
6 mo	17	11.1±6.1	17	15.5±7.1	16	11.6±7.7	0.14
Psychosocial adjustment							
Baseline	24	31.0±19.7	22	41.4±17.0	19	32.9±15.3	0.17
6 mo	17	18.9±7.9	17	40.1±19.9†	16	32.3±21.2	0.007

Higher scores indicate increased anxiety and/or depression; lower scores indicate increased psychosocial adjustment.

*$P<0.01$. Significance levels refer to the comparison of each of the intervention groups with the control group by paired t tests.

†$P<0.001$.

Clinical Trial

If CPR is to be taught to families of cardiac patients, the intervention must be enhanced to reduce the deleterious psychological effects on the patient or family noted in our preliminary study. We hypothesized two additions to CPR training that might reduce its stressful psychological effects. First, CPR combined with didactic instruction about cardiac risk factors should enhance the sense of predictability, thereby increasing feelings of control in both patients and families. Second, CPR followed by a support group intervention should enhance the expression of feelings in the CPR-trained person, thereby reducing the stress associated with training. Specifically, the social support intervention was designed to reduce family members' anxiety about the occurrence of future cardiac emergencies and the frustration that they might experience in feeling responsible for the patient's well-being 24 hours a day.

Therefore, we conducted a randomized clinical trial comparing these two methods with the usual method of teaching CPR without such content.[26] The aim was to identify the psychological impact of various methods of CPR training for family members of patients at risk for a future cardiac arrest. We hypothesized that the most positive effects would be seen with CPR combined with social support and that the most negative effects would be seen with CPR-only training.

Four hundred fifty-three patient-family pairs were recruited from six large metropolitan area hospitals on the West Coast and randomized to one of three CPR intervention groups or to a control group. Seventy-four percent of the enrolled subjects (N=674, or 337 pairs) completed all instruments at baseline, 2 weeks after CPR training, at 3 months, and at 6 months. Data from these subjects were used in all analyses.

Patients and family members who completed the study were compared with those who dropped out on sociodemographic characteristics (ie, age, sex, marital status, race, work status, and education level) and baseline dependent variables. No differences were noted. Family members with incomplete data were significantly more anxious, more depressed, and younger (mean, 55 versus 59 years) than family members who completed all data collection ($P<0.05$). Finally, there were significant differences by family member occupational status; ie, a larger proportion of homemakers was seen in the incomplete data group and a larger proportion of retired persons was seen in the complete data group ($P<0.05$).

The majority (317, or 94%) of the 337 participating family members were spouses of the patients. The remaining 20 family members were adult children or live-in partners. On average, patients were middle-aged (mean age, 63 ± 10 years), male (84%), employed, white, and in New York Heart Association functional class I or II. Family members were predominantly middle-aged (mean age, 59 ± 11 years), female (83%), and white.

Protocol

All subjects in the three CPR intervention groups attended a single CPR training class of ≈90 minutes. Classes were attended by two to six family members at a time to ensure maximal individual attention and time for practice. All classes were taught by cardiovascular clinical nurse specialists certified by the American Heart Association as Basic Life Support instructors. Classes were structured to maximize learning and retention of CPR skills, and subjects demonstrated appropriate CPR technique at the completion of the class. Patients did not attend the classes, and family members were excluded from the study if they had attended a CPR class within the previous 2 years.

Recent American Heart Association recommendations[2] were incorporated as follows: only one-person CPR was taught, the teaching of CPR was divided into discrete segments emphasizing the individual components, and each segment was practiced and reinforced before new segments were taught. A videotape was used to ensure consistency among classes and instructors. The tape was designed to be stopped as each discrete skill was shown, with subsequent demonstration by the instructor and practice by the participants on a resuscitation mannequin. At the end of the tape, the instructor demonstrated several CPR sequences, followed by a return demonstration by the participants. Finally, participants were asked to perform CPR for four uninterrupted and uncoached cycles.

The CPR-Social Support group received CPR training as above, followed by a 30 to 45-minute group discussion led by the same clinical nurse specialist who taught CPR. The group discussion addressed family members' psychological responses to having learned CPR. The goals of the support group were to help families identify and reduce inappropriate feelings of responsibility for the outcome of a cardiac emergency and to reduce potential negative emotional responses by identifying anticipatory grief responses and acknowledging the normalcy of these feelings. Group facilitators began the discussion with specific questions intended to elicit the participants' feelings regarding CPR instruction.

The CPR-Education group also received CPR training per protocol and also watched a didactic videotape presentation about heart disease and cardiac risk factors. The videotape was stopped at regular intervals so that the clinical nurse specialist could clarify any misconceptions and answer questions. The discussion included information about atherosclerotic heart disease, risk factors, and heart attack warning signs. The CPR-Only group received CPR training as described above without any additional intervention. The control group completed all questionnaires, but family members did not attend any intervention class.

All subjects, both patients and family members, completed a series of research questionnaires at baseline, 2 weeks, 3 months, and 6 months after CPR training to measure psychological and social adjustment. Control subjects completed questionnaires in this same time frame. Psychological adjustment was defined as anxiety, depression, and hostility and was assessed with the Multiple Affect Adjective Checklist, and psychosocial adjustment was tested with the Psychosocial Adjustment to Illness Scale.

Results

A multivariate analysis of variance (ANOVA) for repeated measures revealed a significant group effect ($P=0.005$) when the four patient groups were compared on all dependent variables over time. The psychological adjustment of patients was negatively affected when family members learned CPR without a social support intervention (Table 2). Patterns of change were similar across the dependent variables. Univariate ANOVA revealed significant differences at 3 months in total psychosocial adjustment to illness scores ($P=0.02$) and at 6 months in anxiety ($P=0.04$), hostility ($P=0.007$), and total psychosocial adjustment to illness scores ($P=0.003$). See Figures 1 and 2 for illustration.

To determine the influence of potential confounding variables on the differences seen between the four patient groups, we analyzed the following characteristics using multifactorial ANOVA: previous CPR training by family member, sex, education (using 14 years as the median split), and marital adjustment (using the median of the Spanier Dyadic Adjustment Scale). No significant interactions were noted.

Examination of the trends across time in family groups showed that psychosocial trajectories were more negative than in the patients and, at 6-month follow-up, mirrored those of the four patient groups (Table 3). However, there were no statistically significant differences between CPR groups on any dependent variables when family members were compared at each time point.

TABLE 2

Summary of Comparisons Among Patient Groups

	Control (n=99)	CPR–Social Support (n=74)	CPR–Education (n=74)	CPR-Only (n=90)	P*
Anxiety					
Baseline	6.3±4.7	6.1±4.7	7.3±4.6	6.6±4.6	NS
2 wk	6.9±4.6	5.8±4.8	7.1±4.7	7.0±4.9	NS
3 mo	5.8±4.2	5.6±4.3	7.2±4.7	7.3±4.6	NS
6 mo	5.6±4.1	5.2±4.6	7.2±4.8	7.4±4.9	0.004†
Depression					
Baseline	11.8±7.0	12.4±6.4	11.8±5.5	12.9±7.1	NS
2 wk	12.5±7.8	11.3±7.4	11.8±6.2	13.2±7.9	NS
3 mo	11.4±6.5	11.8±7.3	12.1±5.6	13.3±7.1	NS
6 mo	11.0±6.4	11.3±7.2	12.2±5.9	13.5±8.0	NS
Hostility					
Baseline	7.4±4.3	8.1±4.5	8.4±4.2	8.7±4.8	NS
2 wk	8.2±4.4	7.6±4.4	8.3±4.0	8.7±5.0	NS
3 mo	7.5±4.5	7.6±4.2	8.6±3.9	8.8±5.2	NS
6 mo	7.2±4.4	7.0±4.4	8.3±4.1	9.3±5.8	0.007‡
Psychosocial Adjustment to Illness					
Baseline	42.6±10.0	40.0±9.4	42.8±1.9	45.4±12.5	NS
3 mo	41.6±10.5	39.0±9.9	41.5±10.2	45.2±12.9	0.02§
6 mo	41.3±9.2	38.2±9.0	40.6±9.5	45.4±13.3	0.003¶

*P value for univariate ANOVA.

†P=0.03 CPR-Only vs CPR–Social Support; P=0.04 CPR-Only vs Control.

‡P=0.02 CPR-Only vs CPR–Social Support; P=0.02 CPR-Only vs Control.

§P=0.005 CPR-Only vs CPR–Social Support; no significant differences for other group comparisons.

¶P=0.001 CPR-Only vs CPR–Social Support; P=0.03 CPR-Only vs CPR–Education; P=0.03 CPR-Only vs Control.

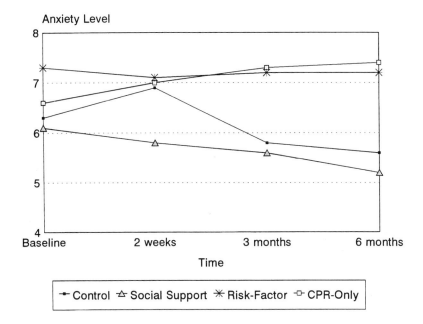

FIGURE 1. *Comparison of patient anxiety level by intervention groups across time.*

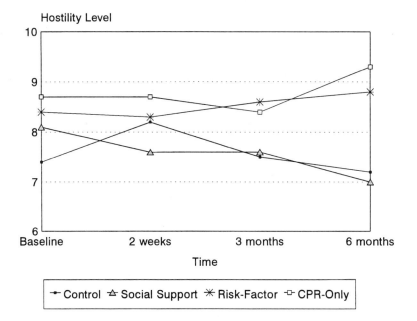

FIGURE 2. *Comparison of patient hostility level by intervention groups across time.*

TABLE 3

Summary of Comparisons Among Family Groups

	Control (n=99)	CPR–Social Support (n=74)	CPR–Education (n=74)	CPR–Only (n=90)	P
Anxiety					
Baseline	7.4±4.7	6.8±4.4	8.0±4.7	6.9±4.5	NS
2 wk	7.7±4.2	6.8±5.0	8.0±4.8	7.6±4.6	NS
3 mo	7.8±4.3	7.2±5.0	7.5±4.7	8.0±4.9	NS
6 mo	7.4±4.8	7.5±4.9	8.3±4.7	7.8±4.5	NS
Depression					
Baseline	11.8±6.1	12.3±6.3	13.2±6.8	13.1±7.1	NS
2 wk	13.1±6.7	12.9±7.6	14.4±6.1	13.9±7.4	NS
3 mo	12.9±6.3	12.4±7.5	12.4±7.2	12.4±7.2	NS
6 mo	13.1±7.5	13.6±8.6	14.5±6.4	13.7±7.5	NS
Hostility					
Baseline	7.4±4.1	8.0±3.9	8.4±4.4	8.1±3.9	NS
2 wk	8.2±5.0	7.7±5.1	8.4±3.8	8.3±5.0	NS
3 mo	8.0±3.7	7.6±4.1	7.9±4.1	9.8±4.8	NS
6 mo	8.5±4.9	8.8±5.4	9.2±4.8	9.4±4.8	NS

Attitudes of Family Members Toward Learning CPR

Of the 238 family members who learned CPR in the clinical trial, 172 (72%) were contacted for a structured telephone interview ≈2 years after CPR training (mean, 21±6 months).[27] The majority of respondents were female (85%) spouses (98%), with a mean age of 59±11 years and 14 years of education.

The majority (89%) reported feeling positive or very positive about having learned CPR. Those who were more ambivalent, worried that they would not be able to perform CPR adequately if called upon to rescue someone. Only 8% said that learning CPR conferred too much responsibility and that they felt burdened by knowing CPR. The majority (82%) also expressed unequivocal willingness to use CPR in the future. Those who expressed concerns about using CPR to rescue someone focused primarily on their fears that they would not be able to perform CPR adequately.

Discussion

Teaching CPR to family members of cardiac patients is controversial. On the one hand, immediate family members of patients at high risk for sudden death are a readily identifiable, logical target group for CPR training because the majority of sudden cardiac deaths occur in the home rather than in the hospital or at the workplace, and spouses or other family members are the individuals most likely to be bystanders to a witnessed cardiac arrest. On the other hand, most physicians and nurses are reluctant to discuss with their patients the possibility of cardiac emergencies occurring in the home and do not recommend CPR training of family members for fear of increasing the psychological burden of family members and, indirectly, of patients. This fear is not inconsequential given recent studies in which negative psychological and social states in patients with cardiac disease resulted in higher levels of morbidity and mortality.[28-33]

In an early study,[20] we found that CPR training of family members of high-risk cardiac patients had negative psychological consequences for patients up to 6 months after family instruction. In a later study, we compared three methods of teaching CPR to family members and contrasted these with a control group who did not learn CPR. We compared the CPR training method currently used in the community, in which CPR instruction is combined with education about heart disease and cardiac risk factors, with a second method specially tailored for family members of cardiac patients. The second method included a social support component. In the third intervention, CPR training alone (without an information or social support component) was used to simulate the method often used in cardiac rehabilitation programs and hospitals to teach family members of patients at high risk for sudden death.

Patients whose family members attended a CPR training session followed by a social support intervention reported significantly better psychosocial adjustment and less emotional distress on follow-up than patients whose family members learned CPR without a social support intervention. These results suggest that the potentially deleterious effects of CPR training on patients can be attenuated with the addition of a short social support intervention as simple as a brief group discussion among participants. The findings add to a growing body of literature about the buffering effect of social support in reducing stress[34–36] and the usefulness of a single support group session.[37]

The finding of more profound effects of CPR training on patients who did not attend CPR classes than on the family members who were the actual participants is intriguing. The families who participated in our studies were, in general, long married. We believe that whatever fears the family member experienced as part of CPR training were related to their awareness of the risk for sudden death in their loved one. CPR training directly undermines the denial used by both patients and family members related to the increased risk of sudden cardiac arrest. Denial is an important defense against anxiety[38] and is more likely to be used if the individual feels that the anticipated event is one over which he or she can exert no control. If it is stripped away without being replaced by another defense mechanism, the individual may experience a sudden increase in anxiety and depression. CPR training evokes the painful realization that the patient is at high risk for sudden cardiac death and that the integrity of the family may depend on the ability of a family member, particularly the spouse, to act quickly and effectively in case of an emergency. By combining CPR training with increased social support, the negative psychological consequences of such training appear to be buffered for both the family member and the patient.

Our findings support the belief that families can learn CPR successfully. Although they can and should learn CPR, specific training strategies should be used to facilitate learning, particularly with those predicted to have difficulty.

Recommendations

CPR instruction for cardiac family members should be tailored so that this instruction does not result in negative psychological consequences for patients. A simple nursing intervention that combines CPR with a brief group interaction to enhance social support is an appropriate and cost-effective way to buffer the negative effects of learning CPR. Based on the current body of literature, recommendations can be made to further tailor CPR training for families in three areas: CPR class content, reinforcement strategies, and retraining requirements. These recommendations are listed in Table 4.

Content for the CPR class should be focused as much as possible on the special needs of this population. For example, only one-person CPR need be taught, since it is unlikely that a cardiac arrest occurring at home will be witnessed by more than one family member trained in CPR. To enhance learning and retention, the content should be focused as much as possible on responding to a cardiac arrest in the home and should limit other emergency material usually included in community CPR training. In addition, family members of cardiac patients are often elderly and may bring significant anxiety to the training session. Both factors suggest that family members would benefit from content focusing.

To increase learning of skills and to build confidence, the practice time in the initial training session should be the major focus of the class. One possible approach to increasing practice time is to divide the CPR instruction into short didactic segments, each of which is immediately followed by a practice session. This pattern of didatic explanation and practice can be repeated to allow for cumulative practice with each session so that the full resuscitation exercise is practiced at several different intervals.

The special needs of family members should also be considered in structuring the CPR class. Given the potential negative

---

TABLE 4

Strategies for Enhancing CPR Training for Family Members

Teach one-person CPR
Adapt for special needs of elder learners
Arrange for adequate practice time
Allow for discussion during and after CPR training
Emphasize need for annual retraining
Devise home review strategies

psychosocial effects, classes should be limited in size to provide opportunities to address the anxiety and depression that learning CPR may evoke. Self-taught methods should be avoided so that skilled interaction between the instructor and the family member can occur. Classes should be followed by a short discussion to help family members acknowledge and cope with any negative feelings of anxiety, depression, or hostility raised by CPR training. Families need time to express their fears and concerns about the responsibility entailed in learning CPR.

Family members should review the steps of CPR frequently to maintain their knowledge and skill levels. They should be told about the importance of mental rehearsal and be encouraged to post the steps in a place that will be seen each day. Two challenges face nurses in this area: (1) devising effective review strategies that will be used by family members at home and (2) identifying opportunities to publicize the CPR sequence in areas used by family members (eg, hospital cafeterias, physician offices, shopping malls). Finally, CPR programs must be designed to include retraining at 1 year. Family members should be told at the time of initial testing that yearly retraining is required for skill and knowledge retention.

In summary, physicians and nurses should recommend that the family members of patients at high risk for sudden cardiac death learn CPR. The majority of family members can learn CPR successfully and do not feel overburdened by training. However, it is important to tailor classes to the special needs of this population and to encourage annual retraining.

Acknowledgment

The author would like to acknowledge the contributions of Debra Moser, Peter Guzy and Shelley Taylor to the research described in this chapter.

References

1. American Heart Association. *Heart and Stroke Facts: 1995 Statistical Supplement.* Dallas, Tex: American Heart Association; 1994.
2. Emergency Cardiac Care Committee and Subcommittees, American Heart Association. Guidelines for cardiopulmonary resuscitation and emergency cardiac care. *JAMA.* 1992;268:2171–2302.
3. Ritter G, Wolfe RA, Goldstein S, et al. The effect of bystander CPR on survival of out-of-hospital cardiac arrest victims. *Am Heart J.* 1985;110: 932–937.

4. Wik L, Steen PA, Bircher NG. Quality of bystander cardiopulmonary resuscitation influences outcome after prehospital cardiac arrest. *Resuscitation.* 1994;28:195–203.
5. Wilcox-Gok V. Survival from out-of-hospital cardiac arrest: a multivariate analysis. *Med Care.* 1991;29:104–114.
6. Einarson O, Jacobson F, Sigurdson G. Advanced cardiac life support in the prehospital setting: the Rekjavik experience. *J Intern Med.* 1989;225:129–135.
7. Weaver WD, Cobb LA, Hallstrom AP, et al. Considerations for improving survival from out-of-hospital cardiac arrest. *Ann Emerg Med.* 1986;15:1181–1186.
8. Guzy PM, Pearce ML, Greenfield S. The survival benefit of bystander cardiopulmonary resuscitation in a paramedic-served metropolitan area. *Am J Public Health.* 1983;73:766–769.
9. Goldberg RJ, Gore JM, Love DG, Ockene JK, Dalen JE. Layperson CPR: are we training the right people? *Ann Emerg Med.* 1984;13: 701–704.
10. Hejl Z, Petrzilkova Z, Stolz I, et al. Population study of the early phase of acute myocardial infarction and sudden coronary death. *Cor Vasa.* 1976;18:145–153.
11. Pane GA, Salness KY. A survey of participants in a mass CPR training course. *Ann Emerg Med.* 1987;16:1112–1116.
12. Goldberg RJ, DeCosimo D, St Louis P, Gore JM, Ockene JK, Dalen JE. Phsyicians' attitudes and practices toward CPR training in family members of patients with coronary heart disease. *Am J Public Health.* 1985;75:281–283.
13. St Louis P, Carter WB, Eisenberg MS. Prescribing CPR: a survey of physicians. *Am J Public Health.* 1982;72:1158–1160.
14. Nelson KM. Cardiopulmonary resuscitation training for families of cardiac patients. *Cardiovasc Nurs.* 1979;6:28–32.
15. Dracup K, Heaney D, Taylor SE, Guzy PM, Breu C. Can family members of high-risk cardiac patients learn CPR? *Arch Intern Med.* 1989;149:61–64.
16. Moser DK, Dracup K, Guzy PM, Taylor SE, Breu C. Cardiopulmonary resuscitation skills retention in family members of cardiac patients. *Am J Emerg Med.* 1990;8:498–503.
17. Taylor SE, Wayment HA, Collins MA. Positive illusions and affect regulation. In: Wegner DM, Pennebaker JW, eds. *Handbook of Mental Control.* Englewood Cliffs, NJ: Prentice Hall; 1993:325–343.
18. Affleck G, Tennen H, Pfeiffer C, Fifield C. Appraisals of control and predictability in adapting to a chronic disease. *J Pers Soc Psychol.* 1987;53:273–279.
19. Averill J. Personal control over aversive stimuli and its relationship to stress. *Psychol Bull.* 1981;80:286–303.
20. Dracup K, Guzy P, Taylor S, Barry J. Consequences of cardiopulmonary resuscitation training for family members of high-risk cardiac patients. *Arch Intern Med.* 1986;146:1757–1761.
21. Zuckerman M, Lubin B. *Manual for the Multiple Affect Checklist.* San Diego, Calif: Edits; 1965.
22. Zuckerman M, Lubin B, Robins S. Validation of the multiple affect adjective checklist in clinical situations. *J Consult Psychol.* 1965;28:418–425.
23. Derogatis LR. The psychosocial adjustment to illness scale (PAIS). *J Psychosom Res.* 1986;30:77–91.

24. Spanier GB. Measuring dyadic adjustment: new scales for assessing the quality of marriage and similar dyads. *J Marriage Family.* 1976;38: 15–28.
25. Smith RA, Wallston BS, Wallston K, et al. Measuring desire for control of health care processes. *J Pers Soc Psychol.* 1984;47:415–426.
26. Dracup K, Moser DK, Taylor SE, Guzy PM. The psychological consequences of cardiopulmonary resuscitation training for family members of patients at risk for sudden death. *Am J Public Health.* In press.
27. Dracup K, Moser DK, Guzy PM, Taylor SE, Marsden C. Is cardiopulmonary resuscitation deleterious for family members of cardiac patients? *Am J Public Health.* 1993;84:116–118.
28. Moser DK, Dracup K. The impact of anxiety on acute myocardial infarction complications. *Am J Crit Care.* 1995;4:245.
29. Ironson G, Taylor CB, Boltwood M, et al. Effects of anger on left ventricular ejection fraction in coronary artery disease. *Am J Cardiol.* 1992;70:281–285.
30. Rozanski A, Bairey CN, Krantz DS, et al. Mental stress and the induction of silent myocardial ischemia in patients with coronary artery disease. *N Engl J Med.* 1988;318:1005–1012.
31. Frasure-Smith N, Lespérance F, Talajic M. Depression following myocardial infarction: impact on 6-month survival. *JAMA.* 1993;270: 1819–1825.
32. Frasure-Smith N, Lespérance F, Talajic M. Depression and 18-month prognosis after myocardial infarction. *Circulation.* 1995;91:999–1005.
33. Frasure-Smith N. In-hospital symptoms of psychological stress as predictors of long-term outcome after acute myocardial infarction in men. *Am J Cardiol.* 1991;67:121–127.
34. Cohen S, Syme SL. Issues in the study and application of social support. In: Cohen S, Syme SL, eds. *Social Support and Health.* New York, NY: Academic Press; 1985:3–22.
35. Fontana AF, Kerns RD, Rosenberg RL, Colonese KL. Support, stress, and recovery from coronary heart disease: a longitudinal causal model. *Health Psychol.* 1989;8:175–193.
36. House JS, Robbins C, Metzner HL. The association of social relationships and activities with mortality: prospective evidence from the Tecumseh Community Health Study. *Am J Epidemiol.* 1982;116: 123–140.
37. Taylor SE, Falke RL, Hoptaw SJ, Lichtman RR. Social support, support groups, and the cancer patient. *J Consult Clin Psychol.* 1986;54: 608–615.
38. Lazarus R, Folkman S. *Stress, Appraisal and Coping.* New York, NY: Springer Verlag; 1984;117–180.

Chapter 15

Public Access Defibrillation

Barbara Riegel, DNSc, RN, CS

Apparently healthy individuals die every day, victims of sudden, unexpected cardiac arrest with ventricular tachyarrhythmia as the predominant cause. Public access defibrillation is a novel strategy for definitive treatment of such persons with "smart" defibrillators. This pragmatic strategy involves putting specially designed automatic external defibrillators (AEDs) into the hands of the public. Four levels of potential responders have been identified: (1) first responders (trained persons who have a duty to respond to medical emergencies, eg, emergency medical services [EMS] personnel, (2) targeted responders or individuals who are not traditional first responders but who are likely to react to a medical emergency and perceive a duty to respond to such emergencies (eg, firefighters, guards, police, airline stewards), (3) members of the lay public (eg, passers-by), and (4) family members of individuals known to be at risk for sudden cardiac death (SCD). This chapter provides an overview of the proposed public access defibrillation strategy. The experience of previous investigators is reviewed. Issues of perceived need, device design, legislation and regulation, training, and research are explored.

Morbidity and mortality from most cardiovascular diseases have declined steadily over the past 20 years, but SCD remains the exception. The frequently cited rate of 1000 deaths per day from SCD has not changed over the past few decades. Prevention has eluded us, because SCD is typically unexpected, occurring as the first clinical manifestation of previously unrecognized heart disease in 20% to 25% of SCD victims.[1] The majority of SCD events occur in individuals with coronary heart disease but not necessarily those in the highest-risk subgroups, such as patients with heart failure.[2] Because ventricular tachyarrhythmia is usually the cause of SCD,

From: Dunbar SB, Ellenbogen KA, Epstein AE, (eds). *Sudden Cardiac Death: Past, Present, and Future.* Armonk, NY: Futura Publishing Company, Inc.; © 1997.

electrical defibrillation remains the most useful method of treatment. The effectiveness of defibrillation is time-dependent, however, with <10% of victims surviving neurologically intact when ≥10 minutes passes before effective resuscitation.[3]

The American Heart Association has developed a "chain of survival" strategy designed to optimize a patient's chance of survival from sudden, unexpected cardiac arrest (Figure 1).[3] There are four links in the chain: early access, early cardiopulmonary resuscitation (CPR), early defibrillation, and early advanced care (eg, intubation, intravenous administration of medications). Early access means that citizens have been trained to recognize a cardiac arrest quickly and that a system of communications and emergency medical dispatch is in place that will immediately send trained EMS personnel and equipment to the scene. Great strides have been made in providing universal emergency phone access in the United States, with 70% of the geographic area and 90% of the population having access to 911 capabilities. Early CPR by bystanders provides ventilation and circulation, buying precious minutes for the EMS team to arrive with a defibrillator and other advanced cardiac life support equipment. Millions of people worldwide have been successfully trained in the mechanics of resuscitation since it was first taught to the general public in the early 1970s.[4]

As effective as these efforts have been, pockets remain in the United States in which the EMS system is hampered in its attempt to access a sudden cardiac arrest victim in a timely fashion due to distance or density. Further, once access is achieved, there is no guarantee that the EMS personnel will be equipped with a defibrillator. In 1989, only 30% of EMS systems in the United States had defibrillators.[5] State legal barriers still exist that hamper progress in this arena. For example, many states have statutes that define

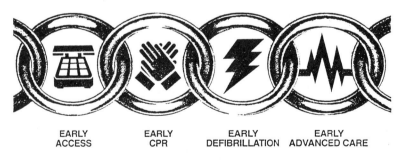

FIGURE 1. *Chain of survival. Reprinted with permission from JAMA. 1992;268:2171–2302. ©1992, American Medical Association.*

AED use as the practice of medicine. These restrictions mean that emergency medical technicians (EMTs) cannot be trained in the use of AEDs in many areas of the country.

In rural, unpopulated areas of the country, EMS personnel may be required to travel many miles to reach the victim and then even farther with the victim to a facility equipped with a defibrillator to provide definitive therapy. In densely populated areas in which high-rise buildings predominate, the time required to negotiate traffic, secure an elevator, and find the victim greatly decreases survival rates because of extended delays from arrest to defibrillation. Survival from sudden cardiac arrest in Chicago was only 2% in 1987, with only 55 of 3221 resuscitation victims leaving the hospital alive.[6] In New York City, only 26 of 2329 victims of apparent cardiac arrest (1.4%) survived to leave the hospital in 1991.[7] The median time to first shock was 12.4 minutes in New York City in 1991, whereas in Seattle, Wash, defibrillation typically occurs within 5 to 7 minutes after the onset of cardiac arrest. Bystander CPR improved the outcome in New York City, but only modestly; survival was 2.9% in the one third of victims who received bystander CPR compared with 0.8% in those who received no bystander CPR. These experiences demonstrate that even if bystander CPR was applied more commonly than it is now, a dismal percentage of victims survive without the addition of definitive therapy for the underlying arrhythmia.

Review of Prior Experience

Previous clinical investigators have explored the feasibility of training the public to use AEDs. Clinical trials of AEDs used by basic EMTs have shown that with few exceptions, this technology is safe and saves lives.[8] For example, field experience from large public gatherings (eg, the Kingdome, World's Fairs) demonstrates that targeted responders can be successfully trained to respond quickly and effectively to witnessed events.[9] A recent meta-analysis of 10 intervention studies of early EMT defibrillation demonstrated an overall effect size of 0.092, indicating a 9.2% increase in survival over the expected rate had the EMTs not intervened.[10]

Interestingly, evidence suggests that providing AEDs to first responders in communities in which CPR is rarely performed by bystanders fails to improve the survival significantly. Kellermann and associates[11] used a crossover design to evaluate the effectiveness of defibrillation by firefighter first responders. Of the 879 persons treated over the 39 months of the study, 431 (49%) were found in ventricular fibrillation. The first responders performed effectively and the AEDs worked reliably, but survival was no higher in those defibrillated than in those not defibrillated on the scene (34% versus 32%), apparently because only 12% had received bystander CPR before the firefighters arrived. The authors warn that early defibrillation alone cannot overcome low community rates of bystander CPR. Other communities also have demonstrated the importance of the CPR link in the chain of survival. For example, in Seattle, 32% of persons with witnessed cardiac arrest survived to leave the hospital when bystanders performed CPR but only 22% of a comparable population survived without bystander CPR.[12]

Weaver and associates[9] demonstrated an increase in survival from 9% to 30% when AEDs were made available to first responders in cities in which CPR training was widespread and EMS response was already rapid. Survival rates soared to 48% (21 of 44 arrest victims survived) when police vehicles in Rochester, Minn, were equipped with AEDs.

Experience with AEDs in the hands of lay bystanders is only anecdotol at this point, with a few studies in progress. Dr. Max Harry Weil, MD in Cochela Valley is currently training all categories of providers, including high school students who cannot be legally certified until age 18 (Weil, personal communication, December 13, 1995). No data on successful use are available as yet, but anecdotal reports suggest that the experience may not be vastly different from that reported by investigators training first responders.

Finally, published reports of the results of home defibrillator use are limited, but successful defibrillation and survival have been reported even though the responder is typically highly emotional, facing the death of a loved one.[13,14]

Issues

Perceived Need

Perhaps most basic to the success of the proposed strategy is an evolution in our perception of the need for AEDs. The public perception is that CPR works. It might be thought that if we could just get more people trained in CPR, we would not need to introduce another tactic. Further, CPR is benign and harmless; damage occurs only when the technique is poorly applied, in which case it is ineffective, and the victim dies. Why put an electrical device into the hands of lay people when CPR is perfectly adequate?

The reality is that CPR is not definitive therapy. Rather, CPR is an effective temporary strategy useful only until a defibrillator is accessed. Prolonged CPR (ie, >30 minutes) is rarely effective because of responder fatigue, inadequate circulation, and/or rhythm deterioration. Timely conversion of ventricular fibrillation is essential to ensure neurologically intact survival (Table 1).

The Device

Is it safe to propose supplying the lay public with electrical devices that deliver ≥200 J to unconscious, defenseless people? Could these devices be used inappropriately or, worse yet, as weapons?

The new generation of AEDs are capable of automatically detecting and treating ventricular fibrillation. Devices are currently designed to walk users through the application and use, and these devices promise to become increasingly "user-friendly." Many AEDs on the market are now passive or fully automated, meaning that they require no interaction by the user after placement on the patient's chest (Figure 2). Most devices currently on the market are semiautomatic or advisory devices.[15] That is, the unit analyzes the rhythm and

---

TABLE 1

Significant Issues Requiring Further Exploration

Perceived need
  Adequacy of CPR alone
Device
  Methods of facilitating correct placement
  Automated rhythm diagnosis
  Design characteristics (eg, size)
  Safety
Legislation and regulation
  FDA requirements
  Advance directives
  Good Samaritan–type statutes
Training
  Desired outcome of training
  Amount of training/retraining
  Ideal method
  Self-confidence
Research
  Sufficient incidence of SCD
  Outcome variables
  Sample size
  Randomization strategies
  Statistical analysis

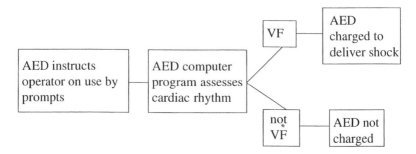

FIGURE 2. Process of AED use. VF indicates ventricular fibrillation.

prepares to deliver a shock, but the rescuer must deliver the discharge by pushing a button. Before 1987, healthcare providers were generally better than AEDs at distinguishing shockable from nonshockable rhythms, but now most newer AEDs outperform trained providers. For example, Cummins and colleagues[16] demonstrated that the AEDs currently on the market are 90% sensitive for ventricular fibrillation and 90% to 95% specific for other rhythms.

Prompts are built into the devices to facilitate correct placement and use. Passive visual prompts are pictorial and/or written directions that are imprinted on the device. Some devices have liquid crystal display (LCD) prompts in which pictorial and/or written prompts are displayed on a liquid crystal screen and selected automatically by the device after computerized algorithms assess the rhythm. Some have voice prompts that are audible through a speaker. A few devices have communication technology that allows the AED to automatically make contact with a medical authority (ie, critical care monitoring team, dispatcher, etc) upon activation of the device by the user, thus allowing direct interaction between the medical provider and the device or between the medical provider and the user. These are referred to as assisted devices, and more complex assisted devices are likely to emerge in the future.

Size, shape, and weight of the AED are important characteristics of devices designed for prehospital use. The ideal device for such use is small for easy storage, lightweight to be carried to the victim, and rugged to withstand being dropped or exposed to weather. AEDs must be low cost so that schools, gyms, apartments, and other public buildings can afford to purchase sufficient numbers to make them easily accessible. Most public access defibrillation devices will be battery-powered, so the ability to easily remove devices from a charging unit is essential. Alternatively, if batteries must be changed, that process must be easy and rapid.

The American Heart Association Task Force on Automatic External Defibrillators is concerned about enhancing the safety of AEDs for the public. Although the manufacturers strive for 100% sensitivity and 100% specificity, such perfection is unrealistic. Some inaccuracy in the diagnostic algorithms will have to be tolerated. The task force has urged manufacturers to design and test devices to avoid potential misuse and to prevent injury should misuse occur. Suggestions include the use of voice chips to deliver prompts to a rescuer opening or activating an AED (eg, "Shake the victim. If he groans or moves his arms or legs, do not attach the electrodes; call 911"). A "wake-up" shock is another option. This approach would involve the administration of an unpleasant but harmless shock after analysis of the arrhythmia by the proprietary algorithm. A wake-up shock would ideally stimulate a patient who was intoxicated or in a deep sleep, thereby warning the rescuer not to deliver the full-strength defibrillating shock. One drawback to the "wake-up" shock approach is that it might not be effective for metabolic or hypoglycemic causes of unresponsiveness.

Legislation and Regulation

The most significant obstacles to public use of AEDs are the regulatory requirements of the FDA. Defibrillators are currently labeled as intended for use by first responders or on prescription by a physician. Prescriptive authority is given for specific situations, so public use of an AED will be inhibited unless the FDA is willing to amend its requirements.

Another FDA rule is that informed consent be given by patients on whom the device is used. Presumably any patient requiring defibrillation will be unconscious and therefore unable to give informed consent. Related to this is the issue of advanced directives, which remains unresolved. Even if an individual who chose not to be resuscitated were to wear a bracelet or necklace announcing his/her wishes, it is conceivable that a well-meaning bystander might resuscitate him or her. This issue requires further discussion and problem-solving.

Lay users may fear the threat of a personal injury claim after using an AED on a SCD victim who is a stranger. When one person aids another, the assumed-duty doctrine requires the rescuer to exercise reasonable care. If the victim fails to survive or is somehow harmed, the survivors (ie, family) could sue the rescuer. The argument that the victim was clinically dead when the AED was used may effectively protect the rescuer, but such a defense has not been attempted. Legislative expansion of Good Samaritan statutes could cover AED users and motivate laypersons to use the device. Good Samaritan–type statutes protect someone acting in good faith in an emergency by allowing the rescuer to be liable only for gross negligence, not ordinary negligence.

The need for legislative change is being addressed by Representative Gerry Studds (D-MA-10) in proposed federal legislation, the Cardiac Arrest Survival Act, HR 3022. The legislation, introduced March 6, 1996, calls for the Secretary of Health and Human Services to establish a program to circulate recommendations aimed at decreasing resistance to AED use at the state and federal level. If the legislation is passed, the Secretary of Health and Human Services will be asked to make specific recommendations to the states regarding implementation of the chain of survival. States will be asked to evaluate the merits of training first responders in lifesaving first aid. Finally, states will be asked to remove barriers to the use of AEDs and to determine the merits of training additional health professionals and first responders in the use of AEDs. The bill requires the development of federal policies relative to federal facilities and employees and addresses tort reform issues.

Training

Training needs will most likely differ for the four groups specified (ie, first responders, targeted responders, laypersons, and family) because of prior experience, perceptions of duty or responsibility, and emotional context.[17] Important training issues that need to be investigated include the educational effectiveness and optimal use of various instructional materials, classroom study, practice, and mass media. CPR training has been based on the premise that skill demonstration is an essential outcome, but thousands of individuals use fire extinguishers annually without ever having been shown how to activate the device or giving a return demonstration. Although advocated by investigators, the need for formal training in the use of AEDs has not yet been clearly demonstrated.

The amount of initial training and retraining needed to achieve and maintain skill proficiency is unknown. A limited amount of time and practice may be adequate in preparing targeted responders to safely and effectively use a public access AED on a victim of sudden, unexpected cardiac arrest. Effectiveness refers to the success of an intervention under "real-world," not ideal, conditions. Unique methods, amounts, types, and combinations of user training may effectively minimize human error and facilitate safe and effective use of AEDs by the public.

The methods (eg, group training, self-learning techniques, hands-on practice) and duration (eg, 2 hours, 4 hours, 8 hours over a period of 1 or 2 days) of training also may vary with the group being trained. Small group face-to-face training with an instructor with the addition of hands-on training with the device, much like the CPR training advocated by the American Heart Association, may be the ideal training method. But programmed learning modules or computer-based modules need to be tested. The effectiveness of computer or television-based education remains unknown, especially in retraining, but recent data from Eisenberg et al[18] demonstrated that videotape CPR training of laypersons was not effective. If knowledge is assumed to be the appropriate outcome variable, a norm-referenced knowledge test with a predetermined success rate of ≈75% would be needed. Once the ideal format for education is determined, the minimum number of hours of training must be identified. Prior experience suggests that 3 to 4 hours of training is sufficient if given in two sessions to reinforce instruction, that face-to-face group training is effective, and that hands-on practice with an AED is essential (M.H. Weil, MD, 1995, personal communication; W.D. Weaver, MD, 1995, personal communication).

The social context in which learning, practice, and use of the device occurs may influence outcomes, as shown by Dracup and colleagues[19] in the context of CPR training. Among family members, at least, learning about CPR and thereby assuming responsibility for the life of their loved one caused poor psychological adjustment among the patients—not among those trained in CPR—at 3 and 6 months after training. Support groups may be an essential complement to AED training of family members.

In terms of training, the outcome variable of most relevance needs to be debated. Knowledge of how to use the device probably is not sufficient for successful AED use. Unpublished data from a survey conducted by Suzanne Thompson, PhD, in 1994 demonstrated more public support for training family members of cardiac patients in AED use (68%) than for training the general public (24%).[20] Marked hesitancy to resuscitate a stranger was noted in this convenience sample from southern California. Myriad reasons exist that would deter a stranger from using an AED on an apparent victim, including fear of a lawsuit, fear of harm from the device, and inability to perform a complex motor skill while under emotional duress.

Formal training with the device may not even be necessary if knowledge is not the essential outcome variable. An outcome more important than knowledge may be desire and self-confidence in one's ability to perform a specific behavior in a particular circumstance. The media have been shown to effectively influence values and may be the intervention of choice to influence the desire to find and use an AED if a sudden cardiac arrest victim is encountered.[21] Since the majority of the population goes through life without ever witnessing a cardiac arrest, perhaps mass media may be the preferred method of motivating individuals to seek out and use an AED when the necessity arises.

Self-confidence may be best influenced through a single return demonstration without the need for retraining. Investigators in the field report that hands-on training effectively convinces people that they can use the device if necessary (M.H. Weil, MD, 1995, personal communication). It may be unnecessary to expect individuals to learn and relearn how to activate the device when the devices are designed to require minimal skill. Data from Moser and colleagues[17] demonstrated that four of five family members trained in CPR but deferring retraining after a year still successfully performed the skill when needed.

Research

Large-scale trials of AEDs in the hands of the public are greatly needed. Organizations such as the National Heart, Lung, and Blood Institute are currently being solicited to fund such research. Design issues abound with such a trial. The foremost issue is simply finding a naturally occurring situation in which the incidence of sudden, unexpected cardiac arrest is sufficient to allow the study to be conducted. If we assume, as the American Heart Association has assumed with CPR training, that retraining at some interval is necessary, the individuals trained to use the AED must have the opportunity to use those skills while they remember them. Further, for the strategy to be effective, such events must be witnessed and the witness must be willing and able to perform the intervention. A recent phone survey of investigators in the field worldwide conducted by the AED Task Force suggested that ≈60% (range, 50% to 82%) of events are witnessed.

Unpublished data recently compiled by Stiell suggest that the incidence of SCD is not as high as previously thought. Data from 23 communities reveal a weighted combined incidence of only 0.62/1000/year (personal communication, Ian Stiell, MD, March 1, 1996). If the population of the United States is 250 million, a rate of 0.62/1000 translates to 155 000 per year and only 425 per day, rather than 1000 per day. Clearly, these rates contradict the widely publicized numbers, but it is important to recognize the difficulty encountered by communities as they compile their rates for submission to the National Center for Health Statistics. If little more than half of unexpected deaths are witnessed, as previously argued, the retrospective determination of cause of death is understandably questionable. The data from Stiell cited above were gathered from investigators working in SCD in typical communities across the western hemisphere and may be more realistic.

A primary outcome variable in any study of resuscitation is neurologically intact survival, which is fairly straightforward to measure. However, effectiveness of the strategy is not sufficient in this era of cost containment. Assessment of the cost-effectiveness of public access defibrillation is needed before communities can be expected to implement such a strategy. A wide variety of fixed and variable costs need to be considered, such as equipment, wages, quality assurance, number of devices needed to successfully cover and protect a community, training, and education. Implementation costs (costs of putting an AED system in place) and the costs of equipment maintenance, retraining, etc. need to be accounted for. Additional direct and indirect costs might include those of wages for targeted responders, but these costs would be significantly reduced in communities using the lay public as providers. Other costs include those of hospitalization for individuals successfully resuscitated, costs of the cardiac care received or averted (irrespective of whether they are directly related to the intervention), costs of noncardiac diseases affected by changes in cardiac prognosis, and costs of lost economic productivity. A societal perspective on a cost-effectiveness analysis would facilitate comparison with competing interventions.

Cost-effectiveness analysis typically includes a measure of quality-adjusted life years. Studies of quality of life after resuscitation suggest some subtle differences that may be difficult to detect unless careful attention is paid to measurement issues. For example, when studying survivors of out-of-hospital cardiac arrest, Callicot and colleagues[22] documented good to excellent health-related quality of life among 32 persons studied an average of 2.5 years (range, 0.02 to 5.5 years) after the event. Hsu and associates[23] found that only 25% of 28 SCD survivors rated their quality of life as worse than before the arrest when studied an average of 18 months after arrest. Patients resuscitated during hospitalization may be assumed to experience the best results, but Miranda[24] documented work dysfunction and poor psychosocial functioning among 477 individuals resuscitated during hospitalization compared with 500 control patients.

Technical issues of sample size and statistical analysis are challenging in any large clinical trial, but a study of AEDs poses some unique problems. An intervention trial would require randomization of communities shown to have a higher than normal incidence of SCD (eg, senior citizen communities). Randomizing communities rather than individuals poses a problem because individuals, not communities, are treated. Such difficulties require a sophisticated knowledge base and some creative solutions.

Summary

This chapter provides an overview of a novel strategy for decreasing death due to unexpected cardiac arrhythmia—public access defibrillation. Consistent with the strategic plan of the American Heart Association, PAD represents the third of four links in the chain of survival: rapid defibrillation. Public access defibrillation is the most aggressive strategy proposed by the American Heart Association to date, and many clinical, education, legal, and ethical issues remain that require debate, commitment from manufacturers, legislative and regulatory changes, and large-scale clinical trials.

References

1. National Center for Health Statistics. *Advance Report of Final Mortality Statistics, 1990. Monthly Mortality Statistics Report.* 1993;41(suppl 7). Hyattsville MD: US Public Health Service.
2. Myerburg RJ, Kessler KM, Castellanos A. Sudden cardiac death: epidemiology, transient risk, and intervention assessment. *Ann Intern Med.* 1993;119:1187–1197.
3. Cummins RO, Ornato JP, Thies WH, Pepe PP. Improving survival from sudden cardiac arrest: the "chain of survival" concept. *Circulation.* 1991; 83:1832–1847.
4. Paraskos, JA. History of CPR and the role of the national conference. *Ann Emerg Med.* 1993;22(pt 2):275–280.
5. US Congress, Office of Technology Assessment. *Rural Emergency Medical Services: Special Report.* Washington, DC: 1989: report OTA-H-445.
6. Becker LB, Ostrander MP, Barrett J, Kondos GT. Outcome of CPR in a large metropolitan area: where are the survivors? *Ann Emerg Med.* 1991;20:355–361.
7. Lombardi G, Gallagher J, Gennis P. Outcome of out-of-hospital cardiac arrest in New York City: the Pre-Hospital Arrest Survival Evaluation (PHASE) Study. *JAMA.* 1994;271:678–683.
8. Eisenberg MS, Horwood BT, Cummins RO, Reynolds-Haertle R, Hearne TR. Cardiac arrest and resuscitation: a tale of 29 cities. *Ann Emerg Med.* 1990;19:179–186.

9. Weaver WD, Hill D, Fahrenbruch CE, et al. Use of the automatic external defibrillator in the management of out-of-hospital cardiac arrest. *N Engl J Med.* 1988;319:661–666.
10. Watts DD. Defibrillation by basic emergency medical technicians: effect on survival. *Ann Emerg Med.* 1995;26:635–639.
11. Kellermann AL, Hackman BB, Somes G, Kreth TK, Nail L, Dobyns P. Impact of first-responder defibrillation in an urban emergency medical services system. *JAMA.* 1993;270:1708–1713.
12. Cummins RO, Eisenberg MS, Hallstrom AP, Litwin PE. Survival of out-of-hospital cardiac arrest with early initiation of cardiopulmonary resuscitation. *Am J Emerg Med.* 1985;3:114–119.
13. Chadda KD, Kammerer R. Early experiences with the portable automatic external defibrillator in the home and public places. *Am J Cardiol.* 1987;60:732–733.
14. Eisenberg MS, Moore J, Cummins RO, et al. Use of the automatic external defibrillator in homes of survivors of out-of-hospital ventricular fibrillation. *Am J Cardiol.* 1989;63:443–446.
15. ECRI. *Health Devices.* August-September, 1995;24:8–9.
16. Cummins RO, Stults KR, Haggar B, Kerber RE, Schaeffer S, Brown DD. A new rhythm library for testing automatic external defibrillators: performance of three devices. *J Am Coll Cardiol.* 1988;11:597–602.
17. Moser DK, Dracup K, Guzy PM, Taylor SE, Breu C. Cardiopulmonary resuscitation skills retention in family members of cardiac patients. *Am J Emerg Med.* 1990;8:498–503.
18. Eisenberg M, Damon S, Mandel L, et al. CPR instruction by videotape: results of a community project. *Ann Emerg Med.* 1995;25:198–202.
19. Dracup KA, Guzy PM, Taylor SE, Barry J. Cardiopulmonary resuscitation (CPR) training: consequences for family members of high-risk cardiac patients. *Arch Intern Med.* 1986;146:1757–1761.
20. Weisfeldt ML, Kerber RE, McGoldrick RP, et al, for the Automatic External Defibrillation Task Force. American Heart Association Report on the Public Access Defibrillation Conference December 8-10, 1994. *Circulation.* 1995;92:2740–2747.
21. Becker MH. Theoretical models of adherence and strategies for improving adherence. In: Schumaker SA, Schron EB, Ockene JK, eds. *The Handbook of Health Behavior Change.* New York, NY: Springer Verlag; 1990.
22. Callicot CA, Valenzuela TD, Spaite DW, Clark LL. Survival and quality of life after cardiac arrest. Presented at the SAEM Annual Meeting, 1995. Abstract.
23. Hsu JWY, Callaham M, Madsen CD. Formal quality-of-life testing of survivors of out-of-hospital cardiac arrest correlates poorly with commonly used neurologic outcome measures. Presented at the SAEM Annual Meeting, 1995.
24. Miranda DR. Quality of life after cardiopulmonary resuscitation. *Chest.* 1994;106:524–530.

Chapter 16

Quality-of-Life Issues in Survivors of Sudden Cardiac Death Entering Treatment

Louise Sherman Jenkins, RN, PhD

Survivors of sudden cardiac death (SCD) experience various physiological and psychosocial responses after cardiac arrest during the early recovery phase. In addition to undergoing a multitude of necessary tests, they are also confronted with participation in decision making regarding ongoing treatment attempting to prevent another such episode.[1] What is known about the quality of life of these patients in the immediate postarrest period—ie, the hospital stay when treatment is instituted and soon after discharge? This question is important to clinicians who care for SCD survivors and support their family members during what is clearly an emotional and difficult period in the recovery process.

The body of literature with this focus is surprisingly small in contrast to the large number of reports on the impact of living with treatment options, particularly with an implanted cardioverter-defibrillator (ICD). Two major criteria were used to select the published research reviewed to address the above question: (1) data were gathered during the immediate postarrest period, and (2) data were obtained directly from the patient. When spouse/family data were also available from this time period, those data are included. In addition, two studies were included even though data were collected later in postarrest recovery because of their contribution to understanding of the topic by comparing SCD survivors with others not having the experience.

From: Dunbar SB, Ellenbogen KA, Epstein AE, (eds). *Sudden Cardiac Death: Past, Present, and Future.* Armonk, NY: Futura Publishing Company, Inc.; © 1997.

Background

Incorporation of physical, mental, and social well-being into the World Health Organization's definition of health in the mid-1970s was really a catalyst for moving to a biopsychosocial model of patient care. This model supports study of the increasingly frequently used term "quality of life." Such study is challenging because quality of life is individually perceived, with meaning varying from individual to individual.

In commentary addressing the "state of the art" of the study of quality of life and health status in clinical research, Bergner[2] noted a dramatic difference between the levels of conceptual clarity in these two constructs. There is some consensus on what constitutes the dimensions of health status (eg, disease state, disability or handicap state, social/physical/cognitive function, mental condition). In addition, she points out that several conceptual frameworks for health status exist that have been disseminated and discussed and provide a theory base for some instrument development.

In contrast, quality of life is generally more broadly conceptualized. Some of the evolving perspectives include considering quality of life as what the individual says it is, what the individual is able to do, the impact of an illness/condition on the patient's life, or the difference between what the patient expects and what actually happens. Aspects of quality of life are viewed as domains or dimensions such as life satisfaction, health perceptions, and symptoms.

Specific aspects or dimensions tailored to a particular population can be identified and measured. For example, such domains for an SCD survivor might appropriately include being able to care for oneself, resuming roles such as return to work, and being able to drive. If the SCD survivor is treated with an ICD aspects of the device firing or not firing would be among relevant dimensions appropriate to consider.

Although there is growing consensus that quality of life is a multidimensional construct, it is difficult to compare results across studies because of different conceptualizations and measures being used. Regrettably, very few reports provide the definition of quality of life that is used in that particular study.[3,4] Although advances are being made, the study of quality of life is clearly at a much earlier stage of development than health status.

In 1989, Bergner noted that often, "well after all aspects of the research [design] have been settled, someone realizes that the therapy may affect aspects of a person's life that are not strictly medical."[2] (p S152) Thus, quality of life becomes a catch-all category of variables composed of various psychosocial aspects and anticipated side effects of the treatment(s) being evaluated; essentially anything that is a nonmedical outcome becomes labeled as quality of life. An exception to this "afterthought" mentality is the emphasis that the National Heart, Lung, and Blood Institute has placed on the study of quality of life in a number of trials for >20 years.[5]

In the years since Bergner's comments, the study of quality of life has continued to evolve. The increasing rigor of contemporary work has moved these efforts toward increased acceptance in the research community,[6] with quality of life being a predetermined end point integrated into project planning such as in the Cardiac Arrhythmia Suppression Trial (CAST)[7] and in the Antiarrhythmics Versus Implanted Defibrillator (AVID) Clinical Trial.[8]

No reported studies were found that claimed to address quality of life per se early in recovery from SCD. The lack of consensus on the definition of SCD extends to the aspects of quality of life in the patient population. Other authors in this publication are dealing with what could be appropriately considered quality-of-life issues. To avoid repetition, specific areas not included in this chapter are coping, the impact of cognitive impairment, and patient decision making. Rather, a variety of psychosocial aspects of quality-of-life issues will be addressed.

Studies Comparing SCD Survivors With Non–SCD Survivors

Three early studies compared SCD survivors with patients who had not had a cardiac arrest. These studies are summarized in Table 1.

1. Druss and Kornfeld, 1967. It was only three decades ago that the first study examining the psychosocial aspects of survival of SCD was published by Druss and Kornfeld.[9] They conducted "psychiatric interviews" lasting about 2 hours with 20 male patients being cared for in a "cardiac monitor unit." Half of these patients were SCD survivors (mean age, 55.5 years); the rest (mean age, 52.1 years) had not sustained an arrest but were cared for in the same monitored unit. Diagnosis was not specified in the comparison group, although presumably it was cardiac in nature and required electrocardiographic monitoring.

The site of the interviews is somewhat difficult to sort out from the report. It is stated that 5 of the interviews with SCD survivors were conducted in the hospital, ". . . just prior to discharge."[9] (p 75) Presumably the other 5 SCD survivors were interviewed after discharge from the hospital. It is not reported where the 10 comparison

TABLE 1.

Summary of Published Studies Reviewed: Comparison of SCD Survivors With Other Patients

Study	Quality-of-Life Measures(s)/Method(s)	Quality-of-Life Results
Authors: Druss and Kornfeld[9] Date: 1967 Design: Descriptive Subjects: 20 patients: 10 SCD survivors* and 10 non-SCD cardiac patients Study aim: Exploration of effect of arrest on lives of survivors and comparison of extent of emotional problems with patients not experiencing arrest *5 of the 10 SCD survivors seen during postarrest hospitalization	Psychiatric interviews	In both groups of patients, serious psychological problems were noted. Post–hospital discharge behavior was similar.

Authors: Finkelmeier, Kenwood and Summers[10] Date: 1984 Design: Descriptive (cross-sectional) Subjects: 60 SCD survivors and 40 patients with serious arrhythmias Study aim: Exploration of emotional sequelae of SCD and comparisons with patients with serious arrhythmias but no SCD	Profile of Mood States (POMS) Investigator-developed questionnaire	POMS scores for both groups of patients were generally comparable and higher than normative values for healthy subjects.
Authors: Kolar and Dracup[13] Date: 1990 Design: Descriptive (cross-sectional) Subjects: 19 SCD survivors and 21 patients with ventricular arrhythmias Study aim: Exploration of whether psychosocial adjustment in patients with ventricular dysrhythmias was different in those surviving SCD	Psychosocial Adjustment to Illness Scale (PAIS-SR)	No significant differences were found in psychosocial adjustment.

cardiac patients were interviewed. For the SCD survivors, the timing between the arrest and the interview ranged from 6 weeks to 11 months (mean, 18 weeks). For the comparison cardiac patients, the time between admission to the hospital and the interview ranged from 6 weeks to 12 months (mean, 23 weeks). As was typical for the time, the length of stay in the monitored unit and the total hospitalization were long, as seen below.

	Mean Length of Stay, Days[9]	
	In Monitored Unit	In Hospital
SCD survivors	9.7	38.9
Comparison patients	6.3	41.5

No statistical tests were reported to compare these data between the two groups; the mean scores reflect that SCD survivors were interviewed closer in time to the arrest than the comparison patients were to their hospital admission. Also, although the SCD survivors had longer stays in the monitored unit, their hospital stays were shorter.

A variety of what were called "protective psychological reactions" were described in detail in the SCD survivors, including isolation of affect, displacement, projection, and hallucinations. Although the comparison patients were not described, it was noted that they differed little in their psychiatric states and life patterns after hospitalization. The authors acknowledged that the numerous similarities between the two groups may be influenced by the environmental impact of the monitored unit. Characteristics such as the small and confined physical space, lack of privacy, darkness, monitor lights and noises, minimal contact with visitors, and constant awareness of other patients, whether progressing well or in crisis, certainly may influence patient responses. The authors state that the two patient groups showed serious psychological problems of similar nature and extent.

Violent dreams and feelings of a sense of particular uniqueness in having been brought back from the dead were evident only in the SCD survivors. At the time, surviving SCD outside of the operating room environment was quite a novel happening, and responses of caregivers, family members, and others with whom the survivors had contact after discharge may have contributed to the sense of uniqueness described. Other aspects contributing to the psychological reactions identified could include postresuscitation cognitive impairment and the guarded prognosis for survivors.

2. Finkelmeier et al, 1984. These investigators[10] studied two groups of patients: 60 SCD survivors and 45 patients with "serious arrhythmias" but no SCD episode. The patient groups were not significantly different in age, sex, marital status, underlying heart disease, coexisting chronic illness, type of treatment, inducibility, activity level, and return to work. The SCD survivors (78% were male; mean age, 58 years) had a total of 104 arrests, with 23 patients experiencing more than one. The time from the initial arrest was <1 year for 42% of the SCD survivors.

The SCL-90, a multidimensional symptom inventory, was used to quantify psychopathology in 9 areas: somatization, obsessive-compulsive, interpersonal sensitivity, depression, anxiety, hostility, phobic-anxiety, paranoid ideation, and psychoticism.[11] This instrument focuses on the last 3 months of the patient's experience. SCL-90 scores were essentially the same for the two groups, with both having scores on the General Symptom Index, Positive Symptom Distress Index, and the Positive Symptom Total Scores significantly ($P<0.05$) higher than normal values for a population of normal subjects. The only area in which there were significant differences between groups was that the SCD survivors had lower scores in the area of somatization than the comparison group. The extent of reported symptoms must be considered in the interpretation of these data, because many of the subjects were on antiarrhythmic therapy that can produce side effects.

This study also explored patient recall of the SCD experience. A surprising two thirds of the SCD survivors reported remembering some aspect of the event—typically awareness of caregivers working around them as well as awareness of what was being said. This is in contrast to more recent data in which SCD patients tend to report no memory of the event[12] and may be influenced by data collection being done at a different point in the recovery process.

3. Kolar and Dracup, 1990. A third study[13] used a cross-sectional design to compare psychosocial adjustment in 19 SCD survivors with that in 21 patients with ventricular arrhythmias but no SCD. Groups were generally comparable (although the SCD survivors tended to be younger, with a mean age of 58.8 versus 62.9 years), not retired, and better educated, with three exceptions: patients with ventricular arrhythmias and no SCD were more likely to be taking oral diuretics, to have cardiomyopathy, and to have had more dysrhythmic episodes). As in previous studies, subjects were primarily male (57.9% of SCD survivors and 81% of comparison group). The length of time since the arrest event in the SCD survivors cannot be determined from this report; however, it is re-

ported that the "last event" was a mean of 10.8 months earlier. It is unclear whether the "last event" was indeed the arrest.

The Psychosocial Adjustment to Illness scale (PAIS-SR) of Derogatis and Lopez[14] was used to measure psychosocial adjustment. This instrument has seven domains: healthcare orientation, vocational environment, domestic environment, sexual relationship, extended family relationship, social environment, and psychological distress.

Mean total and all subscale scores on the PAIS-SR were not statistically different between the two groups. Total scores were consistent with those reported in other cardiac populations and well below the level indicating the need for psychosocial intervention. In both groups, mean scores reflected that the best psychosocial adjustment was in the area of vocational environment; however, 26.2% of the SCD survivors and more than half (52.4%) of the comparison group were retired. In the SCD survivors, 42.1% were employed full-time, compared with 28.6% of the comparison group. Scores in both groups reflected that the most problematic areas of adjustment were in healthcare orientation and extended family relationships.

In multiple regression analysis for the combined groups, being married and not having a history of heart failure predicted better scores on the social environment domain. Being married and having fewer dysrhythmic events predicted lower psychological distress scores. The authors note that the time since the cardiac arrest may have clouded any differences that might have been present between SCD survivors and those who had not had that experience. They concluded that ". . . sudden cardiac death is not, in itself, predictive of poor psychosocial adjustment."[13] (p 53)

Summary

Findings from these studies are consistent in that there are similarities between SCD patients and comparison groups. In the Druss and Kornfeld report, the diagnoses of the patients who had not experienced SCD was not specified. Both groups of patients were cared for in a special care unit with cardiac monitoring. Although there was wide variability across patients in the point of recovery at which data were collected, similar and serious psychological problems were noted.

The remaining two studies used widely utilized measures to identify whether patients with ventricular dysrhythmias differed by whether or not they were SCD survivors. In measurements of either aspects of emotional status[10] or dimensions of psychosocial adjustment,[13] the patient groups were comparable. Given the drama of the

SCD experience, this finding is somewhat surprising. One explanation for this lack of difference may be the difference in amounts of time elapsing between the cardiac arrest and data collection.

Studies of SCD Survivors

Three more recent investigations have focused exclusively on SCD survivors; two of these included family members. These studies are summarized in Table 2.

1. Dougherty, 1994. This longitudinal study[15] of 15 SCD survivors and 15 family members began at hospital discharge, with data collected at 1, 3, 6, and 12 months after arrest. Multiple methods were used (quantitative and qualitative). Instruments were used to measure constructs in the areas of (1) psychological reactions: (a) Profile of Mood States (POMS),[16] (b) the State-Trait Anxiety Inventory (STAI),[17] and (c) the Distancing Subscale of the Ways of Coping Checklist-Revised[18]; (2) neurological sequelae: (a) Confusion-Bewilderment subscale of the POMS,[16] (b) Neurobehavioral Cognitive Status Examination,[19] and (c) Trailmaking A and B tests;[20,21] and (3) family adjustment: (a) Dyadic Adjustment Scale[22] and (b) Family Crisis Oriented Personal Evaluation Scales.[23] Family members completed only the POMS, STAI, and measures of family adjustment. Interviews were also conducted at each data collection point.

Subjects were again primarily male (86.6%), with a mean age of 57 years. Mean length of hospital stay was 22 days, with all SCD survivors receiving an ICD. Family members had a mean age of 53 years and tended to be female spouses.

Findings from this study revealed that the levels of anxiety, depression, anger, global stress, and confusion at discharge were higher than at subsequent data collection points. This was also true for family adjustment and dyadic satisfaction. Family members reported less psychological stress than patients. It was noted that the postarrest hospitalization was the most stressful time of the first year after SCD. The only exception to this was that denial increased over time.

2. Dougherty and Shaver, 1995. In this repeated-measures design study,[24] data were collected from 21 SCD survivors at 48-hour intervals during their postarrest hospital stay. The mean time from arrest to the first data collection point was 2.3 days. Several measures were used, including (1) the Profile of Mood States,[16] which focuses on the emotional indicators of anxiety, depression, and anger; (2) a portion of the Ways of Coping Checklist-Revised[18]; and (3) the Mishel Uncertainty in Illness Scale.[25] Cognitive function and

TABLE 2

Summary of Published Studies Reviewed: SCD Survivors

Study	Quality-of-Life Measure(s)/Method(s)	Quality-of-Life Results
Author: Dougherty[15]	Instruments	At discharge: Levels of anxiety, depression, anger, global stress, and confusion were higher than at subsequent data collection points. There were no significant differences between scores of patients and family members.
	Psychological reactions	
Date: 1994	Profile of Mood States (POMS)	
	Spielberger State-Trait Anxiety	
Design: Descriptive and longitudinal	Inventory (STAI)	
	Ways of Coping Checklist (revised)	
Subjects: 15 patients (SCD survivors) and 15 family members	Neurological sequelae	
	Confusion-Bewilderment Scale of POMS	
	Neuro-Behavioral Cognitive Status	
Study aim: Description of impact of SCD survival on patients and family members.	Examination (NCSE)*	
	Trailmaking A and B*	
	Family adjustment	
Note: Part of a larger study of family adjustment, physical recovery, emotional reactions, and neurological impact of SCD during first year	Family Crises Oriented Personal Evaluation Scales (F-COPES)	
	Dyadic Adjustment Scale	
	*Interviews: patients only	

*Interviews: patients only

Authors: Doughtery and Shaver[24]	Interviews: every 24 to 48 hours during postarrest hospitalizations	There were no differences over time in the emotional indicators. Levels of confusion were low, as were levels of anxiety, depression, and anger, although anxiety, denial, and depression were most evident at first interview. Uncertainty was elevated at all data collection points. Neurocognitive deficits were primarily lack of construction ability and impaired memory.
Date: 1995		
Subjects: 21 SCD survivors	Instruments Profile of Mood States (POMS) Ways of Coping Checklist (revised) Mishel Uncertainty in Illness Scale	
Study aim: Identification of emotional, cognitive, and physiological parameters of early recovery.	Neurobehavioral Cognitive Status Examination Trailmaking A and B	
Authors: Doolittle and Sauvé[12]	Qualitative interviews: In hospital and at 6 to 8, 12 to 15, and 22 to 25 weeks after SCD episode	In hospital, the different reference points of patients and spouses were identified: Patients typically had no memory of SCD experience; their focus was prearrest life and returning to it If spouse witnessed the arrest, it became the focus If spouse did not witness the arrest, focus was on postarrest life.
Date: 1995		
Design: Phenomenological and longitudinal		
Subjects: 40 patients (SCD survivors) and 30 spouses		
Study aim: Exploration of psychological and social impact of SCD on patient and spouse. Note: Part of a larger study of cognitive impairment in SCD survivors.		

physiological responses (number of arrhythmias) were also measured. In addition, interviews were conducted.

Subjects were primarily male (85.7%), with a mean age of 60.8 years; just over half (55%) were employed at the time of the arrest. Nearly three fourths (71.4%) had experienced their first episode of SCD.

High levels of denial and uncertainty were documented during this in-hospital phase of recovery. Although the sample size was small and standard deviations of scores obtained were admittedly high, the results show that "On the average, SCD survivors were not excessively anxious, depressed, angry, or confused during hospitalization, but they did report high levels of denial and uncertainty."[25] (p 160) Of note is the finding that scores on these measures did not change significantly over the period of hospitalization, which was a mean of 13.2 days (median, 6 days), although anxiety, depression, and denial were highest at the first data collection point.

3. Doolittle and Sauvé, 1995. As part of a larger study, 40 SCD survivors and 30 spouses of these patients were interviewed.[12] Although the focus was on the extent, prevalence, and natural history of cognitive impairment in survivors of SCD, the social and psychological impact of aborted SCD was considered in a phenomenological design.

Subjects were primarily male (85%), with a mean age of 62 years. The initial interview took place during the postarrest hospitalization. The mean time from arrest to the interview was 10.2 days. Findings from the interview data offer a major contribution to knowledge about understanding SCD survival in their recognition of the different perspectives of patients and their spouses, depending on whether the arrest was witnessed by the spouse, which indeed it was in 70% of the patients.

The three perspectives identified, labeled reference points, were that (1) SCD patients are interested in prearrest life and returning to it; (2) spouses witnessing the arrest use the arrest as a reference point; and (3) spouses who do not witness the arrest use postarrest life as a reference point.

Summary

Collectively, these three reports enrich our understanding of the SCD experience from the patient's perspective and offer glimpses into the impact of the experience on spouse and family members. These data were collected much earlier in the recovery period than in the first group of studies. Generally, the aspects of quality of life considered improve over time, with the most difficulties noted in the very early stages of recovery.

Studies in Progress

Two studies in progress offer information related to the topic of this paper. The first is a longitudinal nursing research study, and the second is a national randomized clinical trial.

1. Adaptation to Living with an Implanted Cardioverter-Defibrillator (ICD) (NIH NINR contract RO1-NR-03046). This prospective, longitudinal study is in the final stages of data collection. Major purposes of this study are to examine coping and adaptive outcomes before and during the 9 months after ICD insertion and to describe the sensations of ICD firing. Key variables include functional status, affective state, cognitive appraisal, coping, dispositional optimism, and patient concerns.

The instruments being used include the Heart Failure Functional Status Inventory,[26] Profile of Mood States,[16] Meaning of Illness Questionnaire,[27] Jalowiec Coping Scale,[28] Life Orientation Tool,[29] and the Patient Concerns Assessment.[30]

Of the 213 patients enrolled, about one fourth (n=49) had experienced SCD. Preimplantation data were analyzed to see whether there were significant differences on any of these measures between SCD survivors and those who had not had the arrest experience; none were found. In addition, 154 family members were also enrolled in the study; the majority of these were spouses. When their baseline, preimplantation data were also examined to test whether scores of family partners of SCD patients were different, again, no statistically significant differences were found. Analysis of data from 9 months of follow-up will reveal whether SCD survivors differ on key study variables at subsequent data collection points.

Preliminary reports from this study have documented the concerns of patients who receive an ICD just before implantation[30] and at 1 month[31] and 3 months[32] after implantation. Although the mean number of concerns reported drops significantly after implantation, fatigue remains the most frequently reported concern over time.

In addition, mood disturbance/affective state has been examined in these patients before[33] and 1 month after implantation,[34] as well as compared with those of family members at 1[35] and 3 months after implantation.[36] As this study is completed, additional information about aspects of quality of life will become available.

2. Antiarrhythmics Versus Implantable Defibrillators (AVID) (NIH NHLBI contract N01-HC-25117). Some patients who have survived one or several episodes of cardiac arrest are being enrolled in a large, multisite, randomized clinical trial comparing two treatments of ventricular rhythm disturbances.[8] The definition of quality of life being used in this study is that it is individually perceived, dynamic, multidimensional, and quantifiable by individual

self-report. The quality-of-life battery includes (1) a single-item life satisfaction rating, (2) the Medical Outcomes Study Short Form-36 (SF-36),[37] (3) the Ferrans and Powers Quality of Life Index (Cardiac Version), and (4) Patient Concerns Assessment.[30] This assessment is administered at baseline in the hospital before randomization to treatment, with sections of the battery repeated at intervals (3, 6, and 12 months and annually thereafter).

Preliminary analysis of baseline data from the first 451 patients completing the quality-of-life assessment was conducted. These subjects represent 75% of patients randomized to treatment in the first 28 months of the trial. These subjects were primarily (81.3%) male, with a mean age of 65.11 years and a mean ejection fraction of 32%. Because whether patients had experienced a cardiac arrest was not tracked as a variable, all quality-of-life scores were compared by the proxy variable of whether the patient had experienced ventricular tachycardia or ventricular fibrillation.

In general, no statistically significant differences were found. The one exception to this was that at entry, the only score that differed significantly was that subjects who had had ventricular fibrillation self-reported more concerns ($P=0.036$) than those with ventricular tachycardia as the index event. Although this difference was statistically significant, the numerical difference in total number of concerns reported was only 1.73, a value that is not likely to be clinically significant.

These findings suggest that quality-of-life perceptions before treatment generally do not vary by type of ventricular rhythm disturbance. AVID seeks to enroll a total of 1200 patients, so it will be interesting to see whether this conclusion holds in the total sample as well as whether it holds over time in the follow-up assessments of quality of life planned in this longitudinal study. Recently, data collection began on quality of life in spouses/partners of AVID patients, so it will be possible to examine their data as well for differences between spouses of patients who survived SCD and those who did not experience SCD.

Summary

From these few studies, several summary statements can be drawn about what is currently known about quality-of-life issues in survivors of SCD. The studies reported have small sample sizes and are not generalizable because of exclusion, by necessity, of those patients who are most seriously ill, particularly in the area of cognitive impairment. Studies in progress will yield data from larger samples but again will exclude the sickest patients.

In qualitative studies, interview data dramatically reflect the SCD experience as fraught with emotional turmoil for both patients and spouses/family members. On quantitative measures, when it is possible to compare SCD survivors with their spouses/family members, patients have higher levels of psychological distress. Comparison groups are rarely available; however, when they are, it appears that in early stages of recovery, levels of psychological distress are higher in SCD survivors than normative sample scores, but when survivors are compared with other cardiac patients with dysrhythmia or selected quality-of-life variables, no statistically significant differences are found. The earlier in the recovery period that quality-of-life issues are measured, the greater the levels of psychological distress.

Much is yet to be learned about quality-of-life issues in SCD survivors, and more systematic study is clearly indicated. Currently, only bits and pieces of knowledge on patient perspectives exist. Although these pieces are few in number, it is important for caregivers to be aware of them during the early phases of recovery, which is demonstrably a particularly challenging time for patients and family members.

References

1. Brooks R, McGovern BA, Garan H, et al. Current treatment of patients surviving out-of-hospital cardiac arrest. *JAMA*. 1991;265:762–768.
2. Bergner M. Quality of life, health status, and clinical research. *Med Care*. 1989;27(suppl):S-148-S-156.
3. Gill TM, Feinstein AR. A critical appraisal of the quality of quality-of-life measurements. *JAMA*. 1994;272:619–626.
4. Kinney MR. Assessment of quality of life in recovery settings. *J Cardiovasc Nurs*. 1995;10:88–96.
5. National Institutes of Health. *Health-Related Quality of Life: Findings From NHLBI-Supported Clinical Research*. US Department of Health and Human Services: NHLBI; 1995.
6. Schron EB, Shumaker SA. The integration of health quality of life in clinical research: experiences from cardiovascular clinical trials. *Prog Cardiovasc Nurs*. 1992;7:21–28.
7. Wiklund J, Gorkin L, Pawitan Y, et al. Methods for assessing quality of life in the Cardiac Arrhythmia Suppression Trial (CAST). *Qual Life Res*. 1992;1:187–201.
8. AVID Investigators. Antiarrhythmics versus implantable defibrillators (AVID): rationale, design, and methods. *Am J Cardiol*. 1995;75: 470–475.
9. Druss RG, Kornfeld DS. Survivors of cardiac arrest: a psychiatric study. *JAMA*. 1967;205:75–80.
10. Finkelmeier BA, Kenwood MJ, Summers C. Psychological ramifications of survival from sudden cardiac death. *Crit Care Q*. 1984;7:71–79.
11. Derogatis LR. *SCL-90 Administration, Scoring, and Procedures Manual-I for the Revised Version*. Baltimore, Md: Johns Hopkins University Press; 1977.

12. Doolittle ND, Sauvé MJ. Impact of aborted sudden cardiac death on survivors and their spouses: the phenomenon of different reference points. *Am J Crit Care.* 1995;4:389–396.
13. Kolar JA, Dracup K. Psychosocial adjustment of patients with ventricular dysrhythmias. *J Cardiovasc Nurs.* 1990;4:44–55.
14. Derogatis LR, Lopez MC. *PAIS Administration Scoring and Procedures Manual.* Baltimore, Md: Clinical Psychometric Research; 1983.
15. Dougherty CM. Longitudinal recovery following sudden cardiac arrest and internal cardioverter defibrillator implantation: survivors and their families. *Am J Crit Care.* 1994;3:145–154.
16. McNair D, Lorr M, Droppleman L. *Edits Manual: Profile of Mood States.* San Diego, Calif: Educational Testing Service, 1981.
17. Spielberger C, Gorsuch R, Lushene R. *Manual for the State-Trait Anxiety Inventory (Self-Evaluation Questionnaire).* Palo Alto, Calif: Consulting Psychologists Press; 1970.
18. Lazarus RS, Folkman S. *Stress, Appraisal, and Coping.* New York, NY: Springer Publishing; 1984:328.
19. Kiernan RJ, Mueller J, Langston W, et al. The neurobehavioral cognitive status examination: a brief but differentiated approach to cognitive assessment. *Ann Intern Med.* 1987;107:481–485.
20. Reitan RM. The relation of the trailmaking test to organic brain damage. *J Consult Psychol.* 1955;19:393–394.
21. Reitan RM, Wolfson D. *The Halstead Reitan Neuropsychological Test Battery.* Tucson, Ariz: Neuropsychology Press; 1985.
22. Spanier GB. Assessing dyadic adjustment: new scales for assessing the quality of marriage and similar dyads. *J Marriage Family.* 1976;38:15–28.
23. McCubbin HI, Thompson AI. *Family Assessment Inventories for Research and Practice.* Madison, Wis: University of Wisconsin Press; 1987.
24. Dougherty CM, Shaver JF. Psychophysiological responses after sudden cardiac arrest during hospitalization. *Appl Nurs Res.* 1995;8:160–168.
25. Mishel MH. Perceived uncertainty and stress in illness. *Res Nurs Health.* 1984;7:163–171.
26. Dracup K, Walden J, Stevenson L, et al. Quality of life in patients with advanced heart disease. *J Heart Lung Transplant.* 1992;11:273–279.
27. Lazarus R, Folkman, S. *Stress, Appraisal and Coping.* New York, NY: Springer Publishing; 1984:117–180.
28. Jalowiec A. Stress and coping in hypertensive and emergency room patients. *Nurs Res.* 1981;30:10–15.
29. Schelier MF, Carver LS. Optimism, coping, and health: assessment and implications of generalized outcome expectancies. *Health Psychol.* 1985;4:219–247.
30. Jenkins LS, Dunbar SB, Hawthorne MH. Patient concerns pre-ICD implantation. *Circulation.* 1994;90(suppl I):I-424. Abstract.
31. Jenkins LS, Dunbar SB, Hawthorne MH, Dudley WH. Patient concerns before and one month post device implantation. *Circulation.* 1995;92(suppl I):I-584. Abstract.
32. Jenkins LS, Dunbar SB, Dudley WH, Hawthorne MH. Living with an ICD: gender differences in early recovery. *Ann Behav Med.* 1996; D109:S240. Abstract.
33. Dunbar SB, Hawthorne MH, Jenkins LS, Porter L. Predictors of affective state in patients with recurrent dysrhythmia. *Circulation.* 1994;90 (suppl I):I-424. Abstract.

34. Porter LA, Dunbar SB, Jenkins LS, Hawthorne MH. Correlates of depressed mood one month after internal cardioverter defibrillator implantation. *Ann Behav Med.* 1995;17:5001–5024, S136.
35. Dunbar SB, Jenkins LS, Hawthorne MH, Dudley WH. Differences in patient and family member mood before and one month after implantable cardioverter defibrillator insertion. *Circulation.* 1995;92 (suppl I):I-585. Abstract.
36. Dunbar SB, Dudley WH, Jenkins LS, Hawthorne MH. Patient and family member mood disturbance after ICD insertion. *Ann Behav Med.* 1996;A011:S133. Abstract.
37. Ware JE Jr, Sherbourne CD. The MOS 36-item short-form health survey. *Med Care.* 1992;30:473–483.

Chapter 17

Coping and Behavioral Responses

Sandra B. Dunbar, RN, DSN, Louise Sherman Jenkins, RN, PhD, Mary Hawthorne, RN, PhD, Laura Porter, RN, PhD, and William N. Dudley, PhD

When patients survive a sudden cardiac arrest or live with the threat of a malignant ventricular dysrhythmia, the psychological reactions are profound. Behavioral and emotional responses to life-threatening dysrhythmia and treatment with an implantable cardioverter-defibrillator (ICD) and coping strategies used to alleviate the distress are reviewed in this chapter. Studies testing interventions to enhance patient outcomes to recurrent ventricular dysrhythmia are reviewed, with a summary of potential directions for future research.

Psychological Responses to Sudden Cardiac Arrest and Ventricular Arrhythmia

Psychological distress in patients who experience serious ventricular dysrhythmias and survive cardiac arrest has been described since the early 1960s, when modern cardiac resuscitation was developed, and has included anxiety, depression, fear, irritability, insomnia, and a sense of helplessness and loss of control.[1-3] Long-term antiarrhythmic medication, changes in work status, advanced cardiac impairment, unmarried marital status, and number of dysrhythmia episodes have been associated with greater distress in recurrent ventricular dysrhythmia patients.[4,5] Self-reported strategies used by patients with serious ventricular dysrhythmias to manage concerns about their illness have included

Partially supported by NIH NINR RO1NR03047, Adaptation to the ICD.

From: Dunbar SB, Ellenbogen KA, Epstein AE, (eds). *Sudden Cardiac Death: Past, Present, and Future.* Armonk, NY: Futura Publishing Company, Inc.; © 1997.

categories of self-reliance, acceptance, diversion, and doing nothing, as well as feeling unable to handle the situation.[6] In one study of 100 patients (84 men, 17 women) with serious ventricular dysrhythmias who were waiting for ICD implantation, we reported that total mood disturbance could be predicted by lower measures of trait optimism, female sex, higher perceived threat, and greater use of evasive coping strategies.[7] Thus, patients with serious ventricular dysrhythmia who are candidates for an ICD bring existing personality traits as well as newly forming sets of appraisals, coping behaviors, and psychological responses to the process of recovery.

Psychosocial Responses After ICD Implantation

Psychological responses in ICD recipients include anxiety greater than in the normal population, depression, global stress, and confusion. Morris and colleagues[8] found that 50% of their sample of ICD patients had some type of psychiatric disorder, identified as transient adjustment disorders, major depressions, and panic disorders. When patients with ICDs were compared with others who had been resuscitated from sudden cardiac arrest and treated with antiarrhythmic medications, few differences in mood were found; thus, it remains unclear whether the anxiety and depression are related more to the underlying cardiac disease or the ICD therapy itself.[9] While some patients with ICDs have reported viewing the device as a source of security, others have voiced concerns over its function.[10] Conflicting results have been found in terms of the relation of anxiety and number of shocks experienced by patients in the recovery period. Greater anxiety has been reported in those experiencing more than five shocks and in younger age groups.[11,12] Keren et al[13] found no difference in the anxiety levels of those who received a shock versus those who did not receive a shock when matched on many factors, including age, although social factors were not matched. Dougherty's[14] study of cardiac arrest survivors (n=15) found that anxiety, depression, anger, and stress levels were higher for patients and family members if ICD shocks were experienced compared with those who received no shock.

Unique Stressors of Recovery, ICD Shocks, and Sensory Experiences

Since the ICD may deliver shocks for a variety of arrhythmias, many of the expressed fears and concerns related to the anticipated sensation of being shocked, device failure, the social context in which the potential shock may occur, possible unsuccessful shocks, multiple shocks, battery failure, uncertainty about what to do, and death.[10,14–19] Lack of control and unpredictability may also contribute to fear, because most patients have no warning symptoms and loss of unconsciousness is unpredictable.[20]

In the only prospective study of ICD shock experiences, it was found that 88% of patients reported postshock nervousness and professed a need to discuss the event.[16] Physical sensations reported during shock included pain, and the most frequent visual analogue rating was 5 on a 1 to 10-point scale, indicating moderate pain sensations. With multiple shocks, sensations escalated and were accompanied by feelings of pain, fear, dread, and helplessness. Although shocks have been noted to occur during sleep and throughout the 24-hour time period for individual patients,[21] the times of day that shocks occurred most frequently were during the early morning hours from 7 to 11 AM and during daytime activities.[16] The circadian rhythm of arrhythmia is discussed elsewhere in this monograph.

In addition to concerns about shocks, patients with ICDs have concerns regarding driving restrictions, medication regimens, costs, time involved in follow-up care, lack of knowledgeable personnel in their home communities, sexual activity, social support, and body image changes.[10,15,22–24] Many report symptoms of fatigue, tiredness, heat intolerance, dizziness, and weakness. In addition to device awareness and pain, sleep disturbance is one of the most common complaints and is usually attributed to the physical discomfort of the generator, fear of getting shocked during sleep, and dreams or nightmares.[25] In summary, patients have numerous concerns during the recovery period that may be amenable to creative nursing interventions.

Behavioral Coping and Neuroendocrine Responses to the ICD

Kuiper and Nyamanthi[17] used a cross-sectional approach to study stressors and coping strategies at 4 to 14 months after ICD insertion. A semistructured interview revealed perceived stressors in physical, psychological, and social areas. Both problem-focused and emotion-focused coping were used, and scores on the Jalowiec Coping Scale revealed high use and perceived effectiveness of "optimistic" strategies and low use of "emotive" (expression of emotions) strategies. Age was negatively correlated with coping strategies of taking action, positive thinking, self-reliance, and expression of emotions. Neither cognitive appraisal nor adaptive outcomes were measured or related to the coping behaviors. The number of ICD discharges was reported but not in relation to other results. Dougherty's[26] longitudinal study of 15 cardiac arrest survivors with ICDs examined denial as a coping strategy and found that it remained high over the 1 year after implantation. Research on coping with ICDs is limited, but data from these and other studies with cardiac patients suggest that greater use of emotion-focused coping may not be effective and may lead to more negative emotions.[27]

Adaptation to the ICD: Preliminary Report

One aim of the project entitled "Adaptation to the ICD" (NIH NINR R01-NR-03047) was to determine the relation between coping and adaptive outcomes for patients with ICDs during the first 9 months after insertion. The following data are reported for the early recovery period or through the first 3 months after ICD implantation. These data were collected with a longitudinal design to follow patients with ICDs from the preoperative period through the first 3 months after implantation. Data were collected at baseline in the acute-care setting, with follow-up data collected by mail and telephone interview at 1 and 3 months after implantation. Figure 1 shows the coping-adaptation conceptual framework derived from Lazarus and Folkman,[28] which guided the study. Patient variables included demographic and clinical data and measures of affective state (total mood disturbance [TMD] score on the Profile of Mood States [POMS]), coping behaviors (Jalowiec Coping Scale), illness cognitive appraisal (Threat and Challenge subscales from the Meaning in Illness Questionnaire), functional status (Heart Failure Functional Status Inventory), and dispositional optimism (Life Orientation Test). Concerns were measured by the ICD Patient Assessment.[25] Audiotaped semistructured telephone interviews regarding experiences and coping behaviors during the recovery process were conducted at 1 and 3 months after implant. Interview data were coded by use of Ethnograph, with interrater reliability established and verified.

Setting and Sample

Subjects were recruited by three clinical centers in the Southeast and Midwest from the five tertiary and community-level hospitals. Two hundred thirteen patients (77% of those eligible) were enrolled. To date, 35 patients (16% of those enrolling) are no longer followed, for the following reasons: 17 withdrew because of deteriorating health, lack of interest, or feelings of stress; 8 were lost to follow-up

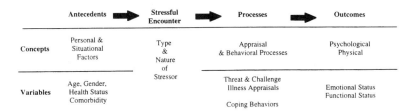

FIGURE 1. *Model of stress-coping process.*

because they received a heart transplant or could not be contacted by mail or phone; and 10 died after hospital discharge. Twenty subjects had incomplete data because of rehospitalizations at follow-up times or failure to return material. The data reported are from the 158 ICD patient subjects who have completed 3-month data collection.

Demographic characteristics of the total ICD patient sample are as follows: The mean age was 59.59±12.82 years (range, 25 to 85 years), with 131 men (83.1%) and 27 women (16.9%). Most subjects were married (79.3%). Mean left ventricular ejection fraction was 32.34±12.71%. Twenty-three percent had been resuscitated from cardiac arrest. The majority (60.7%) had an abdominal surgical approach with transvenous leads (85.7%), although a trend toward pectoral sites evolved toward the end of patient enrollment.

Repeated-measures analyses of variance including entry, 1-month, and 3-month scores (n=158) showed significant change across time for mood disturbance (POMS scores), which decreased slightly but significantly from entry to 1 month, with relative stability from 1 to 3 months (see Table 1). Examination of the subscales of the POMS revealed that declines in TMD scores were primarily due to decreases in the subscale of confusion and slight increases in vigor. Depression and tension subscale scores showed little change. The number of concerns about symptoms decreased from entry to 1 month, followed by a significant increase from 1 to 3 months. At 3 months, the most frequently reported concerns were fatigue, interrupted sleep, fear about one's health and future, reduced activity, and feelings of frustration.[29]

These mean trends reflect the overall recovery process and suggest that the highest mood disturbance is in the acute phase, with some improvement in mood occurring by 1 month and 3 months after implant. The wide variation in recovery response reflected by the range of scores on the POMS requires further analysis. These trends reflect significant time points in the recovery process at which interventions may improve the pattern of recovery for some patients beyond that which occurs by the usual standard of care and individual adjustment process.

TABLE 1

Means and Standard Deviations Across Time

Variable	Entry	1 Month	3 Months
Number of concerns about Symptoms*	10.0±5	6.7±4	7.4±5
POMS*	37.4±36	21.0±33	21.0±35
Range	−21 to 143	−32 to 136	−32 to 135

*Significant change over time for entry, 1 month, and 3 months, $P<0.001$.

Whether outcomes of patients with ICDs in terms of affective state (mood disturbance) can be predicted by dispositional optimism, cognitive appraisal, symptoms, coping behaviors, number of ICD discharges (shocks), cardiac function, and patient demographic characteristics was assessed by a series of multiple regression analyses. Separate hierarchical regression analyses were used to predict TMD by the antecedent and process variables of the model. Personal variables (age, sex, marital status, and Life Orientation Test score) and situational variables (functional status, history of resuscitated cardiac arrest, ejection fraction, and comorbidity index) were entered as the first block and at 1 month accounted for 13% of the variance (F=3.64; $df=9$, 138; $P=0.0004$). The second step entered the 1-month stress appraisal variables (number of concerns about symptoms, fear, threat and challenge scores), problem-focused and emotion-focused coping scores, and number of shocks, which accounted for another 31% of the variance (total adjusted $R^2=0.44$; F=8.9; $df=15$, 132; $P=0.000$). In the full model, threat and challenge appraisal, symptoms, and emotion-focused coping behaviors had β-weights of $P<0.01$, with positive history of cardiac arrest significant at $P=0.05$. For 3-month TMD scores, 18% of the variance was accounted for at step 1, with functional status and optimism scores having significant β-weights. At step 2, the total adjusted R^2 was 0.48 (F=8.15; $df=16$, 110; $P=0.000$), and β-weights were significant for history of SCD ($P=0.05$), optimism ($P=0.02$), threat appraisal ($P=0.0002$), challenge appraisal ($P=0.0004$), symptoms ($P=0.003$), and emotion-focused ($P=0.008$) and problem-focused ($P=0.05$) coping. The direction of the relations in these models suggests that history of cardiac arrest, higher threat appraisal, lower challenge appraisal, greater symptoms, and greater use of emotion-focused and less use of problem-focused coping strategies were predictive of higher levels of mood disturbance.

In summary, patients' adaptive outcomes in terms of mood disturbance were predicted by the proposed theoretical variables. History of sudden cardiac arrest, greater threat and lower challenge appraisals, increased symptoms, and increased emotion-focused coping were consistent predictors of higher mood disturbance at both time points. These findings suggest that interventions aimed at appraisals, reducing symptom distress, and improving use of coping strategies could influence mood disturbance.

The influence of female sex on outcomes of mood disturbance at entry, 1 month, and 3 months was perplexing, given that women were not different from men on objective clinical data of left ventricular ejection fraction, NYHA class, or comorbidity. Men and women at 1 month had significant differences in depression, confusion, and tension subscales on the POMS. Content and thematic analysis of the 1-month interview data revealed significant themes of concerns expressed by women in the areas of body image, role changes, dependency, and activity levels. These data suggest some gender-specific concerns for women with ICDs that could be addressed through more focused intervention.[23] Greater understanding of the role of both sex and culture in adaptation to serious or life-threatening ventricular dysrhythmia and the ICD is warranted.

Potential Interventions

Although few studies have tested psychosocial interventions for patients with ventricular dysrhythmia and/or ICDs, the above studies suggest a direction for further investigation and clinical testing.

Support Groups

Support group interventions for patients with ICDs have been evaluated in two small pilot studies. Badger and Morris[30] compared role functioning and psychological adaptation in 6 ICD patients who self-selected to attend support groups with 6 who did not attend and found no differences between groups. Molchany and Peterson[31] compared the effects of a support group of 11 patients with ICDs and 5 nonattending patients similarly treated. Quantitative measures of anxiety and functional status did not change significantly with support group participation, although qualitative data (anecdotal notes) implied improved perceptions of ability to cope and increased satisfaction with life in group participants. Other anecdotal reports suggest that support groups may be beneficial for ICD patients, yet this strategy has limitations in the early recovery period for many patients who are physically or emotionally not ready to participate. For tertiary care centers with referral patients from a large geographic catchment area, the feasibility of frequent or consistent attendance at support groups is small.

Psychoeducational Interventions

Sneed and Finch[32] reported the effects of a randomized psychosocial nursing intervention on the early adjustment of 34 ICD patients and their caregivers. The intervention involved telephone contacts delivered weekly in the first month and every other week in the second month after implant, in-patient evaluation and counseling by a psychiatric liaison nurse, and participation in an ICD support group. No significant differences between treatment and control groups were found on the POMS or Psychosocial Adjustment to Illness Scale at 4 months after implantation.[32] This type of psychoeducational intervention could be tested for a more targeted patient population, such as those with high anxiety or depression during acute care.

Concrete Objective Information

Concrete objective information (COI) consists of two types of information: sensory and procedural. Sensory information includes typical subjective symptoms or sensations associated with a stressful experience. Knowledge of symptoms, including their frequency, intensity, and duration, can be obtained only from those who have undergone the experience. To reflect typical experiences, COI should include symptoms or sensations experienced by at least 50% of patients.[33] COI has undergone extensive theoretical and research development and is based in self-regulation theory, in which information is processed into a mental schema incorporating expectations and past experiences similar to cognitive appraisal of a situation. Accurate anticipatory sensory information is hypothesized to enhance coping by facilitating a less emotional interpretation of the experience.[34] Procedural information refers to aspects of the experience that can be observed by someone other than the patient, such as when follow-up appointments will be scheduled or when sutures will be removed. Procedural information reduces distress by enhancing congruence between patients' expectations and the actual experience.[33,34]

COI has been effective in several groups, enhancing coping and reducing psychological distress in patients undergoing radiation therapy, endoscopy and other invasive procedures. The effects of COI on cardiac patients have been studied primarily in those having cardiac catheterization. Watkins et al[35] provided preparatory procedural information only (n=29), sensory and procedural information (n=28), and usual standard instruction (n=29) to subjects having cardiac catheterization. Although there were no differences in the information groups in heart rate and blood pressure on arrival at the catheterization laboratory or in anxiety after the catherization, both intervention groups had significantly better outcomes than the control group. Anderson and Masur[36] found that sensory/procedural information before cardiac catheterization reduced levels of autonomic arousal before and during the catheterization and was better than a placebo intervention; and subjects who received an intervention involving modeling and coping skills also demonstrated less anxiety and better adjustment than control subjects. Rice et al[37] compared the responses of cardiac catheterization subjects receiving preparatory COI or usual care. The experimental group reported lower negative mood 1 to 2 hours before the procedure and the first day after the procedure, and they were observed to be less distressed. These studies demonstrate that COI is beneficial for cardiac patients undergoing a highly somatic procedure. No studies have examined the effects of COI on coping with cardiac procedures after hospitalization, such as the ICD population. Adjustment to the ICD involves coping with symptoms and sensations associated with surgery, awareness of the device in the body, and the possibility of an electric shock; thus, providing COI may facilitate the development of appraisals and enhance coping during the recovery process.

Symptom Management Training

Because of the nature of biopsychosocial symptoms experienced by patients with ICDs in the early recovery period and the associated distress, symptom management training may facilitate the patients' ability to manage at home. One model of symptom management involves the symptom experience (perception, evaluation, and response), symptom management, and symptom outcomes.[38] The management component involves assessment of the symptom from the patient's perspective and developing a focus for intervention. Since patients with ICDs report a large number of physical concerns, such as sleep difficulty, pain, incision discomfort, heat intolerance, and device awareness, focused symptom management training and protocols should be developed and tested for their effectiveness in this population.

Cognitive-Behavioral Therapy

Cardiac patients in general and dysrhythmia patients specifically may benefit from cognitive therapy in the form of reframing and coping training interventions.[39] Studies combining cognitive therapy with special counseling of cardiac patients have demonstrated positive outcomes in terms of lower depression and mortality.[40,41] Cognitive behavior interventions have been reported to be superior to patient education in reducing anxiety in patients undergoing cardiac catherization[42] and in patients experiencing cardiac awareness with panic disorder.[43] Although specific data are not reported, Fricchione et al[44] describe psychological approaches in specific ICD patient case studies and suggest that nurse- or psychiatrist-managed cognitive therapy may be highly useful with ICD patients.

Similarities are found between patients with epilepsy and those with serious cardiac dysrhythmia in that both are confronted with unpredictable and potentially devastating physical manifestations of their illness over which they may have little control. Both groups have reported psychological problems of depression, fear, anxiety, anger, and social isolation, and both have complex medication treatment regimens that interact with antidepressant medications.[44,45] Cognitive therapy that included negative thought–stopping, increasing positive cognitions, self-reinforcing statements, and focus on active self-management techniques was effective in reducing depression in a treatment group over a control group of epileptic patients.[46] The relevance of these studies with epileptic patients to patients with arrhythmias is found in the beneficial effects of a psychologically focused intervention in patients with life-threatening health problems and in health situations over which they perceive they have little control.

Family Interventions

Although family members are usually included in psychoeducational interventions such as education or support groups, with the exception of the work of Dracup et al (see chapter 14) no studies have tested the impact of a focused family intervention on outcomes of high-risk dysrhythmia patients or their family members. Clearly, additional research is needed in this area, because the trauma of cardiac arrest and high risk for dysrhythmia recurrence have an effect on the entire family system.[26,47]

Summary

The impact of life-threatening arrhythmia on a patient's mood states may be serious and may include depression, anxiety, and fear. These responses may be provoked regardless of whether or not the individual has experienced a cardiac arrest. Research-based interventions to facilitate psychosocial recovery are sparse and need to be developed and tested. Psychoeducational and family-based strategies hold much promise to improve recovery for patients with serious ventricular arrhythmia. The timing of such interventions may be important in the acute care setting and early recovery period to facilitate adaptation to the threat of recurrent ventricular arrhythmia and its treatment.

References

1. Bergner L, Bergner M, Hallstrom AP, et al. Health status of survivors of out-of-hospital cardiac arrest six months later. *Am J Public Health.* 1984;74:508–510.
2. Finkelmeier B, Kenwood N, Summers C. Psychological ramifications of surviving sudden cardiac death. *Crit Care Q.* 1984;7:71–79.
3. Vlay SC, Ficchione GL. Psychosocial aspects of surviving sudden cardiac death. *Clin Cardiol.* 1985;8:237–243.
4. Dunnington C, Johnson M, Finkelmeier B. Patients with heart rhythm disturbances: variables associated with increased psychologic distress. *Heart Lung.* 1988;17:381–389.
5. Kolar J, Dracup K. Psychosocial adjustment of patients with ventricular dysrhythmias. *J Cardiovasc Nurs.* 1990;4:44–55.
6. Burke LJ, Rogers BL, Jenkins LS. Living with recurrent ventricular dysrhythmias. *Focus Crit Care.* 1992;19:60–68.
7. Dunbar SB, Jenkins LS, Hawthorne MH, et al. Mood disturbance in patients with recurrent ventricular dysrhythmia prior to implantable cardioverter defibrillator insertion. *Heart Lung.* 1996;25:253–261.
8. Morris P, Badger J, Chmielewski L, et al. Psychiatric morbidity following implantation of the automatic implantable defibrillator. *Psychosomatics.* 1991;32:58–64.
9. Vlay SC. The automatic internal cardioverter-defibrillator: comprehensive clinical follow-up, economic and social impact: the Stony Brook experience. *Am Heart J.* 1986;112:189–194.
10. Sneed NV, Finch NJ. Experiences of patients and significant others with automatic implantable cardioverter defibrillator after discharge from the hospital. *Prog Cardiovascu Nurs.* 1992;7:20–24.
11. Luderitz B, Jung W, Deister A, et al. Patient acceptance of the implantable cardioverter defibrillator in ventricular tachyarrhythmias. *PACE.* 1993;16:1815–1821.
12. Vitale MB, Funk M. Quality of life in younger persons with an implantable cardioverter defibrillator. *DCCN Dimensions Crit Care Nurs.* 1995;14:100–111.

13. Keren R, Aarons D, Veltri E. Anxiety and depression in patients with life-threatening ventricular arrhythmias: impact of the implantable cardioverter-defibrillator. *PACE*. 1991;14: 181–186.
14. Dougherty CM. Pyschological reactions and family adjustment in shock versus no shock groups after implantation of internal cardioverter defibrillator. *Heart Lung*. 1995;24:281–291.
15. Cooper DK, Luceri RM, Thurer RJ. The impact of the automatic implantable cardioverter/defibrillator on quality of life. *Clin Prog Electrophysiol Pacing*. 1986;4:306–309.
16. Dunbar SB, Warner C, Purcell JA. Experiences of patients and families after internal cardioverter defibrillator discharge. *Heart Lung*. 1993; 22:494–501.
17. Kuiper R, Nyamanthi A. Stressors and coping strategies in patients with automatic implantable cardioverter defibrillator. *J Cardiovasc Nurs*. 1991;5:65–76.
18. Pycha C, Calabrese JR, Gulledge AD, et al. Patient and spouse acceptance and adaptation to implantable cardioverter defibrillator. *Cleveland Clin J Med*. 1990;57:441–444.
19. Pycha C, Gulledge AD, Hutzler J, et al. Psychological responses to the implantable defibrillator: preliminary observations. *Psychosomatics*. 1986;27:841–845.
20. Kou WH, Calkins H, Lewis RR, et al. Incidence of loss of consciousness during automatic implantable defibrillator shocks. *Ann Intern Med*. 1991;115:942–945.
21. Behrens S, Galecka M, Bruggemann T, et al. Circadian variation of sustained ventricular tachyarrhythmias terminated by appropriate shocks in patients with an implantable cardioverter defibrillator. *Am Heart J*. 1995;130:79–84.
22. Craney JM, Powers MT. (1995). Factors related to driving in persons with an implantable cardioverter defibrillator. *Prog Cardiovasc Nurs*. 1995;10:12–17.
23. Hawthorne MH, Dunbar SB, Jenkins LS, et al. Mood disturbance during early recovery in women after implantable cardioverter defibrillator placement. *Circulation*. 1995;92(suppl I):I–492. Abstract.
24. Vlay SC, Olson L, Fricchione GL, et al. Anxiety and anger in patients with ventricular tachyarrhythmias: responses after automatic internal cardioverter defibrillator. *PACE*. 1989;12:366–373.
25. Jenkins LS, Dunbar SB, Harthorne MH. Patient concerns pre-ICD implantation. *Circulation*. 1994;90(suppl I):I–424. Abstract.
26. Dougherty CM. Longitudinal recovery following sudden cardiac arrest and internal cardioverter defibrillator implantation: survivors and their families. *Am J Crit Care*. 1994;3:145–154.
27. Keckeisen M, Nyamanthi A. Coping and adjustment to illness in the acute myocardial infarction patient. *J Cardiovasc Nurs*. 1990;5:25–33.
28. Lazarus R, Folkman S. *Stress, Appraisal and Coping*. New York, NY: Springer Publishing Co; 1984.
29. Jenkins LS, Dunbar SB, Dudley WN. Living with an ICD: gender differences in concerns in early recovery. *Ann Behav Med*. 1966;(suppl): S240. Abstract.
30. Badger JM, Morris PLP. Observations of a support group for automatic implantable cardioverter-defibrillator recipients and their spouses. *Heart Lung*. 1989;18:238–243.
31. Molchany CA, Peterson KA. The psychosocial effects of support group

intervention on AICD recipients and their significant others. *Prog Cardiovasc Nurs.* 1994;9:23–29.

32. Sneed NV, Finch NJ. Effect of a psychosocial intervention on patients and families with AICD. Abstract. Presented at the Sigma Theta Tau Conference; 1995; Charleston, SC.

33. Christman NJ, Kirchhoff KT, Oakley MG. Concrete objective information. In: Bulecheck GM, McCloskey JC, (eds. *Nursing Interventions: Essentials Nursing Treatments.* 2nd ed. Philadelphia, Pa: Saunders; 1992.

34. Suls J, Wan CK. Effects of sensory and procedural information and coping with stressful medical procedures and pain: a meta-analysis. *J Consult Clin Psychol.* 1989;57:372–379.

35. Watkins LO, Weaver L, Odegaard V. Preparation for cardiac catheterization: tailoring the content of instruction to coping style. *Heart Lung.* 1986;15:382–389.

36. Anderson KO, Masur FT. Psychologic preparation for cardiac catheterization. *Heart Lung.* 1989;18:154–163.

37. Rice VH, Sieggreen M, Mullin M, et al. Development and testing of an arteriography information intervention for stress reduction. *Heart Lung.* 1988;17:23–28.

38. University of California San Francisco School of Nursing Symptom Management Faculty Group. A model for symptom management. *Image.* 1994;26:272–276.

39. Cowan MJ, Kogan HN, Buzaitis A, et al. Self-management biofeedback therapy for sudden cardiac arrest subjects: the use of process variables. In: *Nursing Research and Its Utilization: International State of the Science.* New York, NY: Springer Publishing; 1994:83–90.

40. Frasure-Smith N, Prince R. Long term follow-up of the ischemic heart disease life stress monitoring program. *Psychosom Med.* 1989;51:485–513.

41. Friedman M, Thoresen CE, Gill JJ, et al. Alteration of type A behavior and its effect on cardiac recurrences in post myocardial infarction patients. *Am Heart J.* 1986;112:663–665.

42. Kendall PC, Williams L, Pechacek TF, et al. Cognitive-behavioral and patient education interventions in cardiac catheterization procedures: the Palo Alto medical psychology project. *J Consult Clin Psychol.* 1979;47:49–58.

43. Antony MM, Meadows EA, Brown TA, et al. Cardiac awareness before and after cognitive-behavioral treatment for panic disorder. *J Anxiety Disorder.* 1994;8:341–350.

44. Fricchione GL, Vlay LC, Vlay SC. Cardiac psychiatry and the management of ventricular arrhythmias with the internal cardioverter-defibrillator. *Am Heart J.* 1994;128:1050–1059.

45. Chaplin JE, Yepez LR, Shorvon SD, et al. National general practice study of epilepsy: the social and psychological effects of a recent diagnosis of epilepsy. *Br Med J.* 1992;304:1416–1418.

46. Davis GR, Armstrong HE, Dennis DM, et al. Cognitive-behavioral treatment of depressed affect among epileptics: preliminary findings. *J Clin Psychol.* 1984;40:930–935.

47. Dunbar SB, Jenkins LS, Hawthorne MH, et al. Differences in patient and family member mood before and one month after implantable cardioverter defibrillator insertion. *Circulation.* 1995;92(suppl I):I–491. Abstract.

Chapter 18

Lifestyle and Ethical Issues:
Driving and Occupational Aspects

Andrew E. Epstein, MD

Introduction

Patients may experience complete or partial loss of consciousness when arrhythmias occur. Thus, the safety of both patients and others may be threatened when these individuals engage in such activities as driving. Furthermore, just as arrhythmias themselves may lead to impaired consciousness, antiarrhythmic therapies may alter the cognitive state as a consequence of reactions to drugs, shocks from implantable cardioverter-defibrillators (ICDs), and physical limitations that may follow arrhythmia operations.

One of the questions most commonly asked by patients, families, and society relates to the advisability of driving, because the safety of both patients and others may be threatened when personal or professional activities are performed by individuals with arrhythmias that may impair consciousness. In view of the magnitude of the problem, the American Heart Association (AHA) and the North American Society of Pacing and Electrophysiology (NASPE) cosponsored two conferences to examine the medical, ethical, and regulatory issues related to arrhythmias in the context of their relation to driving and other activities. Although these conferences addressed both supraventricular and ventricular arrhythmias, this chapter reviews the consensus related to only the latter. The full document describing the entire conference is published as a Medical/Scientific Policy Statement of the AHA.[1] This

From: Dunbar SB, Ellenbogen KA, Epstein AE, (eds). *Sudden Cardiac Death: Past, Present, and Future.* Armonk, NY: Futura Publishing Company, Inc.; © 1997.

chapter summarizes the position articulated in this statement regarding ventricular arrhythmias.

Risk of Death Related to Driving

Electrocardiographic recordings at the time of sudden cardiac death in ambulatory patients document that terminal events usually begin with ventricular tachycardia, followed by degeneration to ventricular fibrillation.[2-5] In nonambulatory, often hospitalized patients, such as those with congestive heart failure, bradycardia is more commonly observed.[6] Furthermore, a significant number of sudden deaths do occur as a consequence of noncardiac causes, such as pulmonary embolism, stroke, and ruptured aneurysms.[7]

The actual frequency of death while driving is uncertain. The primary cause of death is even less well known, and how often the event contributes to injury while the patient is driving is incompletely reported. Most importantly in the context of this discussion, the frequency with which ventricular tachycardia or ventricular fibrillation occurs in individuals who have survived a prior event while they are driving and especially their role in causing injury or harm to drivers or bystanders as a result of impaired consciousness of the driver, is completely undocumented. The data that follow illustrate these points.

Despite the anticipated danger of sudden cardiac death at the wheel leading to injury of others, available data do not support the contention that the problem is of large magnitude with respect to the issue of public safety. Norman[8] observed in 1960 that in 220 000 driver-years, only 14 of 46 drivers who lost consciousness at the wheel did so from a cardiac cause. In 12 of the 14 cases, the vehicle was moving, but only three accidents occurred, and no individuals other than the driver were injured. Similarly, Trapnell and Groff[9] reported no accidents in 50 cases of myocardial infarction that occurred in truck drivers. Of interest, 5 of the infarctions were recurrent, 4 occurred at work, and none resulted in an accident, in part because 4 of the individuals had stopped their vehicles beforehand. Herner et al[10] reported that of 44 255 road accidents that occurred in Sweden during the years 1959 to 1963, 41 were probably caused by sudden illness in the driver. Of these, 10 were attributed to epilepsy and 7 to myocardial infarction. Furthermore, 7 events occurred as a consequence of illnesses without loss of consciousness. The remainder were due to miscellaneous causes. Eight of the drivers died at the wheel as a result of their disease, including all 7 with myocardial infarction. However, in the latter cases, no one else was injured, although property damage occurred in 4 instances. From their data, Herner et al[11] estimate that 1/1000 to 3/1000 accidents are caused by driver impairment. There are rare reports of driver-related deaths resulting in the death of others.

In a landmark paper published in 1964, Myerburg and Davis[12] examined the circumstances of 1348 deaths due to coronary artery disease in Florida. Of 122 patients designated as having "hazardous occupations," 75 (61.4%) were responsible for ground transportation (truck drivers, 30.3%; taxi drivers, 16.4%; bus and streetcar operators, 7.4%; and a variety of others including railroad work, ambulance drivers, and chauffeurs). Thirteen (10.7%) were seamen and 8 (6.6%) were airmen (airline transport pilots, 2.5%; Air Force pilots, 2.5%; airline flight engineers, 0.8%; and commercial pilots, 0.8%). Of 52 persons who died while driving private automobiles, 32 had pulled their vehicles to the roadside without an accident. There were 15 minor accidents that resulted in property damage but no bodily injury, and there were no incidences of major property damage or fatalities to others in this series. There were 2 minor accidents related to the 15 deaths that occurred in truck drivers. Finally, 2 pilots died while flying. One was a commercial pilot, but the aircraft was landed by the crew without incident. The other was a young student pilot in a single-engine plane who probably died of myocardial infarction. The notable conclusions were that of 122 persons who died suddenly of coronary artery disease and who had occupations that were potentially dangerous to the public (9.1% of all sudden deaths), no serious accidents occurred as a consequence of the deaths. Similarly, of the 101 persons (7.5% of the population) who were performing a hazardous activity at the time of death (including 52 who were driving automobiles), no serious injury occurred to others.

The rarity of injury as a consequence of impaired driver consciousness has been reported by others.[13-17] All driver-related fatalities examined at the Office of the Chief Medical Examiner in Baltimore, Md, during the 4-year period 1956 to 1960 were reviewed by Peterson and Petty.[13] Of 81 deaths (80 drivers and 1 passenger), 36 drivers collapsed at the wheel as a consequence of an antecedent medical illness and had an accident. The remaining 45 individuals were dead or moribund at the wheel of an automobile that had not been in an accident. Of the drivers with accidents, 28 of 36 deaths were the result of heart disease (24 atherosclerotic). Other causes of death were dissecting aortic aneurysms in 2, a ruptured aortic aneurysm in 1, and stroke in 5. For the 36 drivers who collapsed, there were 21 accidents that resulted in damage to fixed objects or parked automobiles. In 6 cases, there were a total of 10 passengers accompanying the deceased driver. Of these passengers, only 1 was hospitalized for injuries. In 13 cases, moving vehicles were hit, and in 2 others the automobile left the road and hit no other object. In none of these instances was a person in the target vehicle injured.

Hossack[14] reported in 1974 that of 102 deaths of drivers at the wheel of their automobiles, 10 were probably due to coronary artery disease and 1 to aortic dissection. Five of the drivers had stopped their automobiles before death, thereby preventing injury. For the other 5, accidents, when they occurred, were minor and there was no injury to others. Öström and Eriksson[16] reported 126 sudden deaths in Swedish drivers. The majority (112/126) were due to ischemic heart disease. Among at least 31 individuals thought to be placed at risk during the driver's loss of consciousness, 2 suffered minor injuries, and no other road users were hurt. Similarly, Christian[17] reported 267 patients who died within 2 hours of arrival at an emergency room after a "road incident." Most drivers who died were able to stop their automobiles before their collapse. The only death of another person in addition to the patient occurred in a head-on accident in which the driver of the other vehicle was killed instantly. However, when other cars were hit, they were usually parked or traveling slowly, and there was no recorded injury to any of their occupants.

The incidence of injury associated with impaired consciousness while driving must be placed in the context of other risks associated with driving. Grattan and Jeffcoate[18] concluded in 1968 that in only 0.5%, at most, of 593 injury-related traffic accidents could chronic disease be considered contributory to the event. To assess the role that impaired consciousness has on driving, Parsons[19] in 1986 analyzed 131 press reports and the records of 92 patients who attended a neurological clinic. Almost 80% of the events were attributed to epilepsy, coronary artery disease, or falling asleep at the wheel. Whereas drivers with epilepsy and coronary disease frequently had warning before loss of consciousness, those who fell asleep did so without warning. Although these patients accounted for only 27% of the series, they accounted for 83% of the deaths attributed to trauma. This translates into a risk for traumatic death of 0.05 per incident in patients with a coronary disease cause of collapse and of 1.55 per incident when falling asleep was the cause of collapse, supporting the observation that falling asleep and fatigue represent much greater risks for injury than does sudden death due to coronary artery disease.

Alcohol is also a major contributor to deaths that occur during driving. West et al[11] recognized in 1968 that 648 of 871 drivers

(74%) who died as a result of an accident had blood alcohol levels averaging 0.19g/100 mL. Of 1026 drivers in the study, 155 (15%) died of natural causes at the wheel. Blood alcohol levels were measured in 96 patients, of whom 20 had "positive" tests, with 18 having levels >0.1 g/100 mL. Furthermore, high blood alcohol levels in the driver increased the risk of death to others. In the 155 accidents, 1 passenger was killed and 18 passengers were injured, 4 seriously. High blood alcohol levels were recorded in 4 of 5 drivers in whose vehicles passengers were killed or injured. No determination was made in the fifth.

Another point of comparison is the risk of having an accident as a function of age relative to the risk related to the presence of heart disease or a previously documented ventricular arrhythmia. In Oregon, individuals 16 to 19 years old have an average accident rate of 0.9%/mo (ie, 0.9 accidents per 100 drivers per month), compared with survivors of ventricular tachycardia and ventricular fibrillation, who have 1.8% and 1.1% average monthly risks, respectively, for experiencing an event that could impair their ability to operate a motor vehicle (recurrent ventricular fibrillation, poorly tolerated hemodynamically unstable ventricular tachycardia, syncope, sudden cardiac death, or ICD discharge).[20] In the 8 to 12 months after hospital discharge for treatment of ventricular arrhythmias, the accident rates were only 0.8% and 0.4% for survivors of ventricular tachycardia and fibrillation, respectively, similar to that of all licensed Oregon drivers (0.4%) and not different from the risk for teenage drivers. Conversely, an increased risk for death among the elderly has been recognized for years. In 1967, Waller[21] reported that healthy individuals 30 to 59 years old had 9.1 accidents per 1 million miles driven. In contrast, "healthy" individuals ≥60 years old had accident rates of 12.1 per 1 million miles driven, and patients with senility, cardiovascular disease, or both had accident rates of 19.3, 14.7, and 36.2 per 1 million miles driven, respectively. A similar distribution of increased fatalities for young and older drivers was documented in 1993.[22]

Anderson and Camm[23] extended these observations and made assumptions that allowed the incidence of sudden incapacitation in patients with ICDs to be estimated. The authors assumed that the presence of an ICD increased the risk of sudden incapacitation 100-fold and extrapolated that if 2/1000 fatal accidents were caused by such an event, there would be only a 0.5% rise in fatal accidents from sudden incapacitation. This translates into a net rise in fatal accidents of 0.001%. Stated in absolute terms, even when patients with ICDs die while driving, only 1 in 10 fatal events could be potentially attributable to an arrhythmia or the defibrillator.

The composite data support the following observations: First, sudden death due to a cardiac cause is a rate event during the performance of potentially dangerous activities and rarely results in injury to others when it does occur. Second, an increase in the overall death rate as a consequence of ventricular arrhythmias in patients with ICDs performing potentially dangerous activities is probably low. Nevertheless, it is unknown how these older data can be extrapolated to the present, when driving habits, automobile safety features, and the management of coronary disease and arrhythmias are all different. In regard to the latter, it is possible that the increased use of thrombolytic and β-blocker therapies, for example, may have decreased the risk of sudden death in drivers to levels even below those observed in earlier years. Furthermore, the frequency with which proarrhythmia due to either antitachycardia pacing or lower-energy shocks (causing ventricular fibrillation) contributes to the loss of consciousness and danger to the public is unknown.[24] If ICDs are used in lieu of antiarrhythmic drug therapy, the recurrence rate of sustained ventricular arrhythmias that impair consciousness could even be increased.[25]

Ethics of Regulation

It must be recognized that it is impossible to achieve a 0% risk to others when any activities are performed in society. Indeed, society has multiple precedents for accepting degrees of risk affected by certain members of the population. For example, we license the young and elderly to drive, allow measurable blood alcohol levels for people operating motorized vehicles, and legalize speed limits at which the risk of death in the event of an accident is clearly increased. What constitutes an acceptable risk is a function of the setting and activity in question. For example, although an individual may have a quantifiable risk for arrhythmia recurrence and a possible accident, consequences of arrhythmia recurrence will be different depending on whether the person is driving on a deserted country road or on an expressway at 70 mph. For activities that may affect the health of the public, society has legislated what it sees to be acceptable risks. For example, although blood alcohol levels fall on a continuum, "acceptable" risk is based on state-by-state assessments. Similarly, specific degrees of visual impairment preclude individuals from obtaining driver's licenses. On the other hand, it is much more difficult to legislate against activities that can be affected by illnesses that occur paroxysmally, such as arrhythmias, for which simple measurements (such as a blood alcohol level or vision test) cannot be used to assign risk. Because attendees of the AHA/NASPE Consensus Conferences felt constrained by the limitations of the data available on which to make recommendations, and since the rights of individuals, including the acceptance of personal risk, seem to compete with society's right to legislate a level of risk that it considers acceptable, a discussion of ethics was incorporated into their analysis.

Medical ethics deals with issues that relate to medical practice in the care of patients and their families, medical research, and public policies related to medical issues that impact on society. In the case of limiting activities in patients with arrhythmias, ethical considerations are even more important because guidelines are based, by necessity, on incomplete scientific data and risk cannot be absolutely eliminated. Since most individuals do not want to harm others and "virtuous" individuals (private drivers, pilots, or bus drivers) would want to remove themselves from activities that place others at risk, a tenable position is that society should have the power to restrict certain individuals from activities that may place others at risk of harm. However, individuals with and without arrhythmias must be treated equally, and any regulation that limits an individual's activity must be applied equally to all such individuals with a given condition.

Expectations of doctor-patient confidentiality further complicate the ethics of regulation. On the one hand, medical information is usually released to third parties only when patients give authorization. On the other hand, if a patient wishes to withhold medical information from an organization to preserve his job and security and if the physician knows that the patient's condition may place the individual and others at risk if the individual remains in the job, one school of thought believes that it is unethical to withhold this information. At the very least, the physician should try to persuade the patient to give permission for release of information, but if the patient refuses, there is an ethical responsibility for the physician to break confidentiality and alert the organization of the potential harm that could occur if the physician remained silent and the patient were to perform a medically unwise activity. Although breaking confidentiality may lead to legal action against the physician, the principle of confidentiality may be outweighed by the ethical principles of beneficence and nonmaleficence in these situations.

Current Regulations

As discussed previously, information on the frequency with which cardiac arrhythmias contribute to or cause automobile accidents is limited. However, recognizing the limitations of available data, the risk of accidents attributable to arrhythmias appears to be relatively low. For example, the Medical Control Unit of the State of

Virginia Department of Motor Vehicles examined the records of 3000 cases, of which only 6% were deemed to be related to cardiovascular disease, and of these, only 14% appeared to be associated with a cardiac arrhythmia.[26] It is unknown whether the subset of patients with ventricular arrhythmias is responsible for a higher frequency of arrhythmia-related accidents than those with supraventricular arrhythmias. In the United States, regulations concerning driver fitness are determined by individual states. For example, some states have laws relating to syncope of any cause, whereas others have specific laws related to arrhythmias, seizure disorders, and other syncopal syndromes. In Canada, the Canadian Cardiovascular Society has made recommendations related to commercial and personal driving.[27]

The risks of driving are probably different for private and commercial situations. Whereas private drivers may use their car only to travel to a country store, US commercial truckers, for example, accrued 288 billion road miles in 1992.[1] It is of interest that the Ontario Provincial Police records suggest that 50% of all commercial vehicular accidents are attributable to failure to follow rules such as the speed limit, right of way, etc. Only 5% appear to be due to loss of control such as might be experienced during an acute medical incident. Even in these cases, separating factors of fatigue, alcohol, illicit drugs, and other medical causes may be difficult.[1,11,18,19]

Medical standards for US interstate commercial drivers with cardiovascular disease were last reviewed in 1986. For patients with ventricular arrhythmias, classification was based on the Lown grading scheme.[28] Lown grade 3 arrhythmias and above (including multiform premature ventricular complexes, couplets, 3 or more ventricular beats in succession, and R-on-T phenomena) disqualified individuals from driving unless approved by a cardiologist on a case-by-case basis. Both sustained and nonsustained ventricular tachycardia, irrespective of symptoms, were considered disqualifying. The consensus, furthermore, indicated that patients who had survived a cardiac arrest were considered unfit for commercial driving indefinitely irrespective of subsequent therapy. ICD treatment was not considered in this report.

Basis for AHA/NASPE Recommendations

Before recommendations on limiting the activities of patients with ventricular arrhythmias are made, the risk of arrhythmia recurrence and consequences of recurrence on consciousness must be examined. Literature exists related to the time course of arrhythmia recurrence in patients with ventricular arrhythmias treated with

ICDs.[29–32] Early work classified shocks as "appropriate" or "inappropriate," depending on whether or not syncope or presyncope occured at the time of device therapy, and indicated that ≥70% of patients receive at least one "appropriate shock" during the first several years after implantation. Most shocks occur in the first year after ICD implantation, after which the risk of recurrence decreases. For patients who experience shocks during follow-up, only 10% have syncope in association with therapy. An additional 10% may have presyncope severe enough to impair voluntary motor activity. Unfortunately, there are no clinical markers to prospectively identify patients who will or will not have syncope at the time of ICD therapy.

It must also be recognized that the event of syncope or impaired consciousness during arrhythmia recurrence does not necessarily translate into either death or injury of the driver, a passenger, or bystander. The 501 patients discussed earlier, as reported by Larsen et al,[20] all had ventricular arrhythmias, the majority (92%) treated by nondevice therapies. The event rate for recurrent ventricular fibrillation, poorly tolerated and hemodynamically unstable ventricular tachycardia, syncope, sudden cardiac death, or ICD discharge for the entire population was 17% at 1 year. The rate was highest in the first month after hospital discharge (4.22% per month), intermediate in months 2 through 7 (1.81% per month), and lowest in the subsequent 8 to 12 months (0.63% per month). Although recommendations were made regarding driving, incomplete data are available regarding the frequency and risks of motor vehicle accidents in this study population.

Curtis et al[33] surveyed 742 physicians who cared for patients with ICDs. They were questioned as to the size of their practice and the numbers of fatal and nonfatal accidents known to them. A total of 30 motor vehicle accidents were reported by 25 physicians over a 12-year period from 1980 through 1992. Among these, there were 9 fatalities, including 8 patients with an ICD and 1 who was a passenger. Notably, no bystander was fatally injured. The authors concluded that since the fatality rate for patients with an ICD (7.5/100 000 patient-years) is significantly lower than that of the general population (18.4/100 000 patient-years), excessive restrictions or a total ban on driving seem to be unwarranted.

Recommendations[1]

Three categories, referred to as classes A, B, and C, form the basis of the recommendations. No restrictions are recommended for patients with a class A categorization. Those classified as class B are restricted from driving for a defined period of time (denoted in Table 1 by the number qualifier associated with the B categorizations) without arrhythmia recurrence, with the implication that a therapeutic intervention has been made. Patients classified as class C are totally restricted from performing hazardous activities.

Recommendations were modified depending on the circumstances of driving (eg, personal or commercial) because of anticipated differences in the time spent driving and the potential risk to others depending on the type of driving performed. For example, loss of consciousness in a patient driving a school bus would have potentially very different consequences than syncope in a patient driving a private vehicle on a country road. Furthermore, not only the number of miles driven per year and hours spent behind the wheel but also the weight of the vehicle affect risk.[27] The Canadian Consensus Conference indicated that loss of control of a heavy vehicle does result in a more devastating accident than loss of control of a private automobile. Because of these modulating factors, the AHA/NASPE guidelines were intended to be guidelines and not practice standards. The authors of the Medical/Scientific Policy Statement encourage physicians to use personal judgment when deciding whether or not a patient's particular situation warrants him or her to be included in the private or commercial driving category.

Since there is no a priori reason to make different recommendations for patients treated with drug, surgical, or ICD therapy, the guidelines presented apply to all patients with ventricular tachycardia or fibrillation irrespective of how they are managed (Table 1). It is recommended that patients with nonsustained ventricular tachycardia be restricted from neither noncommercial nor commercial

TABLE 1

Guidelines for Driving in Patients With Ventricular Arrhythmias

	Noncommercial Driving	Commercial Driving
Nonsustained VT	A[†], B3*	A[†], B6*
Sustained VT	B6, B3[‡]	C, B6[‡]
Cardiac arrest/VF	B6	C

A indicates no restrictions; B, restrict for defined period (indicated by number in months); C, total restriction; VT, ventricular tachycardia; VF, ventricular fibrillation; *, symptoms of impaired consciousness with arrhythmia; †, no impairment of consciousness with arrhythmia; and ‡, idiopathic VT (normal coronary arteries, normal left ventricular function, and no symptoms of impaired consciousness).

driving if there is no impaired consciousness with the presenting arrhythmia. On the other hand, if symptoms are present, patients are restricted from driving to document a symptom-free/arrhythmia-free interval of 3 months for noncommercial driving and 6 months for commercial driving. It is recommended that patients with sustained ventricular tachycardia be restricted from noncommercial driving for 6 months to document an arrhythmia-free interval and totally restricted from commercial driving. However, for the special subset of patients with idiopathic ventricular tachycardia and structurally normal hearts who experience no impairment of consciousness with their presenting arrhythmia, the restrictions are 3 and 6 months for noncommercial and commercial driving, respectively, again to document an arrhythmia-free interval before driving. Finally, patients with ventricular fibrillation are restricted from noncommercial driving for 6 months to document an arrhythmia-free interval and totally restricted from commercial driving.

There are instances in which exceptions to the above guidelines can be considered. For example, some patients with antiarrhythmic devices may have multiple episodes of asymptomatic ventricular tachycardia that on follow-up are repeatedly shown to be terminated by antitachycardia pacing with no episodes of acceleration.[34] In this situation, the rules proscribing driving may be adjusted. In general, however, if any arrhythmia occurrences are documented, the 6-month period of driving abstinence is started again to provide sufficient time to again judge whether any alterations in medical therapy have adequately suppressed arrhythmia occurrence.

Rarely, ICDs may be implanted in patients who have never experienced a sustained ventricular arrhythmia.[35] These might include individuals with long-QT syndrome or hypertrophic cardiomyopathy and a strong family history of sudden death. There may also be patients in protocols comparing ICD and drug therapy who have never experienced symptoms related to an arrhythmia. In all of these circumstances, it is recommended that there be no restrictions from private driving.

Other Considerations

Regardless of the consensus recommendations presented above, liability and other considerations may take precedence. For example, it is unlikely that a school board would assume the liability of allowing a patient with an ICD to drive a school bus. Trucking companies may be similarly unwilling to assume liability. Licensing agencies have often relied on a physician's input to make specific recommendations for individual patients.

Another potential tension in the management of patients with life-threatening arrhythmias relates to the interactions between members of the family and friends. On the one hand, patients need support when limitations are prescribed by physicians or a disease process limits activity. On the other hand, encouragement is required for patients to overcome depression, disability, and physical limitations. Denial may complicate the ability of patients to accept limitations and make responsible decisions about what activities are pursued. Ongoing counseling is a prerequisite for successful therapy for such individuals.

Tensions may also be expected from employers and insurance carriers, both of which have a complex group of competing responsibilities. Employers must consider the benefits and compensation required in the event of injury on the job and their economic impact. The employer also may have a liability for personal injury and property loss to third parties when workers are injured as a result of acts by a patient arising out of a medical condition. Whether or not insurance is paid will also be determined by regulations and practice guidelines. Finally, physicians are also affected by medical malpractice and feel not only a social responsibility but also personal liability when allowing patients to perform certain activities that may be hazardous to the health of the patient or others.

Summary

Ultimately, physicians have the responsibility to define and estimate the risk of arrhythmia recurrence and loss of consciousness, recognizing that no 0 % risk is achievable. Regulators have the responsibility to translate the data and recommendations into law or widely applied guidelines. Tension between the individual and society, the physician and the patient in regard to confidentiality, employers and patients, and insurance carriers and patients all require ongoing dialogue to be resolved. As new information on outcomes becomes available, the guidelines outlined herein will almost certainly be revised.

References

1. Epstein AE, Miles WM, Benditt DG, et al. AHA/NASPE Medical/Scientific Statement. Personal and public safety issues related to arrhythmias that may affect consciousness: implications for regulation and physician recommendations. *Circulation*. 1996;94:1147–1166.

2. Nikolic G, Bishop RL, Singh JB. Sudden death recorded during Holter monitoring. *Circulation.* 1982;66:218–225.
3. Lewis BH, Antman EM, Graboys TB. Detailed analysis of 24 hour ambulatory electrocardiographic recordings during ventricular fibrillation or torsade de pointes. *J Am Coll Cardiol.* 1983;2:426–436.
4. Pratt CM, Francis MJ, Luck JC, et al. Analysis of ambulatory electrocardiograms in 15 patients during spontaneous ventricular fibrillation with special reference to preceding arrhythmic events. *J Am Coll Cardiol.* 1983;2:789–797.
5. Panidis IP, Morganroth J. Sudden death in hospitalized patients: cardiac rhythm disturbances detected by ambulatory electrocardiographic monitoring. *J Am Coll Cardiol.* 1983;2:798–805.
6. Luu M, Stevenson WG, Stevenson LW, Baron K, Walden J. Diverse mechanisms of unexpected cardiac arrest in advanced heart failure. *Circulation.* 1989;80:1675–1680.
7. Manolio TA, Furberg CD. Epidemiology of sudden cardiac death. In: Akhtar M, Myerburg RJ, Ruskin JN, eds. *Sudden Cardiac Death: Prevalence, Mechanisms, and Approaches to Diagnosis and Management.* Baltimore, Md: Williams & Wilkins; 1994:3–20.
8. Norman LG. Medical aspects of road safety. *Lancet.* 1960;1:989–994, 1039–1045.
9. Trapnell JM, Groff HD. Myocardial infarction in commercial drivers. *J Occup Med.* 1963;5:182–184.
10. Herner B, Smedby B, Ysander L. Sudden illness as a cause of motor-vehicle accidents. *Br J Industr Med.* 1966;23:37–41.
11. West I, Gilmore AE, Ryan JR. Natural death at the wheel. *JAMA.* 1968; 205:266–271.
12. Myerburg RJ, Davis JH. The medical ecology of public safety, I: sudden death due to coronary heat disease. *Am Heart J.* 1964;68:586–595.
13. Peterson BJ, Petty CS. Sudden natural death among automobile drivers. *J Forensic Sci.* 1962;7:274–285.
14. Hossack DW. Death at the wheel: a consideration of cardiovascular disease as a contributory factor to road accidents. *Med J Aust.* 1974;1: 164–166.
15. Kerwin AJ. Sudden death while driving. *Can Med Assoc J.* 1984;131: 312–314.
16. Öström M, Eriksson A. Natural death while driving. *J Forensic Sci.* 1987;32:988–998.
17. Christian MS. Incidence and implications of natural deaths of road users. *Br Med J.* 1988;297:1021–1024.
18. Grattan E, Jeffcoate GO. Medical factors and road accidents. *Br Med J.* 1968;1:75–79.
19. Parsons M. Fits and other causes of loss of consciousness while driving. *Q J Med.* 1986;New Series 58(227):295–303.
20. Larsen GC, Stupey MR, Walance CG, et al. Recurrent cardiac events in survivors of ventricular fibrillation or tachycardia: implications for driving restrictions. *JAMA.* 1994;271:1335–1339.
21. Waller JA. Cardiovascular disease, aging, and traffic accidents. *J Chronic Dis.* 1967;20:615–520.
22. Rigdon JE. Rise in older drivers poses safety risk. *The Wall Street Journal.* October 29, 1993, A8.
23. Anderson MH, Camm AJ. Legal and ethical aspects of driving and working in patients with an implantable cardioverter defibrillator. *Am Heart J.* 1994;127:1185–1193.

24. Lauer MR, Young C, Liem LB, et al. Ventricular fibrillation induced by low-energy shocks from programmable implantable cardioverter-defibrillators in patients with coronary artery disease. *Am J Cardiol.* 1994;73:559–563.

25. Trappe H-J, Klein H, Kielblock B. Role of antitachycardia pacing in patients with third generation cardioverter defibrillators. *PACE.* 1994;17:506–513.

26. US Department of Transportation, Federal Highway Administration. Medical regulatory criteria for evaluation under section 391.41(b)(4). Federal Register. November 23, 1977; revised October 1983.

27. Consensus Conference. Assessment of the cardiac patient for fitness to drive. *Can J Cardiol.* 1992;8:12.

28. Fox SM. Conference on cardiac disorders and commercial drivers. US Department of Transportation report FHWA-MC-88-040, 1987.

29. Fogoros RN, Elson JJ, Bonnet CA. Actuarial incidence and pattern of occurrence of shocks following implantation of the automatic implantable cardioverter defibrillator. *PACE.* 1989; 12:1465–1473.

30. Myerburg RJ, Luceri RM, Thurer R, et al. Time to first shock and clinical outcome in patients receiving an automatic implantable cardioverter-defibrillator. *J Am Coll Cardiol.* 1989;14:508–514.

31. Grimm W, Flores BT, Marchlinski FE. Shock occurrence and survival in 241 patients with implantable cardioverter-defibrillators. *Circulation.* 1993;87:1880–1888.

32. Lessmeier TJ, Lehmann MH, Steinman RT, et al. Implantable cardioverter-defibrillator therapy in 300 patients with coronary artery disease presenting exclusively with ventricular fibrillation. *Am Heart J.* 1994;128:211–218.

33. Curtis AB, Conti JB, Tucker KJ, Kublis PS, Reilly RE, Woodard DA. Motor vehicle accidents in patients with an implantable cardioverter-defibrillator. *J Am Coll Cardiol.* 1995;26:180–184.

34. Higgins JR. Automatic burst extrastimulus pacemaker to treat recurrent ventricular tachycardia in a patient with mitral valve prolapse: more than 2,000 documented successful tachycardia terminations. *J Am Coll Cardiol.* 1986;8:446–450.

35. Levine JH, Waller T, Hoch D, Greenberg S, Goldberger J, Kadish A. Implantable cardioverter defibrillator: use in patients with no symptoms and at high risk. *Am Heart J.* 1996;131:59–65.

Chapter 19

Cognitive Dysfunction After Sudden Cardiac Arrest

Mary Jane Sauvé, DNSc, RN, and John A. Walker, PhD

A major factor contributing to postresuscitation morbidity and mortality in survivors of aborted sudden death (ASD) is brain injury secondary to the insult of global ischemia. In a review of the pathophysiological consequences of sudden circulatory arrest, Safar[1] notes that at normal temperatures, loss of brain oxygen stores and consciousness occurs within 10 to 20 seconds. Within 5 minutes of the arrest, cellular glucose and ATP stores are depleted and the membrane pump is inactivated. Further, the occurrence of calcium shifts, tissue lactic acidosis, increases in free fatty acids, and extracellular amino acids such as glutamic acid creates a cellular environment that fosters reperfusion injuries in vulnerable areas of the brain, such as the hippocampus and the neocortex. These pathophysiological changes that occur within the brain during the arrest and after reperfusion have been associated with a variety of neurological sequelae ranging from mild intellectual impairments to brain death.[2-4] Although the prevalence of severe brain damage, including vegetative states in long-term survivors (>6 months) of ASD is low (1% to 3.9%),[5,6] estimates of full neurological recovery in these patients vary from a low of 25% to a high of 85%, depending on the methods used by the investigators to assess cognitive function.[2,7-10]

This chapter reviews current research on the prevalence and type of impairments described in this patient group, the clinical predictors of cognitive outcomes, the impact of cognitive impairments on the long-term psychosocial recovery of the survivors, and proposals for future research and the clinical management of these patients.

From: Dunbar SB, Ellenbogen KA, Epstein AE, (eds). *Sudden Cardiac Death: Past, Present, and Future.* Armonk, NY: Futura Publishing Company, Inc.; © 1997.

Neurocognitive Outcomes

Despite an impressive array of research on the causes and treatment of ASD, few studies have addressed the quality of survival outcomes in these patients. From a neurological standpoint, postresuscitation outcomes have been addressed either in terms of functional status as determined by neurological examination or in terms of higher cortical functions as assessed with neuropsychological testing.[11] One of the earliest investigations addressing functional outcomes in this patient population was a retrospective study done by Snyder et al.[12] Using data from the survivors' neurological examinations, these investigators categorized the survivors as functional or impaired depending on their ability to carry out activities of daily living. Of the 34 ASD survivors assessed, 21 were categorized as functional and 13 as impaired. Only 2 of the impaired patients lived to hospital discharge, and both of these required total nursing care until their deaths at 18 and 19 months after the arrest, respectively. Among those classified as functional, 19 survived to hospital discharge. Of these, 15 were living at home and independent in activities of daily living after 1 year, and 4 were in nursing homes.

In two prospective studies involving 63 and 50 ASD survivors, respectively, Snyder and colleagues[13] and Caronna and Finklestein[14] continued to define outcomes for those who lived to hospital discharge in terms of the survivors' ability to carry out activities of daily living. An excellent outcome indicated that the individual was able to live at home and carry out activities of daily living without assistance; a good outcome indicated that the survivor needed assistance with some daily activities; and a poor outcome meant that the patient needed total nursing care. In contrast, in the Brain Resuscitation Trials (I, 1979–1984; II, 1985–1989; III, 1989–1993),[1,15] outcomes were defined in terms of the best cerebral performance at any time during follow-up. Five outcomes, adapted from the Glasgow categories, were used: (1) conscious and alert with normal function or slight disability, (2) conscious and alert with moderate disability, (3) conscious with severe disability, (4) comatose or in a persistent vegetative state, and (5) dead. The difficulty in using these functional definitions for determining the quality of survival outcomes is that they tend to underestimate both the prevalence and impact of mild to moderate intellectual impairments on the survivor's ability to return fully to prearrest activities. In addition, unless categories are well defined, interrater reliability becomes an issue even in well-controlled clinical trials.

In a case in point, Earnest and colleagues[2] followed 51 ASD survivors, 21 of whom were still alive 3.5 years after hospital discharge.

These investigators found on careful neurological examination that only 2 of 17 survivors examined (12%) had normal neurological status, whereas 8 (46%) had severe organic brain syndrome, 1 had hemiparesis and aphasia, and 6 had mild organic brain syndrome. Of the 3 living subjects who were interviewed but not examined, 1 had severe intellectual deficits and 2 had returned to work full time. Family members reported that 12 subjects (60%) had significant changes in their personality or mental abilities. Although the results of the limited neuropsychological testing were not given, neurological examination results indicated that the most common intellectual deficits were in immediate and delayed recall (memory). Despite these findings, families also reported that 60% of the survivors had resumed independent social activities and were able to go shopping alone. Thus, independence in activities of daily living, including shopping alone, does not preclude the presence of intellectual deficits that may impact other areas of the survivor's life.

Several studies that have used neuropsychological testing to determine cognitive function in ASD survivors are outlined in Table 1. These studies have uniformly small sample sizes, differing methodologies, and varied use of limited to extensive batteries of neuropsychological tests. However, the findings of these studies present a common neuropsychological profile of the survivors, ie, a general depression of cognitive function, with memory the most severely impaired cognitive area. It is noteworthy that the general depression in cognitive function experienced by these patients is not necessarily severe.[16] Investigators using the Wechsler Adult Intelligence Scales (WAIS) have found that survivors often function within normal range on these tests, but they do so at 1 to 2 SD below their projected premorbid IQ.[16-19] Families therefore become an important source of information regarding changes in cognitive function in these patients.

Reports of cognitive dysfunctions in long-term survivors of ASD when comprehensive neuropsychological testing is done range from a low of 29%[21] to a high of 80%.[9] Differences in incidence rates are generally due to the types of tests chosen by the investigators to assess cortical functions, timing of tests (early versus late in recovery), and whether the survivors were consecutive admissions to the same facility or referrals to the facility for electrophysiological testing and/or defibrillator implantation. In our latest data analysis,[22] we found an incidence of cognitive dysfunction of 46% (28/61) at 6 months after arrest in a sample derived from several regional centers versus the 80% (28/35) for the same follow-up period reported by Grubb et al,[9] whose sample was derived from consecutive admissions to the same facility. Referral bias is very likely a factor in the lower prevalence of deficits in our patient sample.

TABLE 1

Studies Assessing Neuropsychological Outcomes After Sudden Cardiac Death

Author(s)	Design/Sample	Measures	Outcomes
Nielsen JR et al, 1983[3]	Comparative 1–3 years p̄ SCD Matched groups SCD: n=13 AMI: n=13	Psychological interview; visual gestalts, word-pair; digit-span, digit-learning, subtraction, sentence reproduction, text reproduction, abstraction and concept formation test	No difference in dementia symptoms between groups as measured by psychological interview. SCD dementia scores >AMI ($P<0.05$, Mann-Whitney U test)
Reich P et al, 1983[16]	Case study n=6	WAIS; WMS	Functioning below premorbid intellectual capacities. Memory impairments
Kotilla M and Kajaste S, 1984[17]	Repeated measures 3–21 wk p̄ SCD MD 4,5 wk n=10 5–18 mo p̄ SCD MD 7 mo n=9	Not reported	At time, 1, 10 had moderate to severe defects in memory, visual intelligence, and construction; 9 were disoriented At time 2, disturbances milder; 8 had at least one neuropsychological deficit
Volpe BT et al, 1986[18]	*Experimental* 1 year p̄ arrest Matched groups SCD: n=6 Healthy: n=6	Baseline measures; WAIS; WMS; RPM, Token Test; Wisconsin Card Sort; "Famous Faces Test," Oral Word Association Test. *Experiment:* 600 high-frequency one- or two-syllable words	SCD group had moderate to severe memory dysfunction on WMS and "Famous Faces Test," average or above average performance on other tests. *Experimental Outcomes* Intact recognition memory, severely impaired delayed recall

Study	Design	Tests	Findings
Bigger ED and Alfano M, 1988[19]	Comparative 9 mo–4 years p̄ SCD Matched groups SCD: n=12 CHI: n=12	WAIS-R; WMS; Rey Auditory Verbal Learning Test; Rey-Osterrieth Complex Figure Design; Visual Retention–Revised; RPM; Halsten-Reitan Test Battery	Generalized decrease in cognitive function and moderate to severe memory losses. SCD subjects worse on WAIS-R ($P<0.05$) and WMS ($P<0.01$) than CHI subject. Uniform deficits for both groups on Halsten-Reitan Battery
Bertini G et al., 1990[10]	Comparative Mean time: 29.5 mo p̄ SCD (range, 3–57 mo) Matched groups SCD c̄ coma: n=15 SCD s̄ coma: n=15 Prior MI: n=15 Healthy: n=15	Critichon Geriatric Behavior Rating Scale; Eysenck Personality Inventory; Figure repetition test, from WMS; Symbols-Figures Association Test from the WB Scale	Low incidence of neurological and psychological sequelae. Comatose survivors scored worse on WB then noncoma and healthy subjects but not prior MI subjects.
Dougherty CM, 1994[20]	Longitudinal with repeated measures (hospital discharge, 1, 3, 6, and 12 mo) n=15	Confusion-Bewilderment Subscale of Profile of Mood States; NCSE; Trailmaking A and B	Mild to moderate deficits, severe in delayed recall, construction deficits
Sauvé MJ et al, 1996[21]	Longitudinal with repeated measures ≤3 wk, 6–9 wk, 12–14 wk, 22–25 wk n=17	NCSE: Oral Word Fluency Test; Symbol-Digit Modalities Test; Tapping Test; Visual Search; Memory Scan	Deficits in attention and delayed recall

SCD indicates sudden cardiac death; MD, median; CHI, closed head injury; AMI, acute myocardial infarction; p̄, post; c̄, with; s̄, without; WAIS, Wechsler Adult Intelligence Scale; WMS, Wechsler Memory Scale; RPM, Ravens Progressive Matrices; WB, Wechsler-Bellevue; and NCSE, Neurobehavioral Cognitive Status Examination.

Memory deficits in ASD survivors are characteristically described as impairments in delayed recall, eg, the recall of a story or word list 10 to 20 minutes after presentation. However, immediate memory (≤10 seconds), early recall (after distraction or < 5 minutes), and recognition memory in long-term survivors may also be impaired, although not as frequently. In addition to deficits in delayed recall, Roine et al[7] and Dougherty,[20] in their respective studies of 68 and 17 survivors over a 1-year period, have reported deficits in visuoconstructive functions, or the ability to reconstruct designs and patterns, and other investigators have described losses in attention,[21] learning,[16] and the ability to plan and carry out mental activities.[17] Moderate to severe impairments (≥2 SD below normative values) in cognitive function were found in 48% (26/54) of the ASD survivors in study by Roine et al,[7] 37% (13/35) of those reported by Grubb et al,[9] and 30% (18/61) of our own study sample.[22] It should be noted that neither the occurrence nor the severity of impairments reported in these studies was confounded by age, sex, or depression.

Our longitudinal study results indicate that most impairments resolve rapidly during the first 3 months after the arrest event, with no significant increases in cognitive function between 3 and 6 months.[8,21,22] A similar trajectory was described by Roine et al,[7] who assessed patients at 3 and 12 months after the arrest event and found no significant improvements in outcomes between these data points. Figure 1 shows a comparison of the recovery trajectories for impaired and nonimpaired survivors on the four memory outcomes assessed in our study. It should be noted that the very low recognition scores among the impaired survivors is due to the very narrow range of normal for this outcome variable. Hence, reports of excellent cognitive recovery in survivors of sudden cardiac arrest need to be viewed with caution, because up to 80% of these patients may have at least mild memory losses on careful neuropsychological examination.

Predictors of Neurocognitive Outcomes

The search for valid criteria that will predict which patients successfully resuscitated from sudden cardiac arrest will survive and recover good cognitive function has been the object of intensive study for the past 20 years. Objective measures of brain electrophysiology such as electroencephalography and somatosensory evoked potentials have been found to be relatively sensitive predictors of mortality, but these tests are far less prognostic when their results are equivocal, ie, determination of who will die without

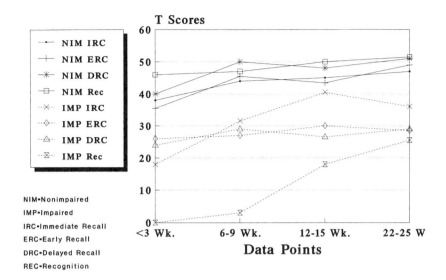

FIGURE 1. *Memory outcomes over time: comparison of nonimpaired and impaired SCD survivors (n = 61), (T score: mean 50; SD ± 10)*

awakening versus entering into a vegetative state. In addition, neither of these tests has the sensitivity to distinguish between those patients who recover completely and those who have varying degrees of motor and/or cognitive impairments.[23] Karkela et al[24] recently reported on the prognostic value of cerebrospinal fluid (CSF) creatine kinase (CK), brain-type creatine kinase isoenzyme (CK-BB), lactate dehydrogenase (LDH) and its isoenzymes, CSF acid phosphatase, and CSF lactate. Kendall rank correlations were used to assess the relation of these laboratory variables to the Glasgow Coma Scale scores of 20 consecutive survivors of out-of-hospital sudden cardiac arrest. Results of this study indicate that the patient's outcome was most reliably predicted by CSF, CK, CK-BB, and CFS lactate concentrations between 28 and 76 hours after the arrest event and by LDH, LDH_1 to LDH_3, and acid phosphatase at 76 hours after cardiac arrest. The authors conclude that these biochemical markers can be used as indicators of hypoxic brain injury and may give additional information about outcome, particularly in those patients who remain comatose.

Clinical markers of outcome after hypoxic cardiac arrest have been the focus of several investigations. In the earliest of these studies, Caronna and Finkelstein,[14] Earnest et al,[25] and Snyder et al[13,26] identified similar clinical signs as predictors of both favorable and unfavorable outcomes. Unfavorable outcomes were associated with the absence of pupillary light reaction, corneal reflexes, and purposeful response to pain during the initial 24 hours after the arrest event and with decerebrate or decorticate posturing at and after 24 hours. Predictors of favorable outcomes included spontaneous and roving eye movements within 12 to 24 hours of the arrest, purposive movement of face, arms, or legs at any time after the arrest, and comprehensible speech and the ability to follow commands within the first 48 hours.

More recent investigations have used multivariate analyses in large data sets to identify neurological predictors of outcomes.[27,28] A major emphasis in these studies has been the identification of clinical neurological signs and the utility of such instruments as the Glasgow Coma Scale for predicting poor outcomes (cerebral performance categories 3 to 5), because the death rate associated with hypoxic ischemic coma is quite high. Levy et al[27] reported a 64% (134/210) fatality rate in these survivors at 1 week, and Edgren et al,[28] reported a fatality rate slightly less than 60% at 1 week for ASD survivors in the Brain Resuscitation Trial I. Both these investigators found the absence of pupillary light reactions on initial examination after the restoration of spontaneous circulation the most accurate early predictor of poor outcome. The second most reliable indicator was the absence of motor response to pain. By postarrest day 3, Edgren and colleagues found that a Glasgow score of <5, a Glasgow-Pittsburgh score of <22, lack of eye opening and motor response to pain, and the absence of pupillary light reaction gave 100% accurate predictions of poor outcomes. However, on multivariate analysis, only absence of motor response to pain was an independent predictor of poor outcome. Neither of these neurological models has been tested prospectively, although the data emanating from these analyses have been adopted clinically in many institutions to make responsible as well as timely decisions regarding limiting or withdrawing further interventions. However, it is important to remember that any neurological model predicting outcomes after ASD, particularly when death is an end point, is confounded by at least two additional factors, ie, age and the extent of underlying cardiac disease. Survivors ≥75 years old have a uniformly high mortality rate after resuscitation,[29] and a good neurological prognosis does not preclude early mortality due to cardiac causes.

Although the emphasis in these multivariate analyses was primarily on predictors of poor outcome, Levy and colleagues[27] also developed an algorithm for positive outcomes. These investigators found, as did Snyder et al[13] and Caronna and Finkelstein,[14] that the single most positive predictor of a good recovery was early awakening, ie, comprehensible speech and/or the ability to follow verbal commands. Earnest and colleagues,[2] in their evaluation of 117 survivors of out-of-hospital cardiac arrest, found that those survivors who were awake on hospital admission and who survived subsequent cardiac or medical complications had a 90% probability of good long-term neurological function and that those who awakened within 48 hours had an 80% probability of good neurological function. Snyder and Tabbaa[30] have reported that survivors who awaken within 72 hours after resuscitation may also do well, although such arousal did not guarantee independent functioning.

Longstreth et al[4] also found that time of awakening after resuscitation was associated with cognitive outcomes in their retrospective study of 459 survivors who had been successfully resuscitated in the community. One hundred eighty patients (39%) never awakened, and 91 of the 279 who did awake had persistent neurological deficits. However, although this study demonstrates a strong correlation ($r=.79$) between time to awakening and the recovery categories of no deficits (188 patients), cognitive deficits only (59 patients), and cognitive and motor deficits (32 patients) as defined by the authors, data for this analysis were collected largely from physician and nursing progress notes and less often from neurological examination or tests of mental status. Given the prevalence of cognitive impairments when neurological examinations or neuropsychological tests are used in the evaluation of hospitalized ASD survivors, it is most likely that the 33% incidence of cognitive deficits reported in the Longstreth study is underestimated.

Time to awakening has also been identified by the American Heart Association's Joint Task Force on uniform reporting for out-of-hospital cardiac arrest as a simple and reliable predictor of postresuscitation cerebral outcomes.[31] Table 2 presents our study results, which show moderate to strong associations between time to awakening, orientation, and all four memory outcomes assessed (immediate recall, early recall, delayed recall, and recognition) over time (≤ 3 weeks to 22 to 25 weeks). Less stable associations were found for attention and problem solving. Hierarchical regression analyses indicated that the cardiopulmonary resuscitation (CPR) variables accounted for a significant portion of the variance in orientation and the four memory outcomes, but only time to awakening contributed uniquely to the variance in each of these outcomes (see Table 3). We recently reported on the associations between the CPR variables of CPR onset, definitive therapy (medication, defibrillation), duration of CPR, and awake times.[8] We found that the earliest awake times (≤ 1 hour) were associated with a pattern of early CPR onset (<4 minutes), definitive therapy (<8 minutes), and

TABLE 2

Relations* Among Cardiac Arrest, Left Ventricular Function, Psychological, and Cognitive Outcome Variables

Independent Variables	Cognitive Outcomes								
	ORI	ATT	IMRC	ERC	DRC	REC	REAS	MSPD	MVAR
Time 1 (n=73)									
Time to CPR		-0.31							
Time to Rx	-0.34	-0.32	-0.33	-0.34	-0.37		-0.29		
CPR duration	-0.49	-0.40	-0.41	-0.45	-0.51	-0.41	-0.40		
Awake time	-0.55	-0.60	-0.58	-0.48	-0.53	-0.50	-0.46		
Time 2 (n=68)									
Time to CPR	-0.27	-0.29		-0.27	-0.25				
Time to Rx	-0.35	-0.26							
CPR duration	-0.36	-0.27	-0.33	-0.41	-0.38	-0.26			
Awake time	-0.53	-0.40	-0.44	-0.59	-0.56	-0.40			
EF							-0.27		
NYHA								-0.41	-0.39

(table continues)

Time 3 (n=63)								
CPR duration	−0.26		−0.28	−0.34	−0.31	−0.36		
Awake time	−0.43		−0.89	−0.51	−0.41	−0.50		
EF		−0.32					0.38	
NYHA							−0.27	
Depression								−0.31
Time 4 (n=61)								
CPR duration	−0.32		−0.28		−0.43	−0.38		
Awake time			−0.33	−0.45	−0.59	−0.57		
EF							0.36	0.30
NYHA							−0.34	−0.35
Anger							−0.36	
Depression							−0.47	−0.37

*Correlations: Pearson's r. Minimum significance level, 0.05. Two-tailed test.

ORI indicates orientation; ATT, attention; IMRC, immediate recall; ERC, early recall; DRC, delayed recall; REC, recognition; REAS, MSPD, tapping speed; MVAR, tapping variability; CPR, cardiopulmonary resuscitation; Rx, definitive therapy; EF, ejection fraction; NYHA, New York Heart Association class I–IV.

TABLE 3

Hierarchical Regression Analyses: Memory–Delayed Recall

	R^2	df	F	P	β	sr^2	df	F	P
TIME 1									
Step 1									
CPR variables	0.37	3.34	10.96	0.000					
CPR onset					0.06	0.00	1.34	0.00	0.950
CPR Rx					−0.08	0.00	1.34	1.36	0.550
Awake					−0.56	0.22	1.34	19.19	0.000
TIME 2									
Step 1									
CPR variables	0.31	3.30	9.84	0.000					
CPR onset					−0.07	0.00	1.30	0.35	0.556
CPR Rx					0.18	0.02	1.30	1.29	0.187
Awake					−0.65	0.29	1.30	24.98	0.000
TIME 3									
Step 1									
CPR variables	0.18	3.00	4.25	0.008					
CPR onset					−0.06	0.01	1.28	.23	0.633
CPR Rx					0.15	0.01	1.28	1.05	0.320
Awake					−0.48	0.16	1.28	10.98	0.000
TIME 4									
Step 1									
CPR variables	0.33	3.28	9.16	0.000					
CPR onset					−0.02	0.00	1.28	0.02	0.879
CPR Rx					0.11	0.01	1.28	.71	0.402
Awake					−0.63	0.27	1.28	22.80	0.000

CPR indicates cardiopulmonary resuscitation; Rx, definitive therapy.

a CPR duration of <20 minutes and the longest awake times (36 to 72 hours) with delays in CPR onset (≥4 minutes), definitive therapy (≥8 minutes), and CPR duration of ≥20 minutes. Intermediate patterns and outcomes were also identified.

Depression, antiarrhythmic drugs with central nervous system toxic side effects, hypoxia due to low cardiac output states, and older age are other factors that may affect cognitive status in ASD survivors, if only transiently. Kennedy and associates[32] found significant associations between cognitive impairment, depression, and subsequent morbidity and mortality ($P<0.01$ to $P<0.0005$) in 88 patients with diverse cardiac arrhythmias. The incidence of cognitive deficits in the total group was 15.7%, as measured by the Cognitive Capacity Screening Examination (CCSE), a global screening test that produces a single score. In the 66 patients with documented ventricular tachycardia (VT) or ventricular fibrillation (VF) in this study, the incidence of cognitive deficits was 21%. Several factors make the interpretation of these data difficult. First, the authors do not differentiate between the patients with hemodynamically unstable VT/VF that necessitated CPR and those whose VT was hemodynamically stable. Thus, it is unclear whether the lower CCSE scores occurred among the patients who had cardiac arrest or whether they were evenly distributed among the two groups. Second, the validity of assessing cognitive dysfunctions with global measures like the CCSE is under question because of the high number of false-negative results with single-score screening methods. Last, although a small ($r=0.29$) but highly significant relation ($P<0.005$) was reported between cognitive impairment and depression, in fact, only 3 of the 14 cognitively impaired patients were also depressed, leaving some doubt as to the strength and stability of this relation.

In our pilot study of cognitive recovery patterns in sudden cardiac arrest survivors,[21] we also found a significant association between depression and impairments in both attention ($r=-0.67$) and delayed recall ($r=-0.74$) at 6 months after resuscitation. In the larger study sample, however, no relations between these variables were found (see Table 2). In addition, no significant associations were found between measures of left ventricular function (ejection fraction; New York Heart Association functional class) and deficits in orientation, attention, memory, or problem solving. In both studies, however, relations were found between these measures of left ventricular function and motor function. Lower tapping speeds and greater intertap variability were consistently associated with depressed left ventricular ejection fractions and higher New York Heart Association functional class, indicating that low cardiac output states are more likely to affect the rapidity of responses rather than accuracy.

The relation of age to cognitive dysfunctions was also assessed in our pilot and subsequent studies. Although the average age (58 versus 61 years) of the ASD survivors increased over the two study periods, no significant relation between age and impairments was found. In contrast, Roine et al[7] reported an effect of decreasing cognitive performance with increasing age at both 3 and 12 months after resuscitation, although their findings also failed to reach statistical significance. Rogove et al,[29] reporting for the Brain Resuscitation Clinical Trial I and II study groups, found a significant relation between older age (>80 years) and 6-month mortality (94%) but no difference in the neurological recovery between older survivors and survivors in younger age groups. Thus, current data would seem to indicate that mortality rates do increase with increasing age, but the chance of achieving a good neurological recovery is unaffected by age.

Cognitive Dysfunctions and Pyschosocial Recovery

Reich and coworkers[16] were the first investigators to associate poor psychological adjustment and employment difficulties after cardiac arrest with mild brain dysfunctions. In a series of six case studies, these authors describe changes in both the personality and mental abilities of patients whose overall test performances on the WAIS and Wechsler Memory Scale, while depressed compared with their estimated premobid IQ capacities, were still within normal range. Yet these patients were apathetic, exhibited poor judgment, had disturbances in insight, impulse control, empathy, and self-awareness. These behavioral changes, which are often associated with head-injury patients, resulted in poor work performance and job losses; strained marital relationships and divorce; and loss of family and community relationships. These authors suggest that there is a need to be alert to the possibility of cerebral dysfunction in survivors of cardiac arrest even in the absence of focal neurological signs or positive evidence of cognitive impairments as determined by neurospychological testing.

Reports of return to work among survivors of sudden cardiac arrest range from a low of 44% reported by Earnest et al[2] to a high of 78% reported by Dobson and coworkers[33] in hospitalized patients with acute myocardial infarction complicated by one or more

VF events. In a previous study, we found an initial return to work (≤6 months) among ASD survivors of 72% (26/36).[34] After a mean follow-up of 21 ± 11 months, 10 of the 26 who had returned to work had either stopped working or were unemployed. As in other studies of cardiac patients, the most frequent reasons for not returning to work or for subsequently stopping work were poor or worsening cardiac status, proximity to retirement, and type of occupation. However, three patients in this investigation were unable to return to work because of mental status changes, and three additional survivors either stopped working or were unemployed because of cognitive dysfunctions during follow-up. In subsequent studies, we did not specifically address the impact of deficits on return to work. However, ≈10% to 25% of the survivors in these studies were either unable to return to work because of their cognitive deficits or had sufficient difficulties with job performance upon return to work that they chose to retire, were asked to retire, or were given positions with less responsibility.

The impact of cognitive deficits on survivor psychological adaptation is less straightforward. As noted earlier, we did not find any significant correlations between deficits in orientation, attention, memory, and problem solving and selected mood states (depression, anger, fatigue, anxiety) in our most recent study sample.[22] In addition, we did not find any significant differences in reports of mood disturbances between impaired and nonimpaired survivors, nor were their reports of mood states different from subjects in the nonpsychiatric normative population. These findings are in stark contrast not only to our earlier study results but also to the realm of studies using similar screening measures to assess psychological distress after acute coronary events. The incidence of major mood disturbances, particularly depression, among patients recovering from acute myocardial infarction[35-37] as well as from ventricular tachyarrhythmias, including ASD, has been well documented.[34,38,39]

Several factors appear to be influencing these outcomes. First, the subjects in this latest study, like patients with cardiac disease in other investigations,may be underreporting negative mood states, particularly depression.[40,41] Second, it is also possible that impaired survivors may not fully appreciate the impact of their deficits on their ability to resume many of their former activities and roles during the initial 6 months after the arrest event. Last, several of the survivors with the most severe impairments were unable either initially or during follow-up to complete the Profile of Mood States,[42] the instrument used to assess affective state in the study. In addition, when the most severely impaired survivors did complete this instrument, they actually reported less distress than unimpaired survivors. Although one could hypothesize that the occurrence of moderately severe cognitive deficits does not necessarily create psychological distress for the individual, it is more likely that the global ischemia accompanying the cardiac arrest resulted in decreased insight, emotional processing, and self-awareness, as suggested by Reich and colleagues.[16]

Differences were found in reports of distress between male and female survivors. Female survivors had higher levels of anger and depression throughout the study period than male survivors. In addition, female survivors reported significant increases in both anger ($P \leq 0.02$) and depression ($P \leq 0.03$) at 6 months after resuscitation, suggesting that some aspects of postresuscitation recovery may be sex-specific. A qualitative analysis of our interview data supported this hypothesis. It was found that female recovery patterns differed from male recovery in three important ways: female survivors resumed family and work roles sooner in their recovery; they received less assistance with activities of daily living and less emotional support; and they reported more body image changes due to implantation of internal cardioverter-defibrillators.[43] Similar differences in female and male recovery patterns after both acute myocardial infarction and coronary artery bypass surgery have been reported.[44,45]

Perhaps the most profound impact of cognitive dysfunctions after aborted sudden death is experienced by the spouses of the survivors. In a qualitative study specifically addressing the emotional experiences of wives of male survivors, Simons et al[46] reported that the anger expressed by the wives was directed not only at the changes in financial or job status resulting from the arrest event but also at the difficulties of dealing with a severely impaired survivor. One wife described herself as "just kind of a keeper." Our own spousal interview data support these findings. Both husbands and wives of survivors with moderate to severe impairments express the belief that their spouse is no longer the person he or she was before the arrest event.[34] Even more distressing for some is the loss of intimacy due to changes in the survivors' emotional responses, ie, lack of empathy and concern for the needs and feelings of others. Our quantitative data analyses substantiate these findings.[47] Spouses of impaired survivors demonstrate significantly increased anger and depression 6 months after the arrest event and report significantly more fatigue than spouses of nonimpaired survivors (see Figure 2).

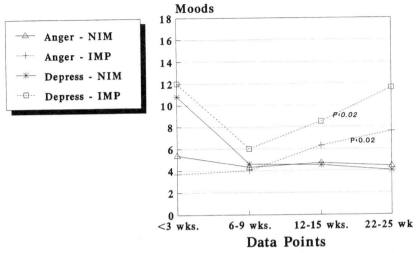

FIGURE 2. *Anger and depression in spouses: impaired vs nonimpaired repeated measures ANOVA.*

Future Research and Clinical Management

Given the consistent reports of mild to severe memory losses in up to 50% of sudden death survivors, it would seem that the next logical step in the research process is the development of intervention strategies designed to determine whether cognitive retraining is possible in this patient group. Currently, the literature dealing with cognitive retraining programs among head-injured and stroke patients is more anecdotal than substantive. In addition, it is unclear whether improvements in function as measured by neuropsychological testing also transfer to some of the more difficult behaviors associated with cognitive dysfunctions. Other areas that need to be explored more thoroughly include the impact of cognitive dysfunctions on factors such as work return and spousal/family distress. In addition, other mechanisms for assessing and measuring negative mood states in the more severely impaired survivors need to be explored and/or developed.

Although the clinical management of ASD survivors generally focuses on therapies for the control of life-threatening ventricular arrhythmias and maintenance of optimal cardiac function, it is time for both physicians and nurses to begin to address some of the behavioral changes that may occur as the result of the arrest. There is little or no support for spouses of survivors with significant cognitive impairments, either in the form of information about the type of changes to expect or the social/community services necessary to help ameliorate some of the more disturbing aspects of these changes, whether economic or behavioral. For many spouses, returning to work or having to remain in their jobs longer than they had anticipated is difficult, but it is less arduous than dealing with the survivors' erratic or insensitive behaviors. Most distressing when they occur are changes in sexual behavior, including obsessive demands for sex and inappropriate sexual advances to other adults and/or family members. It therefore behooves those healthcare professionals involved in the long-term clinical follow-up of these patients to become informed about the medical and rehabilitation resources within their communities that may be of assistance to these patients and their families.

References

1. Safar P. Cerebral resuscitation after cardiac arrest: research initiatives and future directions. *Ann Emerg Med.* 1993;22(part 2):324–349.
2. Earnest MP, Yarnell PR, Merrill SL, Knapp G. Long term survival and neurologic status after resuscitation from out-of-hospital cardiac arrest. *Neurology.* 1980;30:1298–1312.
3. Nielsen RJ, Gram L, Rasmussen LP, Dalsgaard M, Richardt C, Beck J. Mild chronic brain syndrome in survivors of cardiac arrest. *Acta Med Scand.* 1983;213:36–39.
4. Longstreth WT Jr, Inui TS, Cobb LA, Copass MK. Neurological recovery after out-of-hospital cardiac arrest. *Ann Intern Med.* 1983;98:588–592.
5. Yarnell PR. Neurological outcome of prolonged coma survivors of out-of-hospital cardiac arrest. *Stroke.* 1976;7:279–282.
6. Gustafson I, Edgren E, Hulting J. Brain-oriented intensive care after resuscitation from cardiac arrest. *Resuscitation.* 1992;24:245–261.
7. Roine RO, Kajaste S, Kaste M. Neurophysiological sequelae of cardiac arrest. *JAMA.* 1993;269:237–242.
8. Sauvé MJ, Doolittle N, Walker JA, Paul SM, Scheinman MM. Factors associated with cognitive recovery following cardiopulmonary resuscitation. *Am J Crit Care.* 1996;5:127–139.
9. Grubb NR, O'Carroll R, Fox KAA. Memory function in survivors of out-of-hospital cardiac arrest. *Circulation.* 1995;92(suppl I):I-174.
10. Bertini G, Giglioli C, Giovannini F, et al. Neuropsychological outcome of survivors of out-of-hospital cardiac arrest. *J Emerg Med.* 1990;8:407–412.
11. Mandzak-McCarron K. Cognitive dysfunction following cardiac arrest. *Crit Care Nurs Clin North Am.* 1989;1:175–179.
12. Snyder BD, Ramirez-Lassepas M, Lippert DM. Neurologic status and prognosis after cardiopulmonary arrest; I: a retrospective study. *Neurology.* 1977;27:807–811.
13. Snyder BD, Loewenson RB, Gummit RJ, et al. Neurologic prognosis after cardiopulmonary arrest, II: levels of consciousness. *Neurology.* 1980;30:52–58.

14. Carrona JJ, Finkelstein S. Neurological syndrome after cardiac arrest. *Stroke.* 1978;9:517–520.
15. Brain Resuscitation Clinical Trial I Study Group. Randomized clinical trial of thiopental loading in comatose survivors of cardiac arrest. *N Engl J Med.* 1986;314:397–403.
16. Reich P, Regestein QR, Murdowski BJ, Silver RA, Lown B. Unrecognized organic mental disorders in survivors of sudden cardiac arrest. *Am J Psychiatry.* 1983;140:1194–1197.
17. Kotilla M, Kajaste S. Neurological and neuropsychological symptoms after cardiac arrest. *Acta Neurol Scand.* 1984;69(suppl 98):337–338.
18. Volpe BT, Holtzman JD, Hirst W. Further characterization of patients with amnesia after cardiac arrest: preserved recognition memory. *Neurology.* 1986;36:408–411.
19. Bigler ED, Alfano M. Anoxic encephalopathy: neuroradiological and neuropsychological findings. *Arch Clin Neuropsychol.* 1988;3:383–396.
20. Dougherty CM. Longitudinal recovery following sudden cardiac arrest and internal cardioverter defibrillator implantation: survivors and their families. *Am J Crit Care.* 1994;3:145–154.
21. Sauvé MJ, Walker JA, Massa SM, Winkle RA, Scheinman MM. Patterns of cognitive recovery in cardiac arrest survivors: the pilot study. *Heart Lung.* 1996; 25:172–181.
22. Sauvé MJ. Patterns of cognitive recovery in sudden death survivors: the final report. Bethesda, Md: National Institute of Nursing Research; National Institutes of Health; R01-NR-02525-03.
23. Rothstein TL, Thomas EM, Sumi SM. Predicting outcome in hypoxic-ischemic coma: a prospective clinical and electrophysiologic study. *Electroencephalogr Clin Neurophysiol.* 1991;79:101–107.
24. Karkela J, Pasanen M, Kaukinen S, Morsky P, Harmoinea A. Evaluation of hypoxic brain injury with spinal fluid enzyme, lactate and pyruvate. *Crit Care Med.* 1992;20:378–392.
25. Earnest MP, Breckinridge JC, Yarnell PR, Olivia PB. Quality of survival after out-of-hospital cardiac arrest: predictive value of early neurologic evaluation. *Neurology.* 1979;29:56–60.
26. Snyder BD, Gumnit RJ, Leppik IE, Hauser WA, Loewenson RB, Ramirez-Lassepas M. Neurologic prognosis after cardiopulmonary arrest, IV: brainstem reflexes. *Neurology.* 1981;31:1092–1097.
27. Levy DE, Caronna JJ, Singer BH, Lapinski RH, Frydman H, Plum F. Predicting outcome from hypoxic-ischemic coma. *JAMA.* 1985; 253:1420–1426.
28. Edgren E, Hedstrand U, Kelsey S, Sutton-Tyrrell K, Safar P, BRCT 1 Study Group. Assessment of neurological prognosis on comatose survivors of cardiac arrest. *Lancet.* 1994;343:1055–1059.
29. Rogove HJ, Safar P, Sutton-Tyrrell K, Abramson NS. Old age does not negate good cerebral outcome after cardiopulmonary resuscitation: analyses from the brain resuscitation clinical trials. *Crit Care Med.* 1995;23:18–25.
30. Snyder BD, Tabbaa MA. Assessment and treatment of neurological dysfunction after cardiac arrest. *Mod Concepts Cardiovasc Dis.* 1987; 22:1–6.
31. Cummin RO, Chamberlain DA. Recommended guidelines for uniform reporting of data from out-of-hospital cardiac arrest: the Utstein style. AHA Medical/Scientific Statement. *Circulation.* 1991;84:960–975.
32. Kennedy GJ, Nofer MA, Cohen D, Schindledecker R, Fisher JO. Significance of depression and cognitive impairment in patients undergoing

programmed stimulation of cardiac arrhythmias. *Psychosom Med.* 1987;49:410–421.

33. Dobson M, Tatterfield AE, McNicole MW. Attitudes and long-term adjustment of patients surviving cardiac arrest. *Br Med J.* 1971;3: 207–212.
34. Sauvé MJ. Long-term physical functioning and psycho-social adjustment in survivors of sudden cardiac death. *Heart Lung.* 1995;24: 133–144.
35. Wishnie HA, Hackett TP, Cassem NH. Psychological hazards of convalescence following myocardial infarction. *JAMA.* 1971;215: 1292–1296.
36. Stern M, Pascale JL, Ackerman A. Life adjustment post myocardial infarction. *Arch Intern Med.* 1977;137:1680–1685.
37. Cay E, Vetter N, Philip A, Dugard P. Psychological problems in patients after myocardial infarction. *Adv Cardiol.* 1982;29:108–112.
38. Dunnington CS, Johnson NL, Finkelmeier BA, Lyons J, Kehoe RF. Patients with heart rhythm disturbances: variables associated with increased psychologic distress. *Heart Lung.* 1988;17:381–389.
39. Haggerty TI, Burkett MB, Foster JR. Psychological dysfunction in patients surviving ventricular tachycardia or fibrillation. *Circulation.* 1983;68(suppl III):III-108. Abstract.
40. Ahern DK, Gorkin L, Anderson JL, et al, for the CAPS Investigators. Behavioral variables and mortality or cardiac arrest in the cardiac arrhythmia pilot study (CAPS). *Am J Cardiol.* 1990;66:59–62.
41. Carney RM, Rich MW, TeVelde A, Saini J, Clark K, Jaffee AS. Major depressive disorder in coronary artery disease. *Am J Cardiol.* 1987;60: 1273–1275.
42. McNair D, Lorr M, Droppelman L. *Edits Manual: Profile of Mood States.* San Diego, Calif: Educational Testing Service; 1981.
43. Doolittle N, Sauvé MJ, Walker JA, Massa S. Gender differences in recovery following sudden cardiac death: a qualitative analysis. *Circulation.* 1994;90 (pt2):I-589. Abstract.
44. Rankin SH. Pyschosocial adjustment of coronary artery disease patients and their spouses: nursing implications. Nurs Clin North Am. 1992;27:271–284.
45. King KB, Clark PC, Hicks GL Jr. Patterns of referral and recovery in women and men undergoing coronary bypass grafting. *Am J Cardiol.* 1992;69:179–182.
46. Simons LH, Cunningham S, Catanzaro M. Emotional responses and experiences of wives of men who survive a sudden cardiac death event. *Cardiovasc Nurs.* 1992;28:17–21.
47. Sauvé MJ, Doolittle N, Walker JA. Trajectory of psychological recovery in impaired and non-impaired sudden death survivors and their spouses. Circulation. 1994;90(p 2):I-424. Abstract.

Chapter 20

Sudden Cardiac Death:
Moral Responsibilities of the Patient and the Healthcare Provider

John Collins Harvey, MD, PhD

Moral philosophy, otherwise called ethics, is that branch of philosophy that systematically and formally examines the rightness and wrongness of human acts, the logic used in ethical arguments, and the assumptions on which ethical decisions are based. Medical ethics deals with these issues as they relate to medical practice in the care of patients and their families, medical research, and setting public policies related to medical issues that impact on society and its culture. In a pluralistic society, there are many bases for an ethics applied to medicine. In our culture, we are indebted for the most part to the Scottish and German philosophers of the 18th and 19th centuries for the ethical systems that form the bases of our moral philosophy and medical ethics today, although the great Greek philosopher Aristotle gave us the principles embodying the ethics of virtue in the third century before the common era.[1] John Locke (d. 1704) wrote *A Second Treatise on Government,* and we are indebted to him for a libertarian ethics.[2] David Hume (d. 1776) wrote *An Enquiry Concerning the Principles of Morals,* and we are indebted to him for the concept of autonomy.[3] John Stuart Mill (d. 1873) wrote *On Liberty,* and we are indebted to him for a consequential or utilitarian ethic.[4] Immanuel Kant (d. 1804), the German "philosopher of Königsberg," wrote on the categorical imperative, and to him we are indebted for the ethics of duty or "deontology."[5] One contemporary American philosopher, John Rawls,[6] has given us an ethic of distributive justice, and two others, Beauchamp and Childress,[7] an ethic based on the prima facie principles of autonomy, beneficence, nonmaleficence, and justice. This latter principle-based ethic has

From: Dunbar SB, Ellenbogen KA, Epstein AE, (eds). *Sudden Cardiac Death: Past, Present, and Future.* Armonk, NY: Futura Publishing Company, Inc.; © 1997.

generally been adopted by medical ethicists as their basic guide for practice today. It is a neutral ethic, devoid of the philosophical controversies engendered by one or another of the systems based on utilitarianism, deontology, distributive justice, or a theology that reflects a given religious creed. Principle-based ethics can be used by moral strangers in mutual conversations.

To consider the moral responsibilities of patients and healthcare providers dealing with sudden cardiac death, we must first agree on certain definitions that will permit us to talk clearly with one another. It is imperative that we define carefully what we mean by the term "disease" and what we mean by the term "illness."

Disease is a pathological condition with a specific cause and characteristic symptoms. Often, pharmaceutical or surgical intervention can correct the pathological condition and effect a cure. Sometimes the body's defense and curative powers bring about an amelioration or cure of the condition without medical intervention.

Disease is of two types. One is acute and self-limited. Such pathological processes—an example is pneumococcal pneumonia—usually can be cured and leave no permanent residual change in the functional capacity of the organ or group of organs affected by the pathological condition. Sometimes, of course, the body does not respond to the curative intervention, and death results. Disease can also be of a second type: chronic, noncurable, and resulting in a decrease in functional capacity of an organ or organ system affected by the individual pathological process. Death will eventually occur from the chronic condition, its complications, or an intervening acute disease process. Examples of such chronic diseases are emphysema, rheumatoid arthritis, Parkinson's disease, and generalized arteriosclerosis. Certainly, therapeutic measures such as pharmacotherapy or surgical interventions, as well as palliative measures, may be taken to attempt to ameliorate the pathological condition and to relieve symptoms and/or improve functional capacity, but a cure is really impossible. The healthcare worker's job is to keep the patient comfortable and functioning at the highest level possible.

Illness is quite a different thing from disease. Illness is the response of the individual to the pathological condition—in other words, to the disease—that he or she has. This response may be in the subjective changes caused by the pathological condition and reported by the sufferer. These we call symptoms: such things as pain, loss of appetite, decreased energy, etc. The response may be observable signs that reflect alterations in the physiological functioning of the individual—changes in body temperature or alterations in the functioning of one or another organ or organ system such as the heart, the digestive system, or the neurological system.

These changes can be investigated and measured in various ways. If the response to the pathological condition in the heart is an electrical disturbance, then ventricular fibrillation or cardiac standstill, ie, complete cessation of beat, may result. This we call sudden cardiac death. The response may also be an anatomic one, with easily observable changes at the molecular, microscopic, or gross levels. The response also includes psychological changes of various types—depression, euphoria, denial, etc. Illness includes engendered sociological responses such as inability to work, to earn money, and to support oneself, or one's family. We see then that illness, either acute or chronic, is quite different from disease. This concept is very important in understanding and considering the moral responsibilities of the patient and healthcare provider in dealing with any pathological condition, such as coronary artery disease or primary disease of the pericardium, myocardium, or endocardium, that could result in physiological electrical disturbances that may cause cessation of heartbeat and thus sudden death, the subject of this monograph.

It must be emphasized that illness affects the individual in many ways. The phenomenology of illness includes loss of freedom, inequality of knowledge and power, assault on self-image, irreducibility of trust, vulnerability, exploitability, anger, hostility, and fear. Thus, the healthcare worker must always consider the individual as a person and not just a biological entity.

In evaluating a patient, the healthcare worker must find out what is wrong, what can be done, and what should be done. In the traditional Hippocratic formula, the physician did this to the best of his ability. He practiced paternalistically. In the age of autonomy, some have considered that the patient is supreme; but this, too, is morally wrong. Decision making should be shared by the patient and the healthcare worker so that the patient's values of the good are brought to bear on the treatment decisions. In this, the ethical or moral requirements for the healthcare worker are to seek the truth and to exhibit beneficence. In the established caring relationship, these precepts of beneficence—confidentiality, truth telling, self-effacement, virtuous behavior, and fidelity to trust—must always be demonstrated by the healthcare provider. For the patient, there are of course limits on autonomy, and these are morally binding on him or her—namely, that the autonomous action cannot lead to harm to third parties, conflict with the physician's ethical values, or conflict with the law or violate the internal morality of medicine.

Sudden death is usually the consequence of the development of a cardiac dysrhythmia that cannot support the body economy—eg, ventricular fibrillation or asystole resulting from acute occlusion of blood flow to the myocardium or from other specific cardiac patho-logical processes. These happenings result in anatomic and/or physiological changes to those cells that, when normal, generate and control the flow of electricity in the myocardium so that proper and orderly myocardial function is maintained to support systemic perfusion. Coronary artery disease is a process that can result in not just acute illness and death but also in chronic, long-term ill-ness that leads to progressive myocardial dysfunction (heart fail-ure) and then impaired functional capacity of all organ systems to a degree that body homeostasis cannot be maintained and death of the individual inevitably occurs.

The treatment for the acute illness caused by coronary artery disease is cardiopulmonary resuscitation. Thus, it is morally incum-bant on the healthcare worker to be able to give this type of treat-ment properly and expeditiously. This is a moral requirement for every healthcare worker in the field of cardiology. It is also incum-bent on these workers to see that their coworkers in health care who do not give direct patient care but nonetheless may be the only indi-vidual present when a patient suffers the consequences of the acute illness of coronary artery disease, namely sudden cardiac death, as well as members of the public, are generally trained in these resus-citation techniques. Many lives can be spared if this technique is ap-plied immediately when the fatal illness (dysrhythmia) occurs.

Treatment for the chronic illness caused by coronary artery disease may be directed toward the obstructive plaques responsible for ischemia by use of angioplasty, coronary artery bypass surgery, or medical therapy such as advocated by Brown and Goldstein as a result of their Nobel prize–winning investigations relating lipid dis-orders to coronary atherosclerosis. Thus, it is morally incumbant on the healthcare worker to understand the pathophysiology of dis-ease and when to prescribe one of a variety of appropriate thera-pies. It is a moral requirement that the goals for treatment of both the chronic and acute illnesses caused by coronary artery disease as I have defined them and the way they are or will be applied be clear to the healthcare provider and be made explicit to the patient. These are not always discussed. The decision must be the patient's if he or she is competent, and if not, the healthcare worker should fol-low an ethically acceptable system to arrive at a decision that re-flects the patient's values. Advance directives are useful in this regard, although they do present some problems. When advance di-rectives or a surrogate must be used to make treatment decisions for an incompetent patient, conflicts may arise. These may concern the definition of the patient's good; difficulty in determining the ef-fectiveness, burdens, and benefits ratio of treatment; difficulty in determining quality-of-life assessments; the impact of economic considerations; clear understanding of philosophical, religious, and ethnic influences; and in this time of managed care, the role of the healer and the meaning of the physician-patient relationship. Some moral problems inevitably arise in treating the acute illness episode (sudden cardiac death) when the patient has chronic illness from coronary artery disease. Should resuscitation always be offered? How many times? How should the patient's wishes be evaluated? Who makes the emergency decisions? These are some of the problems that must be considered. Suggested criteria for withdrawing treatment or applying "DNR" orders are the following: terminal state; progress for recovery hopeless; treatment disproportionately ineffective, burdensome and nonbeneficial; and direction by a competent patient, a valid surrogate, or a valid anticipatory declaration to discontinue under defined circumstances.

From the standpoint of distributive justice, it is the moral responsibility of any patient who accepts one or another of the treatments for chronic illnesses caused by coronary artery disease to follow the designated treatment regimens very carefully, to change lifestyle (ie, give up smoking, if a smoker; maintain a diet low in fat, cholesterol, and caloric content), to follow the prescribed cardiac exercise regimen, and to alleviate stress by changing patterns of behavior. Society cannot afford the large investments for these treatments only to have the patients flout the healthcare provider's instructions for treatment of their disease.

It is also a moral responsibility on the part of the healthcare provider from the standpoint of distributive justice to plan any investigation of disease with the greatest care, because money cannot be spent frivolously in pursuit of medical investigations. The financial support for research that was available in the past is simply not there today. It is also a moral responsibility of any investigator who is carrying out clinical research to fully inform the subjects partaking in the research not only of the plans, methods, and expected outcomes but also of any dangers, complications, or deleterious effects that may result from their taking part in the research project.

These, then, are a few of the moral responsibilities of both healthcare providers and patients in considering the subject of sudden cardiac death.

References

1. Aristotle. *Nicomachean Ethics.*
2. Locke, John. *Second Treatise on Government.* (1690). Crawford B. McPherson, ed. Indianapolis, Ind: Hackett; 1980.

3. Hume, David. *An Enquiry Concerning the Principles of Morals.* (1777). 2nd ed. La Salle, Ill: Open Court; 1966.
4. Mill, John Stuart. *On Liberty.* (1859). Indianapolis, Ind: Hackett; 1978.
5. Kant, Immanuel. *Foundations of the Metaphysics of Morals.* Louis White Beck, tr. New York, NY: Macmillan; 1959.
6. Rawls, John. *A Theory of Justice.* Cambridge, Mass: Harvard University Press; 1971.
7. Beauchamp, Tom and Childress, James. *Principles of Biomedical Ethics.* 3rd ed. New York, NY: Oxford University Press; 1989.

Chapter 21

Cardiac Rehabilitation:
Exercise Testing and Training

Gerald F. Fletcher, MD

Cardiac rehabilitation involves exercise and secondary prevention measures in patients with cardiovascular disease. This comprehensive process begins with a complete medical evaluation, including exercise testing.

The cardiac rehabilitation program involves formulation of a prescription for exercise training based on the exercise test. In addition, there should be comprehensive risk factor modification specifically in regard to modifiable coronary risk factors. These are cigarette smoking, blood lipid abnormalities, high blood pressure, physical inactivity, and body weight. Assessment and evaluation of comorbid states, such as obesity and lung disease, should be addressed. This comprehensive process takes place over weeks and months and usually begins within a few weeks after a cardiac event. Cardiac rehabilitation may be done in centers such as hospitals and clinics with supervision, at home, or at distant sites through monitored and nonmonitored programs.

In the special population of sudden cardiac arrest victims who have been successfully resuscitated, cardiac rehabilitation can be initiated in a format similar to that for other patients after a cardiac event.

Exercise Testing

Exercise testing should be done in a carefully supervised manner. Under most circumstances, a physician should be present in the room and involved in doing the test. Certain elements of the testing, however, may be delegated to a nurse or other physician

From: Dunbar SB, Ellenbogen KA, Epstein AE, (eds). *Sudden Cardiac Death: Past, Present, and Future.* Armonk, NY: Futura Publishing Company, Inc.; © 1997.

support person who has proper training in electrocardiogram (ECG) interpretation, clinical symptom assessment, and knowledge of both the physiology and pathophysiology of the cardiovascular system.

Testing should be done with a system that is acceptable to the patient, usually with a motorized treadmill or a cycle ergometer. The testing is similar to that for other patients who are at high risk, for which guidelines have been published by the American Heart Association.[1]

Exercise protocols should be individualized according to the type of subject being tested. Three-minute stages are not necessary to achieve a steady state at a low workload. Performance can be estimated with the oxygen cost of maximum workload rather than by total treadmill time if subjects do not use hand rails, allowing comparison of performance in different protocols. A 9-minute targeted ramp protocol that increases in small steps has many advantages, including more accurate estimates of MET (metabolic equivalent; 1 MET=3.5 mL oxygen consumed per kg body wt) level. It is important to adjust or select the treadmill or cycle ergometer protocol to the subject being tested. The optimum protocol is 6 to 12 minutes, and the exercise capacity should be reported in METs rather than minutes.[1]

Exercise testing should begin with a baseline ECG to assess for certain characteristics. Special note should be made of infarction location (inferior, anterior, anterolateral, or septal) and specific patterns that might be a marker of future events (Table 1). Left bundle-branch block, left anterior fascicular block with right bundle-branch block, and nonspecific intraventricular conduction defects are all patterns of concern that must be placed in the database of a patient with regard to prognosis. Anterior infarction patterns with persistent ST-segment elevation are of concern with regard to aneurysm formation. Inferior infarction patterns with anterior ST-segment changes suggest the possibility of more extensive injury and disease. In some instances, patients will have had an im-

---

TABLE 1

ECG Patterns of Concern After Sudden Cardiac Arrest

Left bundle-branch block
Left anterior fascicular block with right bundle-branch block
Extreme nonspecific intraventricular conduction delay
Anterior infarction pattern with ST-segment elevation
Inferior infarction with anterior ST-segment changes

---

plantable cardioverter-defibrillator implanted after their arrhythmia event. Knowledge of the device and its program type is essential in regard to follow-up.

This discussion will not specifically address issues of patients who have implanted pacemakers or defibrillators. Guidelines for exercise testing are basically fundamental in this population, and testing is done in a format similar to that for other high-risk patients. Assessment of heart rate and rhythm, blood pressure response, ST-segment changes, arrhythmias, and conduction disturbances and the critical rates at which they develop is very important. For those with defibrillators, the exercise heart rate must be maintained below the arrhythmia detection rate. There should be close communication with the patient during the time of the exercise stress with recording of symptoms and level of perceived exertion.

Blood Pressure During Exercise

Blood pressure correlates with cardiac output and peripheral resistance. Systolic pressure at maximum exertion or at immediate cessation of exertion (≤ 1 minute) is considered a clinically useful first approximation of the inotropic capacity of the heart. An inadequate rise or a fall in systolic blood pressure during exercise can occur. Although some normal subjects have a transient drop in systolic blood pressure at or soon after maximum exercise, this finding is frequently associated with severe coronary artery disease and ischemic dysfunction of the myocardium. Exercise-induced hypotension also identifies subjects at increased risk for ventricular fibrillation in the exercise laboratory.[1]

Heart Rate During Exercise

Relatively rapid heart rates during submaximal exercise or recovery may be due to deconditioning, any condition that decreases vascular volume or peripheral resistance, prolonged bed rest, anemia, or metabolic disorders. This finding is relatively frequent soon after myocardial infarction and coronary artery surgery. Conversely, a relatively low heart rate at any point during submaximal exercise could be due to exercise training, enhanced stroke volume, or drugs. The use of β-blockers, which lower heart rate, often complicates interpretation of the heart rate response to exercise. Conditions that affect the sinus node or other causes of chronotropic incompetence can also attenuate the normal response of heart rate during exercise testing. Therefore, abnormalities of exercise capacity, systolic blood pressure, and heart rate response to exercise can be due to either left ventricular dysfunction, ischemia, cardioactive drugs, or autonomic dysfunction.[1]

Oxygen consumption measures to assess functional capacity are important in the sudden cardiac arrest population. However, if the system of expired air analysis interferes with proper communication with the patient or provokes anxiety in the patient, it should be eliminated. End points of perceived exertion or heart rate can be used to designate the exercise prescription.

Prognostic Indicators

Prognostic indicators derived from exercise testing include the duration of test time, ECG ST-segment changes (particularly the onset, degree, duration, and type of change), systolic blood pressure response, and development of angina pectoris (Table 2). All are important in the patient tested but particularly in those who have experienced sudden cardiac arrest.

In subjects with coronary artery disease, exercise-induced ventricular arrhythmias do not usually represent an independent risk factor for subsequent mortality or coronary events. However, recent data suggest that these arrhythmias add independent prognostic information to ^{201}Tl tests, ST-segment changes, and heart rate changes[2,3] and are associated with severe coronary artery disease and wall motion abnormalities. Exercise testing may be of considerable value in the evaluation of drug therapy for ventricular arrhythmias, particularly in subjects with coronary artery disease.

One study suggests that subjects with cardiomegaly, an exercise capacity of <5 METs, or a maximum systolic blood pressure of <130 mm Hg have a better outcome if treated with surgery.[4] In one surgery trial, subjects who had an exercise test response of 1.5 mm of ST-segment depression had improved survival with surgery. Im-

---

TABLE 2

Prognostic Indicators Derived From Exercise Testing

Duration of test (test time)
ECG ST-segment changes: onset, degree, duration, type
Systolic blood pressure response
Development of angina pectoris

---

proved survival also extended to those with baseline ST-segment depression and those with claudication.[5] In another trial, the surgical benefit to mortality was greatest in those with 1 mm of ST-segment depression at <5 METs. There was no difference in mortality in those who exceeded an exercise capacity of 10 METs, and in this group, the prognosis is generally quite good. Generally, in subjects with stable coronary artery disease, studies comparing angiographic findings, cardiac events, and the differential outcome of coronary artery bypass surgery compared with medical therapy have shown the exercise test to have prognostic power. These studies indicate that subjects with marked degrees of ST-segment depression (ie, >2 mm in multiple leads and prolonged into recovery) accompanied by poor exercise capacity, exertional hypotension, ventricular ectopy, angina, or all of the aforementioned are at increased risk of having triple-vessel or left main disease and a poor prognosis.

Pharmacological concerns are often present in survivors of sudden cardiac arrest. Many of these patients will be on a β-blocker, an angiotensin-converting enzyme inhibitor, a calcium channel blocker, class I antiarrhythmic drugs, and/or amiodarone. Many will be on multiple medications, and the assessment of their response to exercise testing in the presence of drugs is very important.

Critical arrhythmia markers (Table 3) that may develop during testing but must be watched for in training are frequent ventricular ectopy, ventricular tachycardia of ≥3 beats, high-grade atrioventricular block, and sinus pulses. Use of all the data derived from the exercise test (especially arrhythmias) to implement the exercise prescription is vitally important in this group of patients.

It is important to counsel the patient and his or her family after the exercise test about results and to relieve their anxiety about the test, especially if they have not previously exercised regularly. All questions must be answered, and the health team must assure patients and families that the exercise training program will be under supervision and carefully monitored for significant changes.

TABLE 3

Critical Arrhythmic Markers After Sudden Cardiac Arrest

High-grade ventricular ectopy
  ≥3-beat ventricular tachycardia
Atrioventricular block, Mobitz 2:1, complete
Sinus pauses (extreme)

Exercise Training

In training patients after being treated for life-threatening arrhythmias, baseline data, as mentioned, must be considered and used as the patient is stratified into a moderate- to high-risk category based on American Heart Association criteria paraphrased from Reference 1 (Table 4). This classification includes individuals with (1) coronary artery disease with the clinical characteristics outlined below, (2) cardiomyopathy, (3) valvular heart disease, (4) exercise test abnormalities not directly related to ischemia, (5) complex ventricular arrhythmias that are uncontrolled with medication at mild to moderate work intensities, (6) three-vessel disease or left main disease, and (7) low ejection fractions (<30%).

The clinical characteristics of patients in the moderate- to high-risk category are (1) two or more myocardial infarctions, (2) New York Heart Association class III or greater, (3) exercise capacity <6 METs, (4) ischemic horizontal or downsloping ST-segment depression of ≥4 mm or angina during exercise, (5) a fall in systolic blood pressure with exercise, (6) a medical problem that the physician believes may be life-threatening, and (7) ventricular tachycardia at a workload of <6 METs. Activity should be individualized with exercise prescription by qualified personnel.

ECG blood pressure monitoring and supervision should be continuous during exercise sessions until safety is established, usually in 6 to 12 or more sessions. All exercise sessions should be medically supervised until safety is established.

Exercise Prescription

These individuals should be medically supervised with ECG monitoring until they understand the level of activity that is safe and the medical team determines that the exercise is safe and effective. Usually 6 to 12 or more sessions are needed.[6]

TABLE 4

Clinical Characteristics of Those at Moderate to High Risk for Cardiac Complications During Exercise

---

Two or more infarctions
Exercise capacity ≤6 METs
Low ejection fraction (≤30%)
Fall in systolic pressure with exercise
Ventricular tachycardia at <6 METs

Monitored sessions should ideally be performed with continuous ECG monitoring by either hardwired apparatus or telemetry. The sessions should be conducted by personnel who understand the basic exercise principles involved and have a practical knowledge of electrocardiography. The sessions should also be supervised by either a physician or a nurse trained in emergency cardiopulmonary resuscitation, preferably with previous experience in intensive cardiac care. Cardiopulmonary resuscitation capability can be demonstrated by completion of an American Heart Association–sponsored course in advanced cardiac life support. Standing orders for management of a complication should be immediately available.

Monitored sessions should also include symptom assessment by the blood pressure recording, the subject's rating of perceived exertion, and instructions to subjects about selection and proper use of exercise equipment. ECG-monitored sessions should include instruction for different modes and progression of exercise. Therefore, these activity programs are needed to provide close medical supervision for individuals who are at particularly high risk for a complication associated with vigorous physical activity.

These exercise classes require careful medical supervision and surveillance to ensure that the activity is well tolerated. A physician should be readily available, although a properly trained nurse in the exercise room is sufficient if a physician is not available. The qualifications of the physician may vary, but experience in internal medicine and cardiovascular disease and in treatment of subjects with heart disease is recommended. Training programs should be medically supervised until the low risk of the prescribed activity has been established. All individuals entering these programs should be screened as described in Table 5.[1]

Nurses and others experienced in acute cardiac care should be available and attend to the patient's needs that may develop. Patients should be trained in a setting with other patients who are both low-risk and moderate- to high-risk to make them feel that they are part of the patient population at large and not an isolated group. Monitoring of patients with symptom assessment, ECG, careful blood pressure monitoring, and assessment of perceived exertion should be done for the 6 to 12 or more sessions. The exact number of sessions is to be determined by individual patient assessment. Further assessment of arrhythmias may need to be done by Holter recording, home event recording, or "instant" ECG recording[7] in the event that arrhythmias are not seen or detected with ECG telemetry monitoring during the exercise session.

Continual assessment of drugs, dosages of drugs, and time of administration of drugs is important during the cardiac rehabilita-

---

TABLE 5

Basic Requirements for Medically Supervised Programs for
Moderate- to High-Risk Patients

Adequately ventilated and temperature-controlled space
Capability to assess patients with blood pressure and ECG analysis
ECG monitoring during initial sessions to ascertain desirable exercise levels
Supervision by either a nurse or physician in the exercise room. If a physician is
    not present, one must be readily available for consultation
Medically qualified staff (completion of an AHA-sponsored advanced cardiac
    life support course or the equivalent and a minimum of two staff members
    present who are trained in cardiopulmonary resuscitation)
Appropriate drugs and equipment (emergency medications as outlined in
    the AHA's *Textbook of Advanced Cardiac Life Support* and
    cardioverter-defibrillator)
Standard orders for the nurse
Written procedures for the following:
    Identification of conditions needed to conduct session
    Management of problems that do not require hospitalization, such as acute,
        well-tolerated arrhythmias and neuromuscular injuries
    Ruling out myocardial infarction and management of problems requiring
        hospitalization, including postresuscitation problems
    Management of cardiac arrest, including procedure for immediate treatment
        and transportation to hospital

Reprinted with permission from the American Heart Association.

tion session. The importance of electrolyte levels, particularly that of potassium and magnesium, must be considered.

Most patients who have survived a cardiac arrest have residual coronary artery disease, and comprehensive risk factor modification is important. In the setting of the supervised rehabilitation, evaluation and management of blood lipid levels, blood pressure, smoking cessation patterns, and body weight should all be addressed.

It is advisable that patients resuscitated from cardiac arrest and in exercise training have an assessment by the medical director of the cardiac rehabilitation program in their first few weeks or months to assess progress and to be certain that the proper communication is present between the patient's primary physician and the health professionals of the cardiac rehabilitation program. With this, a true continuity of medical care will be provided for the high-risk subjects.

Few data are now available on patients in cardiac rehabilitation who have had implantable cardioverter-defibrillators. It is believed that these patients will have no great problem in the rehabilitative process; however, the status of the cardioverter-defibrillator and/or a associated pacemaker and its programming is vital to the good care of the patient.

It is realistic that most patients with life-threatening ventricular arrhythmias will become stable after 6 to 12 weeks of monitoring and be able to exercise in an unsupervised manner. The intensity of exercise should, of course, be lower if done at home or in a program that is not related to a health facility. Such patients should have exercise testing repeated at least yearly and evaluation of heart rate and rhythm assessment as dictated by their primary cardiologist and/or their cardiac electrophysiologist.

Sudden cardiac arrest survivors constitute a population that will be ever growing in the future as our state-of-the-art technology of preventing or reversing sudden cardiac death and using medications to prevent its recurrence evolves. Until more data are available on this particular population, they should be considered at moderate to high risk, and the above-described process of exercise testing and training should be implemented to safely and efficaciously rehabilitate and manage these patients.

References

1. Fletcher GF, Balady G, Froelicher VF, Hartley LH, Haskell WL, Pollock ML. Exercise standards: a statement for healthcare professionals from the American Heart Association. *Circulation.* 1995;91:580–615.
2. Kaul S, Lilly DR, Gascho JA, et al. Prognostic utility of the exercise thallium-201 test in ambulatory patients with chest pain: comparison with cardiac catheterization. *Circulation.* 1988;77:745–758.
3. Marieb M, Beller G, Gibson R, Lerman B, Sanjiv K. Clinical relevancy of exercise-induced ventricular arrhythmias in suspected coronary artery disease. *Am J Cardiol.* 1990;66:172–178.
4. Bruce RA, Fisher LD, Hossack KF. Validation of exercise-enhanced risk assessment of coronary heart disease events: longitudinal changes in incidence in Seattle community practice. *J Am Coll Cardiol.* 1995;5: 875–881.
5. European Coronary Surgery Study Group. Long-term results of prospective randomized study of coronary artery bypass surgery in stable angina pectoris. *Lancet.* 1982;2:1173–1180.
6. Fletcher BJ, Thiel J, Fletcher GF. Phase II intensive monitored cardiac rehabilitation for coronary artery disease and coronary risk factors: a six-session protocol. *Am J Cardiol.* 1986;751–756.
7. Cantwell JD, Fletcher GF. Instant electrocardiography: use in cardiac exercise programs. *Circulation.* 1974;50:962–966.

Chapter 22

Innovative Approaches:
A Psychosocial Therapy for Sudden Cardiac Arrest Survivors

Marie J. Cowan, PhD, RN

Introduction

The majority of sudden cardiac arrests (SCAs) or deaths are due to ventricular fibrillation,[1-3] the mechanisms of which have been associated with sympathetic arousal and/or an imbalance of the autonomic nervous system[4-6] in the context of coronary artery disease.[7-9] In addition, multiple other factors, such as hypoxia, pH changes, anaerobic metabolites, potassium, calcium, and catecholamines, have been identified as affecting the electrical properties of the myocardial cells. Out-of-hospital ventricular fibrillation represents more than one half of cardiovascular deaths, but depending on the adequacy of mobile life support units, there are growing numbers of SCA survivors in the community.[10] There is a high likelihood that SCA survivors will experience recurrent events of ventricular fibrillation. There is no completely reliable long-term treatment to prevent further episodes of ventricular fibrillation. Few studies have described the psychosocial aftermath of SCA, and there are no reports on the efficacy of psychosocial therapies for SCA survivors.

A number of studies, however, have demonstrated the relation of psychosocial distress to mortality in cardiac patients. Studies

This study was supported by a grant, R01 NR01970, Self-Management Therapy Following Sudden Cardiac Arrest (Marie J. Cowan, PI), from the National Institute of Nursing Research, NIH. Dr. Helen Nakagawa-Kogan and Dr. Randal Beaton from the University of Washington graciously shared results from their studies of symptoms of stress in hypertensives and fire fighters, respectively.

From: Dunbar SB, Ellenbogen KA, Epstein AE, (eds). *Sudden Cardiac Death: Past, Present, and Future.* Armonk, NY: Futura Publishing Company, Inc.; © 1997.

using randomized experimental designs, large sample sizes, and advanced statistical analyses have documented a rate of severe depression ≈15% to 18% after a myocardial infarction (MI) and identified severe depression as a predictor of mortality.[11-13] The most frequent causes of death in severely depressed MI patients within 6 months after MI are arrhythmias, reinfarction, and congestive heart failure.

In the Cardiac Arrhythmia Pilot Study (CAPS) of post-MI patients with significant ventricular arrhythmias, defined as >10 ventricular premature complexes per hour or >5 episodes of nonsustained ventricular tachycardia recorded 6 to 60 days after an MI, depression was a significant predictor of mortality or cardiac arrest within 1 year after MI. The relation of depression to mortality was significant even after history of prior MI, ejection fraction, β-blocker or digitalis use, presence of transmural infarcts, and presence of runs of premature ventricular complexes on the 24-hour electrocardiogram at baseline were controlled for.[14]

Six-month follow-up results from the Post-Infarction Late Potential (PILP) study indicated that dyspnea and reinfarction were related to depressive mood states. Twelve cardiac deaths and 17 arrhythmic events occurred, and they were significantly predicted by severe post-MI depression; the evidence was stronger for predicting death than for arrhythmic events.[15-17] A number of additional studies, such as the Multicenter Diltiazem Post-Infarction Trial,[18] the Beta Blocker Heart Attack Trial (BHAT),[19] and others[20] have demonstrated that social isolation and lack of support are associated with increased mortality following an MI.

More is known about psychosocial distress after an acute MI than after SCA. Dougherty[21] reported that anxiety, depression, anger, and stress levels were higher for both survivors and family members of SCA survivors who received internal cardioverter shocks than those who did not receive shocks. Denial was high in all SCA survivors the first year. Conversely, Sauvé[22] concluded that regardless of significant decreases in physical functioning and reports of mild to moderately severe cognitive impairments, only a small percentage of SCA survivors were severely psychologically distressed. The differences in these findings may be due to differences in sample sizes and definitions of distress.

Very few studies have described the efficacy of psychosocial interventions in cardiac patients. Carney et al[23-25] successfully used cognitive behavioral therapy, according to the Beck[26] model, for mild to moderate depression commonly observed in cardiac populations. Frasure-Smith[11] reported a significant decrease in mortality in psychologically distressed patients post-MI after a psychosocial intervention that involved telephone calls and home visits by nurses. There have been no studies describing the efficacy of psychosocial interventions for SCA survivors.

The overall goals of this psychosocial therapy are to reduce mortality and morbidity after out-of-hospital SCA. However, this study is in year 4 of a 5-year study, and analysis of the primary end points has not been done. The purpose of this chapter is to describe the effects of cognitive behavioral therapy on an overview of the biobehavioral symptoms of SCA survivors who were randomized to treatment or control groups. The therapy consists of three main components: (1) cognitive behavioral strategies, (2) use of biofeedback for physiological relaxation of responses associated with the autonomic nervous system, and (3) health education. The three objectives of this chapter are to describe the effects of the therapy on (1) symptoms of stress in SCA survivors compared with three other populations: hypertensives, patients admitted to a stress management clinic, and firefighters; (2) a structural equation model of quality of life (including the concepts of psychological distress, functional ability, and health status); and (3) heart rate variability (HRV).

Methods

A randomized, two-group experimental design was used for this study. Data were collected at baseline and at 6 weeks after the intervention. The treatment group received cognitive/behavioral therapy, and the control group received conventional care.

Sample

The sample sizes for the objective to compare symptoms of stress across four populations were the following: 130 survivors of SCA, 60 persons with hypertension, 322 persons who were self-admitted to a stress management clinic, and 2003 firefighters. All the subjects except the firefighters received similar forms of self-management therapy with biofeedback.

The sample size for analysis of the structural equation model of quality of life consisted of 117 persons who had out-of-hospital SCA caused by ventricular fibrillation: 59 persons received cognitive/behavioral therapy, and 58 persons were in the control group. There were no significant differences in the characteristics of the two groups of the sample. The mean age of these SCA survivors was 60 years, 20% were women, 91% were white, 5% were black, 1% were Asian American, 2% were Native American, and 1% were Hispanic

American. The average time from the SCA to treatment was 18 months. More than half of the subjects had a prior MI, mild congestive heart failure, and one or more of the primary risk factors for cardiovascular disease (hypertension, hyperlipidemia, and/or smoking).

The sample size for the results shown for the effects of psychosocial therapy on HRV consisted of six SCA survivors before and after therapy.

Psychosocial Therapy

The treatment consisted of 11 sessions of about 1.5 hours each given twice a week for 6 weeks. The treatment consisted of three components, each of which had several dimensions: cognitive behavioral strategies, physiological relaxation strategies, and a health education component.

The theoretical and conceptual bases of the therapy relied on four behavioral models: (1) cognitive behavioral theory, (2) self-management theory, (3) Lazarus' theory of coping, and (4) stress management. Cognitive therapy alleviates symptoms by teaching the person to identify and correct distorted or negative thoughts and teaches certain strategies to prevent further recurrence of these thoughts, or "triggers," that are linked to symptoms. A basic premise of behavioral therapy is that one cannot change behavior without increasing one's awareness, raising one's consciousness, or noticing a behavior pattern (how one thinks, feels, and behaves and the impact one has on others).[26]

Kanfer and Gaelick-Buys[27] described self-management or self-regulation therapy as psychological processes that assume everyday behaviors are well-learned repertoires that are stored in long-term memory, which become an automatic mode of cognitive processing. When behaviors need to be changed, self-regulation processes are called into play.

Lazarus and Folkman[28] defined coping as the cognitive and behavioral process through which the individual manages the demands of the person-environment relationship that are appraised as stressful and the emotions they generate. Coping is viewed as emotion-focused and problem-solving–focused.

Stress management is considered to be a component of relaxation therapy and self-management therapy to enhance cognitive self-control of emotional, physiological, and behavioral responses and as a strategy to cognitively change autonomic nervous system responses by increasing sympathetic and/or decreasing parasympathetic responses. Relaxation strategies are taught with physiological response biofeedback to enhance training and self-efficacy.[29]

Cognitive/Coping Strategies

This component included three general themes: (1) cognitive restructuring, (2) management of emotions, and (3) problem-solving techniques. Cognitive restructuring included management of internal messages and of distorted thinking. Strategies were presented for depression management, anger management, and anxiety management. Problem-solving techniques included conflict management.

Cognitive restructuring is a process whereby the subject alters the chain of events that leads to the labeling of an event as a threat. The subject changes how he or she perceives the situation. The subject can change preexisting beliefs about the situation. This process occurs for events that are real or not real. There are essentially three steps in the process of cognitive restructuring. The first is the assessment of one's internal messages or distorted thinking. The next step is evaluating the message. The third step is to restructure or change troublesome messages, ie, management of internal messages and management of distorted thinking. Distorted thinking includes such processes as filtering, polarized thinking, overgeneralization, mindreading, catastrophizing, personalizing, fallacies, emotional reasoning, blaming, and being right.

Depression management included strategies involving recognition and awareness of the thoughts and patterns associated with depression; covert assertion, which trains the person to end emotional distress through the development of two separate strategies of thought interruption and thought substitution; contracting with oneself for rewards and reinforcers; use of relaxation techniques such as abdominal breathing and progressing muscle relaxation; problem-solving; and cognitive restructuring.

Anger management included strategies involving combatting distorted thinking, stress inoculation, problem-solving, and covert assertion. Stress inoculation consisted of three steps: first, recognition of the "triggers" for one's anger; second, construction of a list of thoughts and behaviors for coping with anger; and third, perfection of an anger-reducing strategy learned through biofeedback (ie, one of the relaxation techniques).

Anxiety management strategies included self-recognition of the physiological and psychological responses associated with anxiety, awareness of the possible antecedents, and the use of values clarification, cognitive restructuring, deep breathing, progressive relaxation techniques, and/or autogenic relaxation techniques.

Conflict management is posed as a five-step method of problem-solving: recognition of the problem, outline of one's responses, list of one's alternatives, recognition of the consequences, and evaluation of one's results.

Physiological Relaxation Strategies

Four types of relaxation techniques with biofeedback were taught: (1) abdominal breathing, (2) progressive muscle relaxation, (3) the quieting response, and (4) autogenic training. These strategies were aimed at training the individual to cognitively control physiological responses to the autonomic nervous system and to become aware of those responses that are indicative of decreased sympathetic nervous system arousal and/or increased parasympathetic tone, as measured with biofeedback by blood pressure, heart rate, breathing rate, digital temperature, and electromyograph signals.

Abdominal breathing consisted of deep (tidal volume 1 to 2 times deeper) and slow (6 to 8 breaths per minute) breathing, which causes relaxation, specifically during expiration. A deeper tidal volume is achieved with abdominal breathing than with thoracic breathing. This strategy is based on the respiratory sinus arrhythmia, that is, deep, slow breathing causes the heart rate pattern to follow the breathing pattern, thus increasing HRV.[30] This response is aimed primarily at training subjects specifically to increase and decrease heart rate, that is, to increase HRV. Decreased HRV has been shown to be a high predictor of mortality 3 years after an acute MI.[31,32] Abdominal breathing also decreases systolic and diastolic blood pressure, heart rate, and breathing rate. These responses were recorded both in digital form and in analog signals on the computer for the subject to have interactive biofeedback.

In progressive muscle relaxation, various muscle groups are tensed and released in succession. The goal is to learn to release muscle tension when it is present and to learn the difference between tension and relaxation. The subjects were taught to relax the shoulders, hands, forearms, feet, lower legs, head, jaws, lips, and forehead.[33] Progressive muscle relaxation decreases the electromyogram signal and blood pressure, which are recorded digitally for biofeedback. The quieting response is a combination of abdominal breathing and progressive muscle relaxation strategies.[34]

The fourth type of relaxation therapy is autogenic training, which helps the subject to control some physiological responses such as increased temperature to the fingers caused by increased blood flow. The exercises used in autogenic training rely on the slow repetition of phrases that emphasize heaviness and warmth in the extremities.[35] Autogenic training is measured by digital temperature.

Health Education Component

Educational material specific to an event of SCA included material on the autonomic nervous system; the relation of HRV and breathing pattern to SCA; effects of the autonomic nervous system on emotions, blood pressure, heart rate, breathing rate, muscle tension, and blood flow; stress theory; and self-management theory. Also, information was provided about cardiovascular risk factors.

Measurements and Analyses

Three sets of measurements will be described as they are related to the three purposes of this chapter: (1) symptoms of stress, (2) measures used in the structural equation model, and (3) power spectral analysis of HRV.

Symptoms of Stress

The Symptoms of Stress (SOS) instrument was used in the standard database of the Management of Stress Response Laboratory. It is a self-report questionnaire adapted from the Cornell Medical Index. Individuals are asked to indicate the frequencies with which they have experienced physiological, psychological, and behavioral stress-related symptomatology (from 0-never to 4-frequently). The tool yields a total score (derived from 94 items) and 10 subscale scores. Interitem reliability (Cornbach's alpha) of the SOS is quite high ($r=0.96$), with correlational coefficients calculated on the subscales ranging from 0.71 to 0.87. Data from a sample of stress management clients (n=410) indicate a relatively high correlation ($r=0.81$) of the total SOS score with the total score on a widely used psychiatric rating scale, the Symptom Checklist-90R.[36] The Cronbach's alphas on the scale/subscales from the author's current study of SCA survivors (n=93) were for peripheral manifestations, 0.69; cardiopulmonary (a), 0.82; upper respiratory (b), 0.84; cardiopulmonary total (a+b), 0.88; central neurological, 0.77; gastrointestinal, 0.61; muscle tension, 0.90; habitual patterns, 0.85; depression, 0.89; anxiety/fear, 0.83; emotional irritability (anger), 0.91; cognitive disorganization, 0.82; and total, 0.96.

Structural Equation Measures

Multiple measures, referred to as "indicators" in the structural equation literature, were collected for each of the dimensions assessed. Results of factor analyses supported the choice of indicators for each dimension. For all factor loadings, $P>0.01$.

Quality of life was measured by use of three indicators, each of which was a weighted score representing importance and satisfaction with peace of mind, happiness, and life in general. These questionnaire items were selected from the Ferrans and Powers Quality of Life Index (Cardiac III),[37] items 31, 34, and 35. For each item, the respondents were asked, "How important is . . ." and "How satisfied are you with . . .": "peace of mind," "happiness," "being satisfied with your life?" Responses were coded from 1 to 6, from very unimportant or very unsatisfied to very important or very satisfied, respectively. Each item was weighted for importance and satisfaction, so that those items that were unimportant and unsatisfying were not weighted as much as others.

Health status was measured by three indicators representing satisfaction with own health, satisfaction with own energy level, and number of sick days. The first two indicators were weighted questionnaire items selected from the Ferrans and Powers Quality of Life Index (Cardiac III),[37] items 1 and 5, respectively: "How important (weighted with how satisfied) are you with your health?" and "How important (weighted with how satisfied) are you with the amount of energy you have for everyday activities?" The third indicator, days sick, was computed from two items (items 3 and 4) of the Functional Status Questionnaire:[38] "During the past month, how many days did illness or injury keep you in bed all or most of the day?" and "During the past month, how many days did you cut down on things you usually do because of your own illness or injury?" This sum was then logarithmically transformed.

Functional ability was measured by three indicators representing difficulty in walking, doing housework, and doing errands. These questionnaire items were selected from the Functional Status Questionnaire,[38] items 1.5, 1.6, and 1.7, respectively: "During the past month have you had difficulty walking one block or climbing one flight of stairs?" ". . . doing work around the house such as cleaning, light yard work, home maintenance?" or ". . . doing errands such as grocery shopping?" Responses were coded 0 to 5 from "usually did not do because of health" to "no difficulty," respectively.

Psychological distress was measured by use of two indicators representing depression and anxiety. The questionnaire item for depression was selected from the Psychosocial Adjustment to Illness Scale (PAIS),[39] section VII, item 2: "Recently, have you felt sad, depressed, lost interest in things, or felt hopeless?" Responses were coded a to d, from "not at all" to "extremely," respectively. The questionnaire item for anxiety was selected from the Symptom Checklist-90 (SCL-90),[40] item 57: "How much were you distressed by feeling tense or keyed up?"

The EQS 5 (Multivariate Software, Inc, Encino, CA) computer program was used to evaluate the plausibility of the factors for a structural equation model.

Heart Rate Variability

HRV was measured by standardized methods described by Cowan et al.[5,6,41] The autoregressive technique was used for power spectral analysis. The power spectrum of HRV was estimated by use of a 25th-order autoregressive spectral model, AR(25), to fit successive 100-second analysis windows of RR sequences that had been interpolated onto a real-time base. Two power spectra of HRV averaged over all individuals were compared descriptively before and after the psychosocial therapy.

Results

Symptoms of Stress

The same instrument was used to measure symptoms of stress for all four samples. Results indicated that cognitive behavioral therapy significantly reduced depression, anxiety, anger, and cardiovascular symptoms of stress in hypertensives and the Stress Management Clinic clients (Figures 1 and 2). However, the therapy did not have an effect on the survivors of SCA. The baseline pretest values of all symptoms of stress in the SCA survivors were very low. The baseline values of symptoms of stress of the other three samples were in general very high, with some subscales being higher than others.

Model of Quality of Life

The results of tests of model fit for the structural equation model were $\chi^2=257.64$; $df=253$; $P<0.05$; and comparative fit index $=0.96$. Therefore, the model fit was satisfactory. Figure 3 shows the structural equation model of the treatment effects.

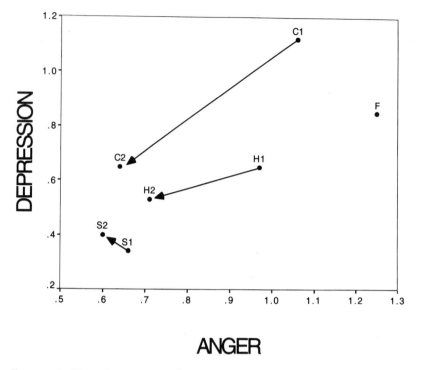

FIGURE 1. *Two Symptoms of Stress subscales, depression and anger, compared across four populations: sudden cardiac arrest survivors (S) (n=130), hypertensives (H) (n=60), stress management clinic patients (C) (n=322), and firefighters (F) (n=2003). The first three groups had similar self-management therapies.*

Cognitive-behavioral therapy had a statistically significant direct effect of decreasing psychological distress, $P<0.05$. Since psychological distress was weighted more heavily by depression, the direct effect of the treatment was to decrease depression in SCA survivors. Cognitive-behavioral therapy did not have a direct effect on quality of life, but it had a significant indirect effect on quality of life through psychological distress, $P<0.05$, since treatment had a significant effect on psychological distress, which in turn had a significant effect on quality of life. Cognitive-behavioral therapy did not have a significant effect on health status or functional ability.

Heart Rate Variability

Figure 4 compares two power spectra for 9 hours of HRV during nighttime sleep, averaged for all subjects before and after 5

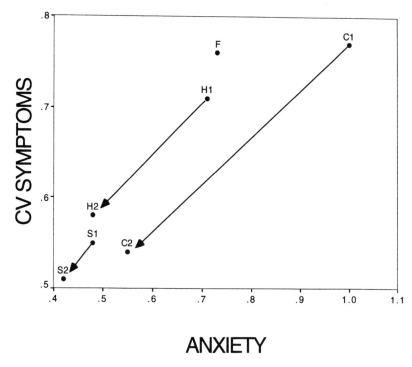

ANXIETY

FIGURE 2. *Two Symptoms of Stress subscales, Cardiopulmonary function and anxiety, compared across four populations: sudden cardiac arrest survivors (S) (n=130), hypertensives (H) (n=60), stress management clinic patients (C) (n=322), and firefighters (F) (n=2003). The first three groups had similar self-management therapies.*

weeks of stress management with biofeedback training. After biofeedback training, the power spectral density is markedly higher in the high-frequency range (0.27 to 0.30 Hz) and slightly lower in the low-frequency range (0.05 Hz).

Conclusions

In conclusion, because of the lack of symptoms of stress in the SCA population at baseline, the cognitive/behavioral and stress management components of the intervention did not and could not further lower their symptoms of stress. This result also explains why there were no significant differences in measuring coping, because the SCA survivors did not perceive a stressor with which it was necessary to cope.

When other factors such as functional ability and perception of

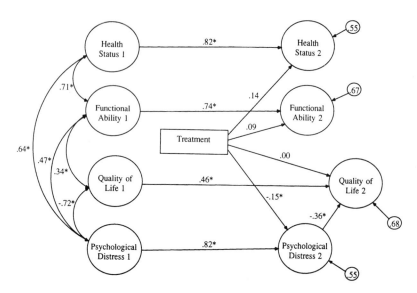

FIGURE 3. *Structural equation model of treatment effects. Goodness-of-fit statistics: $\chi^2=257.64$, df=253, P>0.01, comparative fit index =0.96. *P<0.05.*

health and baseline levels of psychosocial distress were controlled for, the treatment significantly lowered psychosocial distress, of which depression was more heavily weighted than anxiety. However, only ≈15% of the SCA survivors had severe depression, defined as having scores on the depression subscale of the Symptom Checklist (SCL-90) >2 SD above the mean scores. The treatment did not affect quality of life directly; however, if depression was improved, then quality of life improved.

SCA survivors had decreased HRV, usually showing a decrease in the high-frequency range (0.20 to 0.35 Hz) of the power spectrum, indicating decreased parasympathetic tone. The low-frequency range (centered around 0.05 Hz) of the power spectrum, an index of sympathetic tone, was unchanged or minimally affected.[4–6,41,42] Kleiger et al[31,32] reported an association between low HRV and mortality in MI patients within 2 years after the event. This psychosocial treatment increased the power spectrum within the high-frequency range, suggesting an improvement in parasympathetic tone. Most of the physiological relaxation parameters with biofeedback emphasized cognitive control and enhancement of parasympathetic arousal, for example, deep breathing. There is evidence that spontaneous fluctuations in heart rate that occur in relation to the phase in respiration (ie, respiratory sinus arrhythmia) are mediated primarily by the parasympathetic system.[43,44]

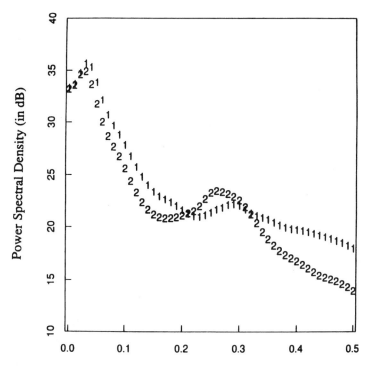

FIGURE 4. *"Pre-post" training contrast of two power spectra of HRV. Average power density spectra of HRV of all subjects (n=6) during 9 nighttime hours. The pretraining spectrum is represented by 1 and the posttraining spectrum by 2. The posttraining spectrum forms a peak in the high-frequency range (0.25 Hz), suggesting an increase in parasympathetic activity. The posttraining spectrum is slightly lower than the pretraining spectrum in the low-frequency range (0.05 Hz), suggesting a slight decrease in sympathetic activity. Reprinted with permission from Reference 5.*

The greatest posttraining increases in the high-frequency peaks of the power spectral densities occurred during the night. Our results are supported by those of Bigger et al.[45] Bigger's group hypothesized that the nighttime heart rate is governed predominantly by the level of parasympathetic activity, except for periods of rapid eye movement.[45] Thus, given our and Bigger's findings of low parasympathetic activity during the night in SCA survivors, one might expect that interventions to increase parasympathetic activity (such as respiration-driven relaxation therapy with biofeedback to induce the respiratory sinus arrhythmia and thus increase HRV during training) would bring about a greater resumption of parasympathetic activity during the night.

Summary

Cognitive behavioral therapy may offer an innovative approach to improving psychosocial and physiological outcomes for SCA survivors, as evidenced in this study by the intervention effect on depression and HRV. As more data on the effect of cognitive therapy become available and are clarified, the ability to define characteristics of responsive SCA survivors will allow more efficient applications of these innovative approaches in clinical settings.

References

1. Bigger JT, Fleiss JL, Kleiger R, et al. The relationships among ventricular arrhythmias, left ventricular dysfunction, and mortality in the 2 years after myocardial infarction. *Circulation.* 1984;69:250–258.
2. Greene HL. Sudden arrhythmic cardiac death: mechanisms, resuscitation and classification: the Seattle perspective. *Am J Cardiol.* 1990; 65:4B–12B.
3. Myerburg RJ, Conde CA, Sung RJ, et al. Clinical, electrophysiologic, and hemodynamic profile of patients resuscitated from prehospital cardiac arrest. *Am J Med.* 1980;68:568–576.
4. Myers GA, Martin GJ, Magid NM, et al. Power spectral analysis of heart rate variability in sudden cardiac death: comparison to other methods. *IEEE Trans Biomed Eng.* 1986;33:1149–1156.
5. Cowan MJ, Kogan H, Burr R, et al. Power spectral analysis of heart rate variability after biofeedback training. *J Electrocardiol.* 1991; 23(suppl):85–94.
6. Cowan MJ, Pike KC, Burr RL. Effects of gender and age on heart rate variability in healthy volunteers and in persons after sudden cardiac arrest. *J Electrocardiol.* 1994;27(suppl):1–9.
7. Baroldi G, Falzi G, Mariani F. Sudden coronary death: a post-mortem study in 208 selected cases compared to 97 "control" subjects. *Am Heart J.* 1979;98:20–31.
8. Reichenbach D, Moss N, Meyer E. Pathology of the heart in sudden cardiac death. *Am J Cardiol.* 1977;39:865–872.
9. Weaver WD, Lorch GS, Alvarez HA, et al. Angiographic findings and prognostic indicators in patients resuscitated from sudden cardiac death. *Circulation.* 1976;54:895–900.
10. Cobb LA, Hallstrom AP. Community-based cardiopulmonary resuscitation: what have we learned? *Ann N Y Acad Sci.* 1982;382:330–341.
11. Frasure-Smith N. In-hospital symptoms of psychological stress as predictors of long-term outcome after acute myocardial infarction in men. *Am J Cardiol.* 1991;67:121–127.
12. Frasure-Smith N, Lespérance F, Talajic M. Depression following myocardial infarction: impact on 6-month survival. *JAMA.* 1993;270: 1819–1825.
13. Frasure-Smith N, Lespérance F, Talajic M. Depression and 18-month prognosis after myocardial infarction. *Circulation.* 1995;91:999–1005.

14. Ahern DK, Gorkin L, Anderson JL, et al. Biobehavioral variables and mortality or cardiac arrest in the cardiac arrhythmia pilot study (CAPS). *Am J Cardiol.* 1990;66:59–62.
15. Ladwig KH, Keiser M, König J, et al. Affective disorders and survival after acute myocardial infarction: results from the post-infarction late potential study. *Eur Heart J.* 1991;12:959–964.
16. Ladwig KH, Lehmacher W, Roth R, et al. Factors which provoke post-infarction depression: results from the Post-infarction Late Potential Study (PILP). *J Psychosom Res.* 1992;36:723–729.
17. Ladwig KH, Röll G, Breithardt G, et al. Post-infarction depression and incomplete recovery 6 months after acute myocardial infarction. *Lancet.* 1994;343:20–23.
18. Case RB, Moss AJ, Case N, et al. Living alone after myocardial infarction: impact on prognosis. *JAMA.* 1992;267:515–519.
19. Ruberman W, Weinblatt E, Goldberg JD, et al. Psychosocial influences on mortality after myocardial infarction. *N Engl J Med.* 1984;311: 552–559.
20. Berkman LF, Leo-Summers L, Horwitz RI. Emotional support and survival after myocardial infarction: a prospective population-based study of the elderly. *Ann Intern. Med.* 1992;117:1003–1009.
21. Dougherty CM. Longitudinal recovery following sudden cardiac arrest and internal cardioverter defibrillator implantation: survivors and their families. *Am J Crit Care.* 1994;3:145–154.
22. Sauvé MJ. Long term physical functioning and psychosocial adjustment in survivors of sudden cardiac death. *Heart Lung.* 1995;24:133–144.
23. Carney RM, Rich MW, teVelde A, et al. Major depressive disorder in coronary artery disease. *Am J Cardiol* 1987;60:1273–1275.
24. Carney RM, Rich MW, Freedland KE, et al. Major depressive disorder predicts cardiac events in patients with coronary artery disease. *Psychosom Med.* 1988;50:627–633.
25. Carney R, Freedland KE, Rich MW, et al. Ventricular tachycardia and psychiatric depression in patients with coronary artery disease. *Am J Med.* 1993;95:23–28.
26. Beck AT, Rush AJ, Shaw BF, et al. *Cognitive Therapy of Depression.* New York: NY: The Guilford Press; 1979.
27. Kanfer FH, Gaelick-Buys L. Self-management methods. In: Kanfer FH, Goldstein AP, eds. *Helping People Change: A Textbook of Methods.* New York, NY: Pergamon Press; 1991:308–314.
28. Lazarus RS, Folkman S. *Stress, Appraisal, and Coping.* New York, NY: Springer Publishing Co; 1984.
29. Nakagawa-Kogan H, Betrus P. Self-management: a nursing mode of therapeutic influence. *Adv Nurs Sci.* 1984;6:55–73.
30. Sroufe LA. Effects of depth and rate of breathing on heart rate and heart rate variability. *Psychophysiology.* 1991;8:648–655.
31. Kleiger RE, Miller JP, Bigger JT Jr, et al. Heart rate variability: a variable predicting mortality following acute myocardial infarction. *J Am Coll Cardiol.* 1984;3:547.
32. Kleiger RE, Miller JP, Bigger JT Jr, et al. Decreased heart rate variability and its association with increased mortality after acute myocardial infarction. *Am J Cardiol.* 1987;59:256–262.
33. Davis M, McKay M, Eshelman E. *The Relaxation and Stress Reduction Workbook.* 2nd ed. Oakland, Calif: New Harbinger; 1982.

34. Stroebel C. Quieting reflex (QR): a conditioned reflex for optimizing applied psychophysiology, biofeedback and self-regulation therapies. In: Basmajian JV, ed. *Biofeedback: Principles and Practice for Clinicians.* 3rd ed. Baltimore, Md: Williams & Wilkins; 1989.

35. Stoyva JM. Autogenic training. In: Basmajian JV, ed. *Biofeedback: Principles and Practice for Clinicians.* 3rd ed. Baltimore, Md: Williams & Wilkins; 1989.

36. Kogan HN, Beaton R, Betrus P, et al. *Therapeutic Manual for Stress Response Management.* Seattle, Wash: Department of Psychosocial Nursing, University of Washington; unpublished, revised 1991.

37. Ferrans CE, Powers MJ. Quality of life index: development and psychometric properties. *Adv Nursing Sci.* 1985;8:15–24.

38. Jette A, Davies A, Cleary P, et al. The functional status questionnaire: reliability and validity when used in primary care. *J Gen Intern Med.* 1986;1:143–149.

39. Derogatis LR, Lopez MC, *PAIS and PAIS SR: Administration, Scoring and Procedures Manual I: Clinical Psychometric Research.* Baltimore, Md: Johns Hopkins University Press; 1983.

40. Derogatis LR, Lipman R, Covey L. The SCL-90. *Psychopharmacol Bull.* 1983;9:13–28.

41. Cowan MJ, Pike K, Burr RL, et al. Description of time and frequency domain based measures of heart rate variability in individuals taking antiarrhythmics, beta blockers, calcium channel blockers, and/or antihypertensive drugs after sudden cardiac arrest. *J Electrocardiol.* 1994; 26(suppl):1–13.

42. Singer DH, Martin GJ, Magid N, et al. Low heart rate variability and sudden cardiac death. *J Electrocardiol.* 1988;21(suppl):S46–S55.

43. Katona PG, Poitras JW, Barnett GO, et al. Cardiac vagal efferent activity and heart period in the cartoid sinus reflex. *Am J Physiol.* 1970; 218:1030–1037.

44. Katona PG, Jih F. Respiratory sinus arrhythmia: noninvasive measure of parasympathetic cardiac control. *J Appl Physiol.* 1975;39:801–805.

45. Bigger JT Jr, Kleiger RE, Fleiss JL, et al. Components of heart rate variability measured during healing of acute myocardial infarction. *Am J Cardiol.* 1988;61:208–215.

Chapter 23

Impact of Managed Care

Gayle R. Whitman, RN, MSN, and Susan M. Daunch, RN, BSN

Accounting for ≈300 000 deaths a year and 100000 annual hospital admissions for the management of recurrent ventricular tachycardia, sudden cardiac death (SCD) remains a major public health problem. Treatment strategies for SCD can include multiple and extensive drug trials, catheter ablation, cardiac surgery, and implantation of a implantable cardioverter-defibrillator (ICD). All of these therapies, their concomitant hospitalization, and follow-up care are not without significant economic impact. Empirical antiarrhythmic therapy has been associated with costs of >$35 000.[1] Pricing for the ICD system ranges from $16 000 to $25 000, and it is estimated that 30 000 devices will be implanted, annually with resultant projected costs of $1.5 billion.[2] Decelerating and controlling the growth in healthcare expenditures has been a major focus in the American healthcare agenda throughout the 1990s. Managed care has emerged as one of the dominant strategies being used to control this growth and to rebalance the national healthcare economic equation. This chapter will focus on some of the resource-controlling strategies that managed care brings to the healthcare market and the actual or potential responses and impact these have on the providers caring for persons who survive a sudden cardiac arrest (SCA).

Managed Care

Simply defined, managed care is a method of managing the delivery of health care in such a manner that costs are controlled. A managed-care plan or system can at present run the gamut from sys-

From: Dunbar SB, Ellenbogen KA, Epstein AE, (eds). *Sudden Cardiac Death: Past, Present, and Future.* Armonk, NY: Futura Publishing Company, Inc.; © 1997.

tems that have high patient/member choice and thus high costs to low patient/member choice and therefore lower costs. A Preferred Provider Organization (PPO) is an example of a healthcare payment and delivery system with networks of doctors and hospitals who agree to provide services and be paid at negotiated rates. Members can go outside the network of care but are offered a discount if they see providers on the preferred list. The method provides high choice but at a high cost. At the other end of the range is a Health Maintenance Organization (HMO), in which members pay a per-member/per-month charge that will cover all the costs associated with the health care provided to them by one healthcare provider group. If members elect to go outside the provider list or desire treatments or procedures outside the provider's protocol, the members assume all the costs. Within this system, there are the fewest patient choices for provider or level of service but the lowest costs.

Currently, 40 million Americans are enrolled in HMOs, and it is projected that 66 million will be enrolled by 1997.[3] As markets become saturated with these higher enrollments and excess costs of care are eliminated from the care delivery systems, the financial profits for managed-care firms will decrease. To remain competitive, managed-care firms will need to redefine their business and goals. Goldsmith et al[4] suggest that this redefining will ultimately lead to a focus on health improvement and prevention to control costs and maintain profits. Table 1 depicts Goldsmith's three stages in the evolution of managed care. These stages are the event-driven cost-avoidance stage, the value improvement stage, and the health improvement stage. Different goals and objectives are desired in each

TABLE 1

Managed Care Stages of Evolution

	Stage 1: Event-Driven Cost Avoidance	Stage 2: Value Improvement	Stage 3: Health Improvement
Objective function	Price	Value customer satisfaction	Health status improvement
Cost targets	Inpatient days	Resource intensity	Health risks
Locus of control	External	Peer driven	"Contract" with family
Focal point	Inpatient hospital	Physician network	Home neighborhood

Reprinted with permission from Reference 4.

stage, and as managed care evolves through these stages, the financial risk is gradually shifted from the payer or managed-care firm to the patient and community. If providers are to be able to continue to provide quality, state-of-the-art care to patients, it will be incumbent upon them to ensure that their practices appropriately match the evolving goals and objectives of these three stages. Specifically, comparing the goals and objectives of these three stages with the current and potential practice trends of care providers will provide a glimpse into the managed-care future awaiting patients who survive (SCA). Table 2 summarizes the actual or potential responses by providers, which will be discussed in more depth below.

TABLE 2

Potential Responses by SCA Patient Care Providers to Managed Care Evolution

Event-Driven Cost Avoidance	Value Improvement	Health Improvement
External benchmarking to compare LOS and admissions	Manufacturing smaller devices	Cost-effectiveness analysis of SCD therapies
Using outpatient department and observation units	Devices have multiple capabilities	"Quality" of life years yet to be determined
Negotiate competitive pricing for technology	Reprogramming to enhance generator longevity	Genetic research to identify high-risk populations
Limit models and inventory	Identifying and targeting educational and psychosocial needs	Primary prevention programs in community and at work
Consider reuse	Increasing transvenous insertions and decreasing resource utilization	Public access defibrillation
	Developing clinical practice guidelines for use of technology and procedures	
	Prospective randomized trials to determine approaches for secondary and primary prevention of SCD	

Responses to the Event-Driven Cost-Avoidance Stage

In this first stage of managed care, emphasis is placed by the payer on generating revenue and avoiding costs. This is done by securing discounted fees and charges from providers. Additionally, aggressive utilization review to drive down unnecessary hospital admissions and length of stay (LOS), and hence costs, is also applied. Providers use a number of strategies in response to these actions. Reevaluating practice, eliminating unnecessary admissions, and shortening LOS is critical. Using external benchmarks to compare LOS and admission rates provides a quick snapshot of what other providers are doing with utilization. Table 3 lists current Health Care Financing Administration–designated LOSs for diagnosis-related groups relevant to ventricular dysrhythmia patients and patients who survive an SCA.[5] Total hospital inpatient days per 1000 HMO members was 275 in 1995, which was down 12.7% from 315 in 1994. The national average for cardiac inpatient days was 32, and cardiac admissions were 6 per 1000 patients.[6] These rates have continued to decrease over the years, partly because of a shift toward the expanded use of the outpatient department and of 23-hour observation units for selected patient populations, such as those requiring generator replacement.

Technology costs involved in care of patients with ventricular dysrhythmias and survivors of SCA are substantial. Wholesale costs of ICD systems have been reported to be between $21 000 and $25 000.[7] Actual costs to the provider may be negotiated as low as $11 000 to $16 000, depending on the current market. Optimally, providers negotiate these costs separately with the payer to be outside the diagnosis-related group or per diem rate. Costs can also be reduced by minimizing provider inventory and limiting the number of vendors and the types of models providers maintain. Using a competitive bidding strategy between a selected group of two or three vendors can optimize provider pricing. Additionally, short-term contracts with savings early rather than later are economically superior and ensure easier access to newer technologies developed by alternative vendors.

Reusing disposable technology to control costs has also gained acceptance in the past several years. A number of studies have reported on the safe reuse of catheters used for electrophysiology procedures.[8,9] Since 1978, nine countries (Australia, Brazil, Canada, Finland, France, Hungary, Italy, Israel, and the United States) have reported on the safe installation of reused pacemakers.[10-17] Mugica et al,[18] in a 10-year follow-up of 3701 patients, re-

TABLE 3

Health Care Financing Administration's Proposed 1996 LOS for
Dysrhythmia-Related Diagnosis-Related Groups

Diagnosis-Related Group	Description	LOS, days
104	Cardiac valve procedures with cardiac catheterization	16.0
105	Cardiac valve procedures without cardiac catheterization	12.0
112	Percutaneous cardiovascular procedures	5.0
115	Permanent cardiac pacemaker implant with acute myocardial infarction heart failure shock	11.8
116	Other permanent cardiac pacemaker implant or ICD lead or generator procedure	5.9
117	Cardiac pacemaker revision except device replacement	4.5
118	Cardiac pacemaker device replacement	3.4
138	Cardiac arrhythmic and conduction disorders with comorbid condition	5.0
139	Cardiac arrhythmic and conduction disorders without comorbid condition	3.2
141	Syncope and collapse with comorbid condition	5.0
142	Syncope and collapse without comorbid condition	3.5

Reprinted with permission from Reference 5.

ported that there were no significant differences in actuarial survival between patients who received new pacemakers and patients who received reused devices. Because 19% to 58% of patients die within 2 years of pacemaker implantation, the number of reliable pacemakers that could be recovered is significant.[19,20] MacGregor estimated that in 1989, if 19% of all the instruments implanted in Canada could have been reused, it would have saved the Canadian healthcare system $4.2 million. In 1985, the North American Society of Pacing and Electrophysiology (NASPE) supported the reuse of pacemakers.[21] Although it is currently not a widespread practice, the economic opportunity of pacemaker reuse and perhaps even ICD recycling cannot be dismissed. The savings incurred from reuse or the savings derived as vendors reduce the costs of new technology to be able to compete with the costs of reused technology could have a major impact in a managed-care environment.

Responses to the Value Improvement Stage

In the value improvement stage of managed care, the easy cost savings have been achieved, and now competitive pricing and customer service advantages are required. In this stage, initiatives to enhance long-term, high-quality, competitive advantages that limit readmission and complications are critical. Resource utilization across the continuum is now scrutinized, and utilization patterns are altered if necessary. Reengineering patient-flow processes by use of clinical pathways and algorithms, outcome monitoring, and total quality management techniques are all used in this stage. However, more important than just using these strategies is a need to see them link to profitability and improved customer satisfaction, which might result in an increase in market share. Many of these strategies are already evolving in the SCD and dysrhythmia field. The movement of ICD and pacemaker technology to smaller devices with longer generator life is congruent with the need for long-term fiscal and patient-satisfaction competitive advantages, because this limits readmission for generator changes. Currently, ICDs have multiple capabilities, such as antitachycardia and bradycardia pacing, low- and high-energy cardioversion, and sophisticated diagnostic functions and invasive programmed stimulation. This allows clinicians to implant devices that can be adapted over time to manage numerous clinical problems that may evolve without the need for generator changes. Optimizing the schedule of postimplantation visits for generator checks can also decrease costs and enhance patient satisfaction. As Gayle et al[22] demonstrated, reprogramming pulse generators at outpatient visits can extend the estimated pulse generator longevity by slightly more than 4 years at a mean cost of $192 per patient, thus increasing the fraction of patients who will require only one pacemaker for life.

Patient and family satisfaction can be enhanced and costs further controlled by identifying interventions that address quality-of-life and psychosocial issues. Dunbar et al[23] demonstrated that patients and spouses have different recovery patterns after ICD implantation. Specifically, family members had significantly greater decreases in tension, depression, and confusion and increased vigor at 1 month after ICD implantation compared with patients. Hawthorne et al[24] report that women 1 month after ICD placement have higher depression, confusion, and tension scores than men and that single women have higher mood disturbance scores than married women. These authors suggest that given these results, providing different and/or separate education and interventions for these subgroups might be appropriate. Providing tailored education and interventions could enhance patient and customer satisfaction and affect costs through decreasing or eliminating unnecessary follow-up for anxiety or depression.

Resource utilization related to ICD implantation has begun to diminish over the past few years as the trend toward transvenous insertion has grown. Hospital charges for epicardial insertions have been reported to range from $63 000 to $72 000, compared with transvenous ICD charges of $53 000 to $55 000.[25-27] This 15% to 20% global reduction in charges has been achieved largely through a decrease in total hospital LOSs and an elimination of intensive care stays. Reduction in professional fees and ICD system costs have also contributed to this overall fiscal improvement.

Clinical practice guideline development has also begun within this population, as evidenced by the various position statements and guidelines developed by NASPE, the American Heart Association, and the American College of Cardiology, many of which deal with the appropriate indications for the timing and use of various technologies and procedures.[28] General consensus on practice patterns for treating survivors of SCA or patients at high risk for SCD continues to evolve. At present, it is widely accepted that guided drug therapy with electrophysiological testing is the first tier of therapies. If this approach fails to suppress dysrhythmias, ICD implantation is then undertaken. Since the efficacy of antidysrhythmic drug therapy is often disappointing,[29-31] a number of practitioners are advocating or have shown that ICD implantation rather than drug therapy should be the first-choice intervention for secondary prevention in SCD survivors.[32-35] To that end, a number of secondary prevention trials have evolved. The Cardiac Arrest Study Hamburg (CASH),[36] the Antiarrhythmia Versus Implantable Defibrillator (AVID) Study,[37] and the Canadian Implantable Defibrillator Study (CIDS)[38] were all designed to evaluate the effectiveness of drug therapy versus the ICD. Ultimately, demonstration of improved survival with ICD implantation will further the movement toward ICD implantation as first-tier therapy for secondary prevention in SCA survivors. However, an unanswered question from these studies will be, "What is the impact of combining these therapies?"

Since fewer than one third of patients who suffer cardiac arrest are resuscitated and live to be discharged from a hospital, the use of drug and ICD implantation for primary prevention or pro-phylactic use in patients considered at high risk for SCD is also be-ing advocated.[39-41] About two thirds of people who experience SCA have recognized heart disease before the terminal event and could be screened effectively for their degree of risk.[42] Three primary prevention trials (the Multicenter Unsustained Tachycardia Trial [MUSTT],[43] the Multicenter Automatic Defibrillator Implantation Trial [MADIT],[44] and the Coronary Artery Bypass Graft-Patch [CABG-PATCH][45]) were designed to assess the effectiveness of drug or device therapy in reducing mortality in these high-risk pa-tients. Development of indications for initiating therapy in these asymptomatic or minimally symptomatic patients previously not treated will greatly expand the pool of people identified as poten-tial SCA patients. In the future, ICD technology could also be ap-plied to other cardiac diseases, such as atrial dysrhythmias, syncope, and dilated cardiomyopathy, in which a high risk of SCD is suggested.[46]

Within the context of a managed-care environment, this ex-pansion and redefining of common guidelines for practice will add value from the perspectives of both clinical outcome and patient and family satisfaction. Care will need to be taken that costs still re-main controlled, because almost doubling the population of pa-tients now considered eligible for treatment would have significant economic impact. The shifting in identification of potential SCA patients from a crisis point in their disease trajectory (ie, after re-suscitation) to a stable point (ie, ischemic but minimally sympto-matic) might also allow for greater overall control of costs, despite the potential burgeoning increase in the number of patients re-quiring these therapies. Testing and procedures can occur on a planned basis, and patients can be queued into the system. Lau et al[47] demonstrated that in a system similar to a managed-care envi-ronment, patients requiring urgent, semiurgent, and elective pace-maker insertions experienced no adverse events and reasonable waiting times when handled via a triaging system for prioritizing pacemaker insertions in a tertiary referral center. However, experi-ence from Britain regarding the impact practice protocols can have on cost should not be overlooked. In 1991, the British Pacing and Electrophysiology Group released recommendations for pace-maker prescription that recommended more use of sophisticated and hence expensive pacemaker technology in most patients. A ret-rospective audit revealed that total adoption of these recommenda-tions could increase expenditures by 75% to 94%.[48,49] In a healthcare system with limited cash and resources, these recom-mendations could not be totally implemented.

Responses to the Health Improvement Stage

The third and final stage in the evolution of managed care is the health improvement stage. By this time, managed-care markets have reduced costs, reengineered their processes, and begun to reach consensus on clinical practice guidelines. To further differentiate themselves and thus maintain their value, they will need to evolve into a public health business. As such, the organizational focus will shift to high-risk individuals in their catchment pools and the prevention and management of their clinical illnesses over the continuum. Although the clinical practice guidelines developed in the second stage addressed indications and timing of treatments and therapies, concerns related to cost-effectiveness and cost-benefit ratios were not completely addressed. In stage three, issues related to cost-effectiveness will now be scrutinized by payers, providers, and ultimately the community, because they will be assuming the costs of wellness and illness for all of their fellow members via their monthly premium payments. Thus, community standards for the use of resources and the expectations for healthy behaviors will grow. This focus on cost-effectiveness and community standards supports the goal of early prevention. Incentives for providers and patients to manage disease before it flows into illness will be offered. Ultimately, genetic testing and manipulation may assist with identifying high-risk individuals early and perhaps to some degree ameliorate the outcomes of their illnesses.

Movement toward these third-stage goals has already commenced for the SCD population. Cost-effectiveness analysis of ICDs describing the costs per year of life saved (YLS) have been reported by a number of authors[50-52] and are summarized in Table 4. When

TABLE 4

Summary of ICD Cost-Effectiveness Studies

	Cost/YLS
Epicardial ICD[50]	$17 000 (1986 $)
	$28 200 (1993 $)
Epicardial ICD[51]	$41 800 (1995 $)
Epicardial ICD vs amiodarone[52]	$29 200 (1989 $)
	$39 400 (1993 $)
Endocardial ICD,[51] no electrophysiological study	$14 200 (1995 $)

implantation of epicardial ICD generators with a 2-year battery life were retrospectively compared with conventional drug therapy, the cost saving per YLS ranged from $17 000 (1986 dollars) to $41 800 (1995 dollars). In an analysis of endocardial ICD systems (which more accurately reflect current practice), the cost per YLS in a group of patients with ejection fractions >25% decreased to $14 200. Cost-effectiveness analysis (CEA) can be calculated from the following equation[53]:

$$CEA = \frac{Cost\ A - Cost\ B}{Outcome\ A - Outcome\ B} = incremental\ cost\ per\ outcome\ unit.$$

An overall criticism of CEA is that the outcome unit or measure (YLSs or survival years) does not capture the true impact of the therapy, because the goal is not merely to prolong life but also to maintain or improve quality of life. One method that can be used to capture this quality-of-life issue is the cost utility analysis (CUA), in which the "utility" is a quality-adjusted life year. Thus, the equation is somewhat altered:

$$CUA = \frac{Cost\ A - Cost\ B}{Utility\ A - Utility\ B} = incremental\ cost\ per\ utility\ unit.$$

In this equation, the utility is a life year adjusted for quality by the patient. A year of life in perfect health would receive a value of 1.0 year, whereas a year of chronic illness might be judged as 0.7 year by a patient. Further refinement of techniques similar to CUA will allow increasing explication of the value and quality perceived by the patients of the health care advances prescribed for them.

Goldman et al[54] state that a quality-adjusted life year of $20 000 to $40 000 is consistent with other cost-effective programs receiving federal funding, such as renal dialysis. Other reported costs of cardiac therapies reveal that managing hypercholesterolemia with oat bran is estimated to cost $77 800 per YLS;[55] streptokinase administration for myocardial infarction in the elderly costs $27 700 per YLS,[56] and lovastatin therapy for men between the ages of 55 and 64 years with cholesterol <250 mg/dL costs $22 900.[57] Thus, the current costs of $14 200 to $41 800 for ICD therapy are within the accepted financial standard of care.

Aspects of prevention have also begun to spring forward in the SCA patient population. Genetic testing and manipulation for entities such as prolonged-QT syndrome, growth factors related to cardiomyopathies, and genes suspected to affect hypercholesterol states are all currently under investigation. And although the benefits of these preventive measures may not be seen for a number of years, other initiatives that address prevention are currently being actively pursued. Public access defibrillation is one such initiative. In 1993, the American Heart Association published a position statement[58] supporting prompt defibrillation to victims of cardiac arrest with an automatic external defibrillator. With this technology, the American Heart Association envisions rapid performance of defibrillation by laypersons, firefighters, police, security personnel, and the nonphysician providers in the community. Considering that no more than 5% of SCA victims currently survive,[59] the introduction of automatic external defibrillators should have a substantial impact on prevention of SCD. The principles of action and an overview of clinical, educational, and ethical issues surrounding automatic external defibrillators are discussed in another chapter.

Another preventive response to this health improvement stage is the use of comprehensive workplace primary prevention programs in which comprehensive assessment and intervention are applied. Milani and Lavie[60] report that in a program designed to reduce coronary risk profiles, they achieved improvement in coronary risk factors that resulted in a 39% reduction in annual medical costs in the high-risk group of participants and an $\approx23\%$ overall reduction in medical claims for the entire group.

Summary

As the major driving force in today's healthcare environment, managed care has succeeded in creating new paradigms and new forces throughout the market and the clinical practice environments. The final impact of managed care on the healthcare equation in the United States will not be truly visible for a number of years. However, its impact on patients and healthcare providers in the SCD field is somewhat more visible. Although tremendous changes have been required in the delivery of care, the changes have remained manageable and have allowed quality and access to be maintained. As for the future, the current responses of providers to the challenges of managed care portend that their responses to future trends in SCD—a broader base of potential patients, smaller and less expensive technologies, more finely targeted treatment regimens, and primary prevention initiatives—will maintain quality and access throughout the evolution of managed care.

References

1. Ferguson DS, Saksena S, Greenberg E, et al. Management of recurrent ventricular tachycardia: economic impact of therapeutic alternatives. *Am J Cardiol.* 1995;53:533–536.

2. Saksena S, Camm A. Implantable defibrillators for prevention of sudden death. *Circulation.* 1992;85:2316–2321.
3. Beyond HMO's: all that glitters. *Hosp Health Netw.* 1996;70:46–48.
4. Goldsmith JC, Goran M, Nackal J. Managed care comes of age. *Healthcare Forum J.* 1995;36:14–24.
5. Jones M: *St Anthony's DRG Guidebook.* Alexandria, Va: St Anthony Publishing; 1996:47–62.
6. Montague J, Pitman H. Managed care. *Hosp Health Netw.* 1995;69:14.
7. Allen BJ, Brodsky MA. Cost-effective management of congestive heart failure and cardiac arrhythmias in the managed care setting. In: Ott RA, Tanner T, eds. *Managed Care and the Cardiac Patient.* Philadelphia, Pa: Hanley & Belfus: 1995;229–235.
8. Dunnigan A, Roberts C, McNamara M. Success of re-use of cardiac electrode catheters. *Am J Cardiol.* 1987;60:807–810.
9. Avitall B, Khan M, Krum D, et al. Repeated use of ablation catheters: a prospective study. *J Am Coll Cardiol.* 1993;22:1367–1372.
10. Mond H, Tartaglia S, Cole A, et al. The refurbished pulse generator. *PACE.* 1980;3:311–317.
11. Rosengarten MD, Chiu R, Hoffman RH. A prospective trial of new versus refurbished cardiac pacemakers: a Canadian experience. *Can J Cardiol.* 1989;5:155–160.
12. Havia T, Schuller T. The re-use of previously implanted pacemakers. *Scand J Cardiovasc Surg.* 1978;22:33–34.
13. Kovas P, Gomory A, Worum F, et al. Five years experience with reused pacemakers. *PACE.* 1981;4:A54. Abstract.
14. Feruglio G, Petz E, Zunuttini D. Pacemaker reutilization: a 7 year multicenter experience in Italy. *PACE.* 1979;2:A73. Abstract.
15. Amikam S, Feldman S, Riss E, et al. Clinical experience with reused pulse generators. *PACE.* 1979;2:A73. Abstract.
16. Balachander J, Siram R, Selhuramarnk H. Efficacy and safety of refurbished pacemakers: report on collaborative programme with 140 implantations and 6-year follow-up. *Indian Heart J.* 1989;41:430.
17. Aren C, Larsson S. Reuse of hermetically sealed cardiac pacemakers. *PACE.* 1979;2:A73. Abstract.
18. Mugica J, Duconge R, Henry L. Survival and mortality in 3701 pacemaker patients: argument in favor of pacemaker reuse. *PACE.* 1986;9:1282–1298.
19. Pringle R, Leman R, Kratz J, et al. An argument for pacemaker reuse: pacemaker mortality in 169 patients over ten years. *PACE.* 1986;9:1295–1298.
20. MacGregor M. The reuse of cardiac pacemakers. *Can J Cardiol.* 1992;8:697–701.
21. Boal B, Escher D, Furman S, et al. Report of the policy conference on pacemaker reuse sponsored by the North American Society of Pacing and Electrophysiology. *PACE.* 1985;8:161–163.
22. Gayle D, Davis K, Simmons TW, et al. Reprogramming pacemakers enhances longevity and is cost effective. *Circulation.* 1995;92(suppl I): I-511. Abstract.
23. Dunbar S, Jenkins L, Hawthorne M, et al. Difference in patient and family member mood before and one month after implantable cardioverter defibrillator insertion. *Circulation.* 1995;92(suppl I):I-491. Abstract.
24. Hawthorne M, Dunbar S, Jenkins L, et al. Mood disturbance during

early recovery in women after implantable cardioverter defibrillator placement. *Circulation*. 1995;92(suppl I):I-492. Abstract.

25. Williamson B, Ching Man K, Niebauer M, et al. The economic impact of transvenous defibrillation lead systems. *PACE*. 1994;17:2297–2303.

26. Venditti F, O'Connell M, Martin D, et al. Transvenous cardioverter defibrillators: cost implications of a less invasive approach. *PACE*. 1995;18:711–715.

27. Luceri R, Zil P, Habel S, et al. Cost and length of hospital stay: comparison between nonthoractomy and epicardial techniques in patient receiving implantable cardioverter defibrillators. *PACE*. 1995;18:168–171.

28. American College of Cardiology/American Heart Association Task Force. ACC/AHA Guidelines for clinical intracardic electrophysiology and catheter ablation catheters. *Circulation*. 1995;90:675–690.

29. O'Donoghue S, Platia EV, Brooks-Robinson A, et al. Automatic implantable cardioverter-defibrillator: is early implantation cost-effective? *J Am Coll Cardiol*. 1990;16:1258–1263.

30. Klein LS, Miles WM, Zipes DP. Antitachycardia devices: realities and promises. *J Am Coll Cardiol*. 1991;18:1349–1362.

31. Wever EF, Hauer R. Cost effectivness considerations: the Dutch prospective study of the automatic implantable cardioverter defibrillator as first choice therapy. *PACE*. 1992;15:690–693.

32. Wever E, Hauer RN, van Capelle JL, et al. Randomized study of implantable defibrillator as first-choice therapy versus conventional strategy in postinfarct sudden death survivors. *Circulation*. 1995;91: 2195–2203.

33. Mirowski M. The automatic implantable cardioverter-defibrillator: an overview. *J Am Coll Cardiol*. 1985;6:461–466.

34. Echt D, Armstrong K, Schmidt P, et al. Clinical experience, complications, and survival in 70 patients with automatic implantable cardioverter-defibrillator. *Circulation*. 1985;71:289–296.

35. Kelly P, Cannon D. Garan H, et al. The automatic implantable defibrillator (AICD): efficacy, complications and survival in patients with malignant ventricular arrhythmias. *J Am Coll Cardiol*. 1988;11:1278–1286.

36. Siebels J, Kuch K. Implantable cardioverter defibrillator compared with antiarrhythmic drug treatment in cardiac arrest survivors (the Cardiac Arrest Study Hamburg). *Am Heart J*. 1994;127:1139–1144.

37. The AVID Investigators. Antiarrhythmics versus implantable defibrillators (AVID): rationale, design, and methods. *Am J Cardiol*. 1995;75: 470–475.

38. Connolly S, Gent M, Robert R, et al. Canadian implantable defibrillator study (CIDS): study design and organization. *Am J Cardiol*. 1993;72:103F–108F.

39. Bigger T. Prophylactic use of implantable cardioverter defibrillators: medical, technical, economic considerations. *PACE*. 1991;14:376–380.

40. Weaver W, Cobb L, Hallstrom A, et al. Factors influencing survival after out of hospital cardiac arrest. *J Am Coll Cardiol*. 1986;7:752–757.

41. Tedder M, Anstadt M, Wharton J, et al. Prophylactic implantable defibrillator patches in patients at high risk for malignant ventricular dysrhythmias. *ASAIO J*. 1992;38:M261–M265.

42. Gordon T, Kannel WB. Premature mortality from coronary heart disease: the Framingham study. *JAMA*. 1971;215:1617–1625.

43. Buxton AE, Fisher JD, Josephson ME, et al. Prevention of sudden death

in patients with coronary artery disease: the Multicenter Unsustained Tachycardia Trial (MUSTT). *Prog Cardiovasc Dis.* 1993;36:215–226.

44. MADIT Executive Committee. Multicenter automatic defibrillator implantation trial (MADIT): design and clinical protocol. *PACE.* 1991;14:920–927.

45. The CABG-PATCH Trial Investigators and Coordinators. The coronary artery bypass graft (CABG) patch trial. *Prog Cardiovasc Dis.* 1993;36: 97-114.

46. Saksena S. The impact of implantable cardioverter defibrillator therapy on health care systems. *Am Heart J.* 1994;127:1193–2000.

47. Lau C, Nishimura S, MacPherson M, et al. Waiting for a pacemaker in Canada: evaluation of a triage system. *Circulation.* 1995;92(suppl I): I–120. Abstract.

48. Ray S, Griffith M, Jamieson S, et al. Impact of the recommendations of the British Pacing and Electrophysiology Group on pacemaker prescription and on the immediate costs of pacing in the Northern Region. *Br Heart J.* 1992;68:531–534.

49. deBelder M, Linker N, Jones S, et al. Cost implications of the British Pacing and Electrophysiology Group's recommendations for pacing. *Br Med J.* 1992;305:861–865.

50. Kuppermann M, Luce BR, McGovern B, et al. An analysis of the cost effectiveness of the implantable defibrillator. *Circulation.* 1990;81:91–100.

51. Kupersmith J, Hogan A, Guerrero P, et al. Evaluating and improving the cost-effectiveness of the implantable cardioverter-defibrillator. *Am Heart J.* 1995;130:507–515.

52. Larson GC, Manolis A, Sonnenberg FA. Cost effectiveness of the implantable cardioverter-defibrillator: effect of improved battery life and comparison with amiodarone therapy. *J Am Coll Cardiol.* 1992;19: 1323–1334.

53. Warner KE, Luce BR. *Cost-Benefit and Cost-Effectiveness Analysis in Health Care: Principle, Practice and Potential.* Ann Arbor, Mich: Health Administration Press; 1982:7–10.

54. Goldman L, Gordon DJ, Rifkind BM, et al. Cost and health implications of cholesterol lowering. *Circulation.* 1992;85:1960–1968.

55. Kinosian BP, Eisenberg JM. Cutting into cholesterol: cost effective alternatives for treating hypercholesterolemia. *JAMA.* 1988;259: 2249–2254.

56. Krumholz HM, Pasternak RC, Weinstein MC, et al. Cost effectiveness of thrombolytic therapy in elderly patients with suspect acute myocardial infarction. *N Engl J Med.* 1992;327:7–13.

57. Goldman L, Weinstein MC, Goldman PA, et al. Cost-effectiveness of HMG-CoA reductase inhibition for primary and secondary prevention of coronary artery disease. *JAMA.* 1991;265:1145–1151.

58. Weisfeldt ML, Kerber RE, McGoldrick RP, et al. Public access defibrillation: a statement for healthcare professionals from the American Heart Association Task Force on Automatic External Defibrillation. *Circulation.* 1995;92:2763.

59. Eisenberg MS, Bergner L, Hallstrom AP, et al. Sudden cardiac death. *Sci Am.* 1986;254:37–43.

60. Milani RV, Lavie CJ. Reductions in coronary risk profile and total medical costs with comprehensive work-site primary prevention programs. *Circulation.* 1995;92(suppl I):I-510. Abstract.

Index